EARLY EXITS IS A MILESTONE THAT WILL BRING COMFORT TO MANY AND MAY change the way we think about end-of-life care. Each page is filled with a wealth of insights not only into medical assistance in dying but also into the natural, unassisted dying process. *Early Exits* shows that the end of life is not only a physical process but a spiritual challenge as well. This thought-provoking and, ideally, conversation-provoking book should be required reading for anyone dealing with or anticipating the process of dying.

– BRUCE GREYSON, MD
Carlson Professor Emeritus of Psychiatry & Neurobehavioral Sciences
Division of Perceptual Studies
University of Virginia Health System
Author of *After: A Doctor Explores What Near-Death Experiences Reveal about Life and Beyond*

THE ONTOLOGICAL, ANTHROPOLOGICAL, AND THANATOLOGICAL QUESTION of what it means to die, and why it matters how we die, has hardly been addressed, and is, of course, a very adequate question in a pastoral setting. This is a well-informed, honest, and deeply spiritual alternative to the materialistic, individualistic, and autonomy approaches to death and dying. The narratives are impressive, as is the author's courage to swim against the current.

– THEO A. BOER, PhD
Universitair Docent Ethiek,
Protestantse Theologische Universiteit Groningen, Netherlands
Center for Bioethics and Health Law of Utrecht University
Chair, Committee on Bioethics and Biotechnology
of the Conference of European Churches

ONE CANNOT HELP BUT HOLD DEEP RESPECT FOR DAVID'S ROLE AS A chaplain. The individuals who have journeyed with him are incredibly fortunate to have such a knowledgeable, perceptive, talented, experienced, and caring companion to help them navigate the mysteries of the end of life. *Early Exits* is a masterfully argued, well-written, compassionate, and provocative book on a contested issue that will likely continue to be debated.

– DAVID PFRIMMER, PhD
Professor Emeritus for Public Ethics
Martin Luther University College
Author of *The Art of Dying Well: Medical Assistance in Dying (MAID) in Canada A Public Theological Primer*

WITHOUT ROMANTICIZING THE SUFFERING OF DYING, DAVID BOTH challenges and reaches past the framing of "medical aid in dying" as primarily an issue of patient autonomy. With humanistic rigor, powerful stories, and gentle questions, this book invites its readers to a noetic dialogue, where justice for our unique and storied existence in time includes being with ourselves and with each other even unto death, ever-honoring the wisdom and compassion that can come to us from gathering the meanings of our deepest vulnerabilities.

– JANETA TANSEY, MD, PhD, FAPA
Principal, Virtue Medicine
Faculty, Viktor Frankl Institute of Logotherapy

AN HONEST AND THOUGHT-PROVOKING REVIEW OF MAiD IN CANADA, urging readers to consider our approach to living, dying, suffering, and reality itself. This is an immensely significant work that contributes to our ongoing societal dialogue on the dying process. I highly recommend this book to anyone who recognizes the importance of embracing life fully, including its inevitable end.

– KRISTINE LUND, PhD, RP
Professor, Spiritual Care and Psychotherapy
Albert J. Datars Chair
Clinical Director, Delton Glebe Counselling Centre

EARLY EXITS IS A PROFOUNDLY INSIGHTFUL AND COMPASSIONATE BOOK THAT explores an incredibly complex topic with wisdom and sensitivity. Each chapter is enhanced by expertly crafted exercises that encourage personal reflection and deepen our understanding of this challenging issue. Drawing from a wealth of personal experiences and diverse perspectives, David offers a non-judgmental exploration that is both well-researched and deeply heartfelt. His extensive background in working with dying individuals shines through in this remarkable book, overflowing with invaluable insights and resources. This is a thought-provoking and enriching read, shedding light on the profound challenges of transitioning with grace and dignity. Magnificent!

– REBECCA AUSTILL-CLAUSEN MS, OTR/L, FAOTA
Ethics Committee, International Association for Near-Death Studies
Author of *Change Maker: How My Brother's Death Woke Up My Life*

WHEN READING THE CHAPTER ON THE BUDDHIST PERSPECTIVE, IT FEELS David Maginley is inviting us to join the exploration of the abundant spiritual opportunities of the dying process, offering a compelling investigation of how these crucial moments remind us of the truth. With clarity and compassion, we are inspired to reflect on the profound ethical and spiritual questions that arise at the end of life. By that we are receiving essential guidance to our heart of hearts."

– ARNE SCHELLING
Dharma teacher and translator,
Siddhartha's Intent Europe

THIS BOOK IS A MASTERFUL EXPLORATION OF THE FINAL PHASE OF OUR LIFE'S journey. With profound insight, David reveals the transformative and sublime nature of the dying process. He approaches this mystery through multiple lenses – major religions, philosophy, spirituality, and modern science. Drawing from both his vast knowledge of spiritual and philosophical writings and over 25 years of personal experience, this book arrives at a crucial moment as MAiD is increasingly adopted. It offers a thoughtful pause and a chance to reflect on end-of-life decisions, serving as a valuable resource for patients, physician advisors, and policymakers considering MAiD. For all of us reflecting on our shared mortality, this book presents a rich and hopeful perspective on ancient and modern approaches to this often-avoided subject.

– DREW BETHUNE, MD
Retired thoracic surgeon,
Former Senior Medical Director Nova Scotia Cancer Program

ALSO BY DAVID MAGINLEY

Beyond Surviving:
Cancer and Your Spiritual Journey

EARLY EXITS

EARLY EXITS

Spirituality, Mortality, and Meaning in an Age of Medical Assistance in Dying

DAVID MAGINLEY

TRISTAN PRESS

Grateful acknowledgement is made for the following:
The Unbroken, © 1991 Rashani Réa, rashani.com, reproduced with permission.
Illustration of Ego Construction and Deconstruction, from *The Grace in Dying*, © 1998 Kathleen Dowling Singh, reproduced with permission from Harper Collins Publishers.
Illustration of The Wilber-Combs Lattice, from *Consciousness Explained Better: Towards an Integral Understanding of the Multifaceted Nature of Consciousness*, © 2009 Allan Combs, reprinted with permission from Paragon House.

This book was written in Mi'kma'ki, the ancestral and unceded territory of the Mi'kmaq people. I am grateful for their stewardship of the land upon which I work and for their spiritual wisdom, which permeates all aspects of life.

Structural Editor: Christine Gordon Manley, Rosemount Writing and Editing Services
Copy Editor: Margaret MacQuarrie, Wordperson Inc.
Book Design and E-book formatting: Amit Dey

TRISTAN PRESS

Tristan Press
PO Box 155
5675 Spring Garden Rd
Halifax NS B3J 1H1
Printed in USA

Paperback ISBN: 978-0-9958811-3-6

Dedicated to all who support the dying,
especially the healthcare teams
I've had the honour of working with.

CONTENTS

AUTHOR'S NOTE

FOR TWENTY-FIVE YEARS, I HAVE PROVIDED SPIRITUAL CARE AS A staff chaplain in palliative, cancer, and intensive care at the QEII Health Sciences Centre in Halifax, Nova Scotia. I have supported thousands as they've considered death, hundreds as they've died, and now dozens as they've received medical assistance in dying (MAiD), a radical change in the fundamental principles of end-of-life care. What I see causes me moral distress, for a growing number now leave this world in a way I never anticipated, in a manner so kind and respectful on one level yet so impoverished and strange on another. This is about more than the assertion that life is sacred; therefore, MAiD is wrong (too simple). And it's far more nuanced than claims of personal autonomy and the defence of dignity (too shallow). This is about our fundamental orientation to life and death, to suffering in society, and to reality itself.

I offer this book to share my observations and explore critical aspects of MAiD left unarticulated in the conversations currently held at the bedside, in the academic halls, courtrooms, and coffee shops. I know I am diving into boiling water – many will disagree with my perspective. Some may even attack me for it. That's the nature of opinions; offer one, and you get one in return. This is one way in which we stake out a secure and identifying mental territory. Who would I be without an opinion?

Let us share them with respect and honest vulnerability, for in the end, what we desire is a healthy connection, a deeper understanding, and for all to be seen and heard and valued. A moral sledgehammer can only divide, yet this does not mean we acquiesce to get along. When it comes to an issue as serious as this, let us be true to our compass and be able to explain the map upon which we base our measurements.

My measurements lead me to a definitive conclusion: I cannot support MAiD. Surprisingly, this is based not so much on my faith as on my twenty-five years of clinical experience with those dying, sound research, and insights on what happens to us at the end of our journey. I need to state this with honesty, integrity, and transparency, for I live and work in a world of competing sorrows – one in which there is no response to this issue that does only good and not harm. As a spiritual care provider, I have a duty to care for the dying, to help them process what we call "total pain" of mind, body, and soul. Yet now, especially when I've established a deep and therapeutic relationship with the dying person, I harm myself by participating in an act that causes me moral injury. I also harm the patient by not walking with them to the end of their final breath by this procedure. This significantly compromises my care for every patient, leaving me in a moral mess that often sabotages my ability to be fully present with those who suffer.

What this does to me on my days off is typical of healthcare providers experiencing burnout and moral injury: I become disconnected from life, joy, and those I love. Research clearly shows that addiction and depression rates for healthcare professionals are frighteningly high in such a soup. What to do?

As I have an ethical obligation to care for myself so I can care for those who suffer, I no longer participate in MAiD cases when the patient has had their first assessment. But I continue to work with those who provide MAiD. I also continue to support the dying as they wrestle with mortality. This means I have discussions with them on MAiD because most will raise it now that it's on the table. But I can only do that until they are assessed. Then I step back, and upon publishing this book will do so completely. Because of MAiD, I will retire early from a vocation I love. I cannot participate with integrity in a system that increasingly operates on principles so at odds with my own.

I am deeply grateful for the teams I have worked with and even more for the thousands of patients who have taught me what is most important in life – love, authenticity, and the all-too-human inconstancy of the ultimate spiritual assignment: awakening to our true nature. At no time does this happen so acutely and completely as through death. But conscientious objection does not result in a clean conscience – it leaves me torn with a sense of abandoning a person just as they are about to die. Nonetheless, that is an injury I can bear far better than participating in a procedure that deliberately ends a person's life.

Writing this book is part of that healing. I hope these pages, begun in 2018, will raise awareness of fundamental issues that should have been central to the discussions on MAiD from the beginning but never showed up. If it not only supports those who wrestle with meaning and mortality, but also becomes an investment in our culture's spiritual growth and social capital, then I will rest well.

This material cannot help but be coloured by my own experience. Nonetheless, I have strived to pierce that cloud and present perennial and fundamental aspects of the most contentious issue in health care. I trust that what I have written has significance. To check for hubris or ignorance on my part, I have consulted with experts in palliative care, law, bioethics, philosophy, and religious traditions. All confirm it has substance and value, offering novel and central insights yet unarticulated in MAiD discussion. I've even checked the integrity of my perspective with artificial intelligence (AI) to get as unbiased an opinion as possible. It stated, "The argument is well-structured and presents a clear conclusion that supports its overall thesis. The logic of the argument is sound and well-supported by the evidence presented." While that's encouraging, it's useless unless I speak to your heart because this is about grief, fear, dignity, and choice. It's about life and death. It's not about logic.

The cases presented in this book are drawn from actual experiences with patients. Names and details have been changed to honour confidentiality, and some accounts are composites. An incomplete exploration of MAiD is an inevitable risk of writing on such an explosive subject, and I'm sure I'll find out afterwards if I've misunderstood anything. May we come to the table respectful and curious of each other's position and find a way forward to a better society, a better tomorrow, and a better end to our days.

FOREWORD

Dr. Robert Twycross

A FEW MONTHS AGO, I LISTENED TO A WEBINAR FOR HOSPICE STAFF in the United Kingdom about Assisted Dying – the generic term in the medical and ethical literature for medical assistance in dying (MAiD). Much of the discussion focused on what the public thinks about the proposed legislation and its possible financial impact on hospices. For me, this was not the right starting point nor the right direction of travel – it was far too shallow an engagement with so serious an issue. 'Context is everything': nothing can be fully understood if divorced from fundamental philosophical and ethical considerations. In healthcare, these are not abstract notions but are experienced daily in cultural and clinical contexts. Accordingly, I strongly recommend *Early Exits: Spirituality, Mortality, and Meaning in an Age of Medical Assistance in Dying*, a book which does not shy away from addressing the most contentious issue in healthcare. The reader is told upfront that MAiD should be considered within a much broader and deeper context than is generally the case by pro-MAiD activists and by the media. As David says, 'I offer this book to share my observations and explore critical aspects of MAiD left unarticulated in the conversations currently held at the bedside, in the academic halls, courtrooms, and coffee shops.'

As a retired physician with 30 years of experience in palliative care, first as a Research Fellow at St Christopher's Hospice in London with Cicely Saunders, and then in Oxford at Sir Michael Sobell House, a palliative care unit/hospice within the National Health Service (NHS) and attached to

Oxford University Medical School, I have witnessed the profound impact of good end-of-life care. But now I am deeply concerned about the direction in which British society seems to be moving. At present, MAiD is not permissible in any part of the UK. However, unremitting pro-MAiD activism linked to largely supportive media coverage means that some form of MAiD is likely to become lawful within the next few years. I am staunchly opposed to it being integrated into healthcare and applaud any efforts to help the public understand the dangers involved, particularly when done with discernment and compassion as in this book.

Early Exits stems from the author's clinical experiences, who provided spiritual care over many years to patients receiving palliative, cancer, and intensive care in Nova Scotia. He knows this terrain well, having faced a rare, life-threatening cancer four times. Like me, he opposes MAiD, stating, "This is based not so much on my faith as on my twenty-five years of clinical experience with those dying, sound research, and insights on what happens to us at the end of our journey."

However, he is not judgmental of those who opt for MAiD. Indeed, he lists ten reasons why it can seem desirable and demonstrates a deep appreciation throughout the book for why people choose it. Nonetheless, he argues that MAiD is one of the most detrimental actions Canada has taken as a culture, attributing its rise to a society in which individual autonomy is an intoxicant. Furthermore, as most MAiD requests are driven by existential distress, he challenges us to consider it as a medical solution being used to treat a spiritual condition.

A perusal of the chapter headings demonstrates the author's breadth of scholarship, making *Early Exits* a 'must read' for all those involved in palliative care or planning to become so. Indeed, it should also be compulsory reading for senior management and, even better, lawmakers. However, this is not bedtime reading; powerful accounts of dying are found throughout these pages, bookended by the author's mother's dementia diagnosis and her death four years later (chapters 1 and 29), and his father's death, which anchors the centre of the book (chapter 14). These and many other stories enable the reader to appreciate the inner world of the dying and understand better the cultural context and clinical impact of MAiD. They are presented with precision and profound compassion; it is deeply moving material.

How the author addresses dignity and self-determination is particularly relevant to the debate. For those in favour of MAiD, individual autonomy is regarded as the unassailable trump card: 'my life, my death, my choice.' However, in medicine, autonomy is based on a partnership between patients and doctors, each respecting the autonomy of the other. This relational model of decision-making incorporates mutual respect and trust, dialogue, and informed negotiation. It contrasts with 'consumer autonomy' where the patient demands specific interventions from the doctor, regardless of established medical norms. In this circumstance, the doctor is reduced to being an agent for carrying out a patient's preferences ('my legal right') – a technician, no longer a professional. It becomes a transactional relationship (that of purchaser and supplier) rather than a partnership.

Exercising autonomy means making a choice. Informed choice requires reliable information about relevant options. Without this, autonomy is not valid. Disturbingly, official reports do not specify the nature of the palliative care received by those opting for MAiD. David identifies a huge gap in this regard: the existential distress at the heart of MAiD remains poorly addressed. Here is the central role for spiritual and psychosocial professionals in palliative care, but such services are often declined because they are not understood. What is known is that, to varying degrees, quality palliative care is not universally available in jurisdictions where MAiD is permitted, Canada included. Furthermore, the extent to which an autonomously expressed wish for MAiD should be acted on must be balanced against the rights of other people involved, notably family and health professionals. In society, people do not have an absolute right to individual autonomy. Individual rights must be balanced against public safety. In other words, people have the right to self-determination only when their actions do not harm others.

David not only addresses these ethical issues but also explores our culture's impoverished spiritual understanding. Materialism is the prevailing model of reality in the Western world, summarized in the phrase, 'what you see is what you get.' However, a narrow-minded reductionist philosophy doesn't match up to the reality we experience alongside our dying patients. Indeed, as Shakespeare eloquently put it in Hamlet, 'There are more things in heaven and earth, Horatio, than are dreamt of in your philosophy.'

When close to death and if conscious, patients may be seen to undergo a transition into a state of consciousness beyond anxiety and pain – a process David calls 'ego-deconstruction in the service of transformation.' Some patients cross over and return several times, oscillating between time and timelessness. This is one of the reasons why most of those working in palliative care are against MAiD, which arises from a materialistic paradigm which ignores a whole dimension of human reality.

Working with the dying typically results in a sense of awe, of mystery and humility. For many patients, it is a time of "finishing business" - seeking forgiveness, mending broken relationships, and giving thanks. Dying patients experience a range of "otherworldly" phenomena, including vivid dreams and visions of deceased relatives, often of a loved one waiting to accompany them into the afterlife. These experiences are reported by about half of hospice inpatients and are not limited to patients with religious beliefs. Since some of these phenomena are witnessed by others, such as relatives, friends, or nurses, they cannot be dismissed as hallucinations. Such phenomena often lessen the fear of dying and bring comfort to the family. *Early Exits* beautifully normalizes this, but it also challenges us to consider how this ultimate dynamic is lost when choosing MAiD.

In surveys of doctors in the UK and Canada, those working in palliative care are the most strongly against MAiD. If legalized, about 85% of them would refuse to be involved. But why should palliative care doctors be the most strongly against MAiD? After all, they are the ones most likely to witness suffering at the end of life. The answer to this conundrum can be found in a study of Swiss palliative care doctors who indicated that palliative care and MAiD are based on diametrically opposed philosophies. Fortunately, the British Medical Association now supports an "opt-in" rather than an "opt-out" model (www.bma.org.uk/pad). Furthermore, it favors a stand-alone Department of Assisted Dying, completely divorced from the National Health Service (NHS) with separate funding. In other words, healthcare should be a MAiD-free zone. Can the same ever be true for Canada now that MAiD is available?

No wonder David offers *Early Exits* as an "investment in our cultural capital." It comprehensively addresses the clinical, cultural, ethical, philosophical, and theological issues with MAiD. There is little one can add to the argument! Even so, in conclusion, I offer four reasons from a medical perspective why I believe that palliative care, in particular, should not be involved in MAiD:

1. It will result in more suffering. Even without MAiD, some people decline referral to palliative care due to the fear of being "drugged to death" despite severe pain or distressing symptoms. This fear is well-known to palliative care professionals and will be heightened if MAiD is legalized. (Note: Palliative care typically prolongs survival by improving comfort, sleep, appetite, and holistic support.)

2. There is a need for a coercion-free sanctuary for dying patients. Coercion – both subtle and explicit – is inevitable if MAiD is legalized. It would further narrow down what is viewed as a worthwhile life, with some people's lives being considered merely an economic drain on society. To avoid being a burden to their family or others, patients might feel they have a duty to die. Pressure to opt for MAiD would further increase as health budgets are further squeezed. Patients need to know that MAiD is definitely not part of palliative care. (Note: MAiD is cheaper than palliative care.)

3. The imposition of MAiD onto palliative care causes moral distress for those opposed to it. In palliative care, there is an unspoken commitment to continuity of care and non-abandonment: 'Whatever happens, we will stay beside you every step of the way. Together we will get through this.' This is the essence of palliative care, and it is very difficult, if not impossible, to work looking in two diametrically opposed directions.

4. Patients change their mind when in receipt of quality holistic palliative care. This relates in large part to the staff's commitment to non-abandonment: 'You are still, and always will be, a person of worth.' It counteracts a patient's feelings of isolation and worthlessness. In such an environment, virtually all patients lose their wish to actively hasten death.

Finally, a quote from the Swiss Academy of Medical Sciences:

> The true role of physicians in the management of dying and death… involves relieving symptoms and supporting the patient. Their responsibilities do not include offering [MAiD], nor are they obliged to perform it. It is not a medical action to which patients could claim to be entitled, even if it is a legally permissible activity.

Undoubtedly, *Early Exits* will generate much discussion by challenging present widely held assumptions and raising issues central to this ultimate decision. Be prepared for an engaging, insightful, and heart-felt exploration of what we must all eventually face: our death.

Robert Twycross MD

June 2024

Emeritus Clinical Reader in Palliative Medicine

Oxford University

THE UNBROKEN

by Rashani Réa
(www.rashani.com)

There is a brokenness
out of which comes the unbroken,
a shatteredness
out of which blooms the unshatterable.
There is a sorrow
beyond all grief which leads to joy
and a fragility
out of whose depths emerges strength.

There is a hollow space
too vast for words
through which we pass with each loss,
out of whose darkness
we are sanctioned into being.

There is a cry deeper than all sound
whose serrated edges cut the heart
as we break open to the place inside
which is unbreakable and whole,
while learning to sing.

INTRODUCTION

How would you like to die? It's a surprisingly simple question, and while you may hear some pretty interesting answers when the conversation is light and lubricated, it gets serious when you've got a terminal disease. Then it's weighted with the worry for loved ones, the real possibility of death, and some sense of when and how it will unfold. Will I suffer? Will I writhe in pain, struggle for breath? Will I end up hooked to machines that do the living for me? The one fate worse than death is being trapped in limbo while it takes its sweet time.

How would you like to die? Whether death is real or abstract, most will say the same thing: while I'm sleeping. I want to close my eyes here and wake up there. I want to slip into sweet slumber, comfortably medicated if needed, and not even know it's happened. Perhaps that's the key: a good death is one we don't see coming, one that gets about its business when it arrives. We don't want the reaper hanging around, leering and loitering. Let it be as if I've awoken from a dream. Let it be gentle and kind for my heart and my family. Above all, let it be quick.

Medical assistance in dying grants that wish. It gives one agency over the ultimate, the ability to decide time and place, method, and mental awareness. No wonder it's so effective at diminishing existential distress – that earthquake in the bedrock of your being which shakes the foundations of identity. Dying makes everything you've built and become crumble before you. MAiD gives you the power to ensure that disintegration happens on your terms.

Ray Cole, suffering from lung cancer at seventy-two and dependent on painkillers, spoke of this relief in being approved for MAiD and the expectancy of what lay beyond: "I've got ten grandchildren. I got to say goodbye to them all, standing up… hug them… It was wonderful… I have no regrets. I have no problem with going to the other side." Then, he added, "I'm really excited because I'm going to know the answers."[1]

Who would not want such an end? It appears so kind, so compassionate, and so sensible. Would not any act that can take what we dread most and make it manageable, even comfortable, be a good thing? Yes, this is medical professionals causing death, but are they not also preventing unnecessary suffering? These questions surface at the beginning of one's consideration of assisted dying and are not easily answered. At best, they lead to better questions and deeper conversations on dignity, personal rights, and core beliefs at the end of life. Most significantly, they guide us to the ultimate matters of life and death – to the spiritual dimensions of MAiD.

I'd like to have that conversation with you. It will be a difficult discussion if it is to be a good one. But since you opened this book, I trust your efforts to engage the spiritual dimensions of MAiD at least as much as I have had to muster the courage to write about it.

We live in anxious times. As these words are penned, we are three years into a pandemic, the United States has experienced an attempted insurrection, politics has become schismatic, and ongoing police brutality against people of colour has emphasized how racism is rampant. Globally, oppressed populations are rising in protest, and Russia has invaded Ukraine. In Canada, the mass graves of Indigenous children unearth generational traumas while our ice caps melt and the world slides toward another recession. All this, on top of epidemic stress, crime, depression, greed, and staggering disparities in health and wealth.

Thanks to social media, every citizen of the planet can feed this frenzy. We have never been more "connected" yet we've never felt more disconnected and alone.[2] That's exponentially so for the dying, who, thanks to advancing medical technology, live into their days far longer than before. However, they do

[1] CTV News, "A rare look at Canada's growing demand for medical assistance in dying." Written by Avis Favaro. https://www.ctvnews.ca/mobile/w5/a-rare-look-at-canada-s-growing-demand-for-medical-assistance-in-dying-1.5854612. Accessed April 12, 2022.

[2] Cacioppo, John T., and Stephanie Cacioppo. "The growing problem of loneliness." *The Lancet* 391.10119. 2018, p. 426.

so in a community that no longer honours its elders or gathers at the bedside, bringing casseroles and comfort. Arguing about MAiD and the autonomy of the individual, personal dignity, the sanctity of life, or the slippery slope, will be irrelevant without appreciating how we no longer gather as a village to usher the dying to their transformation. In the context of advancing technology within the anthropology of assisted death, this is all the more so as we head to a future marked by either staggering transformation or sudden destruction.

Along with this new world is the perennial awareness of our mortality. The fearsome fact of our finite nature unconsciously shapes our lives. **Who** we are in this brief passage is planted by efforts to build the existential exoskeleton of ego-identity through experiences, achievements, and possessions, only to helplessly watch it all crumble with our bodies at the end. Yet **what** we are is revealed through this same disintegration through death. As all beings do, we will return to the universe of which we are such a small and fleeting expression. Our bodies are dragged across the stage of the cosmic play toward nothing or everything. When we identify so strongly with the rational, decision-making aspect of the personality, the ego, death anxiety can only increase in such a setting.

Is MAiD not an understandable outcome of this phenomenon? Advances in science and medicine have painted us into a corner – now you can live into your dying far longer with chronic disease and consider experimental and extreme options that, with many conditions, render you aware but awash in suffering. With MAiD, we now have an empowering action that places you back in the driver's seat and ensures you avoid technocratic and paternalistic dying. It circumvents a lonely death in a hospital, waiting in bed, or hooked into life support that needlessly stretches the dying process out for weeks or months. No wonder MAiD feels like an act of mercy at the ultimate moment of life – its end. However, there is a deeper dynamic at play, one Western culture and leaders in medicine, law, and bioethics are not addressing.

As we weave through the labyrinth of life to arrive at the still point of death, I would emphasize that those on both sides of the issue are striving to help people. While I am exploring the matter as practised in

Canada, it's worth echoing the opening paragraph of the American Medical Association's web page on physician-assisted death:

> "Thoughtful, morally admirable individuals hold diverging, yet equally deeply held and well-considered perspectives about physician-assisted suicide. Nonetheless, at the core of the public and professional debate about physician-assisted suicide is the aspiration that every patient come to the end of life as free as possible from suffering that does not serve the patient's deepest self-defining beliefs. Supporters and opponents share a fundamental commitment to values of care, compassion, respect, and dignity; they diverge in drawing different moral conclusions from those underlying values in equally good faith.[3]

A BRIEF HISTORY

THOSE "DIVERGING, YET EQUALLY DEEPLY HELD AND WELL-CONSIDERED perspectives" have been part of difficult conversations for a while. While Bill C-14, which amended the Canadian criminal code allowing MAiD, came into law in 2016, the story began years earlier.

Sue Rodriguez was living a nightmare. A loving forty-two-year-old mother, her life was shattered by amyotrophic lateral sclerosis (ALS). The disease gradually paralyzes you, scraping away the ability to move and imprisoning you in a tomb of living flesh. It was 1993, and there was little hope for anyone so afflicted. Sue wanted to die but could not bring herself to suicide. Could not a doctor stop her heart? Could not the medical system ensure she could end her life safely? She took her case to the Supreme Court and argued that the prohibition of assisted suicide was contrary to the Canadian Charter of Rights and Freedoms. Rodriguez felt that her right to "life, liberty, and security of the person" was violated by not being allowed to die by assisted suicide. The law sentenced her to suffer when

[3] "Physician-Assisted Suicide." American Medical Association, Ethics. https://www.ama-assn.org/delivering-care/ethics/physician-assisted-suicide. Accessed April 17, 2022.

death could free her from it. It was her life and her body. Should it not be her choice? The court disagreed and declined her petition in a five-to-four decision.[4]

But context and culture change. In little more than twenty years, the Netherlands, Belgium, Luxembourg, and the states of Oregon, Washington, and Vermont passed legislation that allowed assisted dying in certain circumstances. Quebec then legalized "medical aid in dying" in 2014. A year later, cases like Gloria Taylor, also suffering from ALS, and Kay Carter, struggling with degenerative spinal stenosis, changed the court's perspective: Canadian adults could request MAiD. The court's statement was infused with respect and consideration for those who suffer as death approaches.

> It is a crime in Canada to assist another person in ending her own life. As a result, grievously and irremediably ill people cannot seek a physician's assistance in dying and may be condemned to a life of severe and intolerable suffering. A person facing this prospect has two options: she can take her own life prematurely, often by violent or dangerous means, or she can suffer until she dies from natural causes. The choice is cruel.[5]

It's unfortunate the court's decision was so binary, as there is a third choice, an effective choice already part of Canada's medical system: palliative care. Research in this field does not substantiate that the suffering of advanced disease is irremediable. On the contrary, there is an enormous body of literature on active, positive ways to respond compassionately to relieve suffering.[6,7] Training programs are already available to support providers as they learn to recognize suffering, communicate

---

[4] "Rodriguez v. British Columbia (Attorney General), [1993] 3 SCR 519, 1993 CanLII 75 (SCC)." CanLII. September 30, 1993. www.canlii.org. Accessed April 23, 2023.

[5] Constitution Acts 1867 to 1982. Justice Laws Website. https://laws-lois.justice.gc.ca/eng/Const/page-15.html. Accessed Feb. 24, 2019.

[6] Dunlop, Robert. *Cancer: Palliative Care*. Springer Science & Business Media, 2012.

[7] Schulz, Richard, et al. "Patient suffering and caregiver compassion: new opportunities for research, practice, and policy." *The Gerontologist* 47.1 (2007): pp. 4–13.

empathy, encourage patients to share their struggles, and thereby decrease the burden.[8]

But the ruling held, and since then, almost 50,000 Canadians have died through MAiD. The first six months of 2018 saw 1,523 people, a 30 percent increase over the previous six months.[9] 2019 had another 26 percent rise to 5,631 assisted deaths,[10] then over 34 percent to 7,595 in 2020, and a 32 percent increase in 2021 to 10,604.[11] In 2022, 3.3 percent of all deaths in Canada were by MAiD – a small but growing number that may reflect the increasing normalization of assisted dying. In addition, changes were made that expanded access to MAiD people who are not nearing the natural end of their lives but met the other MAiD criteria, so the number of cases will likely increase significantly.[12] Given the rise I've seen in my own hospital, I wouldn't be surprised if the figures triple by 2030.

---

[8] Cassell, Eric J. "The nature of suffering and the goals of medicine." *Loss, Grief & Care* 8.1-2 (1998): pp. 129–142.

[9] *CBC News* "Number of Canadians choosing medically assisted death jumps 30%." Written by Kathleen Harris. Aired June 21, 2018. https://www.cbc.ca/news/politics/MAiD-assisted-death-increase-1.4715944 Accessed Feb. 24, 2019.

[10] *Global News* "Medically assisted deaths rose by 17% in 2020, continuing upward trend: Health Canada." Written by Joan Bryden. Posted June 8, 2021 2:01 a.m. https://globalnews.ca/news/7930055/assisted-dying-statistics-2020/. Accessed Oct. 31, 2021.

[11] *Second Annual Report on Medical Assistance in Dying in Canada 2020.* Canada.ca. https://www.canada.ca/en/health-canada/services/medical-assistance-dying/annual-report-2020.html#3_1. Accessed March 26, 2020.

[12] As of March 17, 2021, persons who wish to receive MAiD must meet the following eligibility criteria:
1. be 18 years of age or older and have decision-making capacity
2. be eligible for publicly funded health care services
3. make a voluntary request that is not the result of external pressure
4. give informed consent to receive MAiD, meaning that the person has consented to receiving MAiD after they have received all information needed to make this decision
5. have a serious and incurable illness, disease or disability (excluding a mental illness until March 17, 2024)
6. be in an advanced state of irreversible decline in capability
7. have enduring and intolerable physical or psychological suffering that cannot be alleviated under conditions the person considers acceptable

Government of Canada, Department of Justice, Electronic Communications. 2024. "Canada's Medical Assistance in Dying (MAiD) Law." March 1, 2024. Accessed March 14, 2024. https://www.justice.gc.ca/eng/cj-jp/ad-am/bk-di.html#:~:text=As%20of%20March%2017%2C%202021,the%20result%20of%20external%20pressure

You may shrug and reflect, why not? Alzheimer's and dementia are rapidly increasing, surpassed only by the rise in cancer incidence.[13] The prospect of your faculties and form fading away can be dreadful. No wonder the public predominantly supports MAiD, and most dying patients consider it as their ability to engage in meaningful activity diminishes. They do not like what dying does to them; they cannot imagine anything of value or purpose in further suffering. MAiD ensures that the critical moment in their final flight is free of such turbulence.

This presents an entirely new challenge for spiritual care practitioners (chaplains). Our specialty is existential distress, especially at the end of life. (Existential, simply put, refers to the nature of our identity and existence in the world. Existential distress is marked by fear of suffering, loss of dignity, meaning, and purpose, and a profound sense of being a burden. Nothing causes existential distress like the end of your existence!) Chaplains engage it as a functional process of forgiveness, reconciliation, release, and surrender that completes one's life. So, while MAiD enables the dying to detour the ultimate suffering they imagine will come, in doing so, they are significantly compromised in engaging the ultimate homework of the soul – integration and release of the ego-identity and opening to one's actual identity. We will explore this complex process shortly.

I realize it sounds crude and harsh, but MAiD allows one to circumvent the tough stuff by having someone shut them off. And it is incredibly tough stuff – unbearable to the mind and heartbreaking to the core. It manifests as lament, worry, death anxiety, and a quiet terror of the suffering and pain as one dies. Now, I know what that pain looks like. I have seen people writhe in agony as cancer dissolves their bones. I have held them while they bled out, pressing a towel to their mouths to absorb the flow. I have heard the wails. I know the nightmares you are imagining. But these are rare. Most people will have episodes of difficult pain, but there is no need to endure that with today's medication. Regretfully, in the most challenging cases, palliative sedation may be

---

[13] "How dementia impacts Canadians." Canadian Institute for Health Information. https://www.cihi.ca/en/dementia-in-canada/how-dementia-impacts-canadians#:~:text=Dementia rates are very low for those younger than 65,24.6% for seniors 85+. Accessed June 15, 2022.

the only option. It's available, and it works, but time and time again, I see people refuse that because they want to maintain communication with their loved ones. They want to continue to feel alive. And they do not want to descend into what may as well be death, in their eyes. This, like MAiD, stems from the fear of death, of no longer being who and what you have always known yourself to be. In the reports from Health Canada, there is no clarification of inadequate pain control or concern about how it could be managed. There is only a brief reference to the main problem: the worry, the imagination, the spectre in the shadows. This is no light matter, for imagined suffering adds significantly to present suffering. It can increase physical pain. It can shatter composure and connection to others. This is why, disturbingly, 34 percent reported that the perceived burden on family, friends, or caregivers was behind their request for MAiD, and 13 percent said it was isolation or loneliness.[14]

As much as people may not care to identify this as spiritual suffering, it is nonetheless, for spirituality is "the aspect of humanity that refers to the way individuals seek and express meaning and purpose and the way they experience their connectedness to the moment, to self, to others, to nature, and the significant or sacred."[15] A healthy spirituality results not so much from faith in God as from the depths of life, belonging, and meaning. It is a fundamental, relational experience of self. Since we are who we are through our relationships, they become a mirror of the soul. Can you gaze at that image without flinching at life's end? Can you do so with kindness, in such a way that loved ones and caregivers willingly, albeit heavily, share in your suffering as a privilege, as a sacred trust? Must such an honour always be phrased as "the burden of care"?

I recognize this may not sound like the pastoral perspective a chaplain should embody, but let's not shrink back from what this is about: our inability to see anything good, purposeful, meaningful – let alone dignified – in

---

[14] Government of Canada, Department of Jusitce. 2020. Medical Assistance in Dying in Canada: Annual Report 2020. Ottawa: Government of Canada. Accessed March 14, 2024. https://www.canada.ca/en/health- canada/services/maid.html.

[15] Puchalski, Christina M., et al. "Improving the spiritual dimension of whole person care: reaching national and international consensus." *Journal of palliative medicine* 17.6 (2014): pp. 642–656.

suffering to the end. And I cannot promise that I will be able to see it when I die, either! I would also state that our culture's inability to grasp this is entirely understandable, given the medicalization of death (which, ironically, is the ultimate spiritual experience in life), our emphasis on individual autonomy, and the fact that few live in multigenerational households anymore to witness death as a natural part of life.

All this, on top of the poverty of modern spiritual intelligence. Western religions continue to emphasize that God is something external and that reality is dualistic: there's the material world and the spiritual world. We still speak in archaic terms, increasingly out of step with modern insights in cosmology and consciousness. And we are increasingly becoming strangers to the most natural and ultimate event, one which calls on the community to gather and enfold the dying and their loved ones with compassionate care. But few have such a community anymore. No wonder death has become emptied of its wonder, void of meaning for so many. Besides, who would suffer to the end when an alternative allows you to regain control of the ultimate agenda, choose your time of exit, gather those you love around you, and be sent off with a song and final words complete?

Who would suffer natural death in the face of that? Well, most people. While a 2020 Angus Reid poll found that 80 percent of Canadians support MAiD (33 percent being "enthusiastic supporters" and 48 percent being "cautious supporters"),[16] these were people going about their lives.[17] That preference is not found among the dying, for whom this is not an abstract question. As stated earlier, 3 percent of patients received MAiD.[18] The majority, I suspect, do consider it, however. It's on the table; it's on their minds because it is now allowed.

---

[16] Pennings, Ray. "Broad Support for MAiD in Canada Has Caveats and Concerns." Cardus. https://www.cardus.ca/research/health/reports/broad-support-for-MAiD-in-canada-has-caveats-and-concerns/. Accessed March 10, 2022.

[17] Of course the poll depends very much on how the question is asked. A Policy Options poll found the consensus is hardly what it appears to be. See Pennings, Ray, et al. "Canadians' Views on Assisted Dying Are Complex." Policy Options. Apr. 15, 2021. policyoptions.irpp.org/magazines/december-2020/canadians-views-on-assisted-dying-are-complex. Accessed Dec. 26, 2022.

[18] And yes, it is climbing, so that may be 4 or 5 percent by the time of publication.

Finally, there is what this does to the practice of medicine itself. Causing death has always been understood as a severe distortion of the healing relationship. Dr. Ira Byock, a palliative physician, author and advocate, explains this well.

> To protect patients' vulnerability and preserve the special trust of this relationship; there are some things that doctors must not do. The big three are no sex, no personal gain, and no killing. No sex is obvious. Doctors possess the unique authority to observe, touch and probe people in intensely intimate ways. The prohibition against sex allows patients to be vulnerable and protected from even subtle manipulation. No personal gain means that the generous compensation physicians receive for their services is enough; they must refrain from accepting personal gifts or requesting donations for their clinical centre or their research project.... No killing means just that. While alleviating suffering and, when death is near, allowing someone to die gently are our duties; even in jurisdictions where physician-assisted suicide is legal, it is beyond the scope of medical practice.[19]

An increasing number of doctors are no longer sure of that, which may be evidence that their good hearts are overflowing with a desire to alleviate suffering, but their hands have felt tied to do what their patients request... until MAiD was passed in 2016. Some have described it as empowering to their practice. Isn't that a good thing? Here is a way to do something instead of standing by and witnessing the descent into death. Is that not compassionate? Is that not merciful? Or is this act clouding their clarity on what medicine is for?

---

[19] Byock, Ira. "Love and Boundaries in Medicine." The Hastings Center, June 22, 2018, https://irabyock.org/wp-content/uploads/2018/07/Byock-Love-Boundaries-in-Medicine-Hastings-Bioethics-Forum-June-22-2018.pdf

WHAT TO EXPECT IN THIS BOOK

MAiD arises from a culture in an age when autonomy is an intoxicant. We cherish self-determination and champion technological progress, all against the backdrop of a consumer ideology of the good life and the good death. Addressing assisted dying without addressing these underlying aspects of identity, purpose, culture, and our connection to life will be an incomplete discussion. And addressing MAiD solely from a moral or religious perspective will be utterly impotent in changing the views of critics of the faith traditions. If we bring that element in, we must do more than preach to the choir. We need to offer a robust and contemporary framework for what we call the "sanctity of life," something the ancient wisdom traditions have claimed about consciousness for thousands of years – that it continues after the body does not and that it is the ultimate mystery in which we all participate, and to which we all give ourselves at death. The spiritual question is not only if and how MAiD affects that process but how it affects humanity as we support those who suffer.

Clearly, I have a lot of material to cover! Central to that is why the Canadian Hospice Palliative Care Association refuses to incorporate assisted death as a response to suffering and the frustration this elicits in the dying.[20] Do you not add to my misery by suppressing my autonomy to end my life? Well, autonomy is a construct that lives in tension with the other bioethical principles. In that tension is the unpleasant growth that evolves a culture to engage suffering with greater insight. Anything that challenges us also causes us to grow, so suffering, as hard as it is, is a potent teacher. We are astonishingly adaptable, far beyond our ability to imagine.

Bioethical debates on the right to die often center on a dichotomy: individual freedom versus the constraints imposed by culture and society. And while the voice of religious professionals (clergy) has mainly been reactionary, the voice of spiritual care practitioners (chaplains) has been… well… modest. Mute, even, as we watched the debates play out in the formation

[20] Canadian Hospice Palliative Care Association, CHPCA's Position Statement on MAiD – 2023 Update (Ottawa: Canadian Hospice Palliative Care Association, 2023). Accessed October 18, 2024, https://www.chpca.ca/wp-content/uploads/2024/07/CHPCAs- Position-Statement-on-MAiD---2023-Update.pdf.

of Bill C-14, the act that introduced MAiD in Canada, and its subsequent revisions.[21] So, what I present in this book is as much a challenge to my own professional body as to anyone else. I will explore why **not** involving spiritual care professionals increases distress among patients and the health care team. I would even assert that any desire to hasten death expressed by a patient should result in an automatic referral to spiritual care.[22] That's a tough sell when an increasing percentage of patients are disconnected from any spiritual tradition and, when asked if they'd like to receive spiritual care, decline, assuming we are religious salespeople, not psycho-spiritual therapists. (Perhaps we should be called spiritual coaches. Ugh!)

In addition, to examine the spiritual dimensions of MAiD, we must move beyond the practice itself and engage ultimate matters of the soul – specifically, the nature of this animating life force we call consciousness and how the final stages of dying allow us, if even momentarily, a glimpse of the mystery that awaits. It's called nearing-death awareness, a seemingly esoteric yet incredibly common phenomenon that is critical to explore if we're going to engage assisted dying seriously. In fact, I believe MAiD disrupts that process of waking to this deeper dimension of consciousness. This is the final stage of human development while we are here in physical form, but it is compromised because of the ego's control over the very process that requires its deconstruction.

Hopefully, I'll be able to present this material grounded in some fascinating research and models of consciousness that speak intelligently to that phenomenon and to you. I will explore death as the ultimate moment facilitating emergence into the final stage of human development, the transcendent or transpersonal apex of consciousness, drawing upon psychology and the insights of the world's most ancient spiritual traditions. They

---

[21] Bill C-14 "create[s] exemptions from the offences of culpable homicide, of aiding suicide and of administering a noxious thing, in order to permit medical practitioners and nurse practitioners to provide medical assistance in dying and to permit pharmacists and other persons to assist in the process." "Bill C-14 (Historical)" openparliament.ca. openparliament.ca/bills/42-1/C-14. Accessed Apr. 23, 2023.

[22] Kukla, Helena, et al. " 'My life became more meaningful': confronting one's own end of life and its effects on well-being – a qualitative study." *BMC Palliative Care* 21.1 (2022): p. 58.

all point to one truth: there is no way to this final state of consciousness except by completely surrendering the personal sense of self. Your ego must be deconstructed. You can delay this all you want, but that will only increase your suffering. Or you can give yourself to this process and discover grace and something far greater.

Based on the best clinical and spiritual practice, practical tools and methods will be offered to work wisely with the distress accompanying death. This is essential for our exploration, as the main reason people request MAiD is existential distress, not physical pain.[23] Those wanting MAiD cannot stand how life has disintegrated, cannot bear the anticipated suffering ahead as they die, and cannot imagine fading away in a bed, whether at home, a hospital, or a long-term care facility.[24] Frankly, most of us don't know what we're doing at the end of life. We're just trying to be human. We're just trying to get through the most challenging thing we've ever faced. It's killing us, literally. All we want is to feel safe. It's a harrowing experience to have self-determination and the foundations of well-being eroded as we approach the end of life. These dynamics at the core of our identity are aching to be addressed, and there are excellent ways to do so as we die. One, in particular, has been described as a miracle pill, effective with only a single dose: psychedelics. While its application for death anxiety is far removed from how traditional cultures have used it throughout the centuries, it may become a standard aspect of palliative care, fuelled in no small part by MAiD.

To best engage this daunting topic, I've structured the book into four parts, with most chapters having a case example and ending with an exercise. These are meant to move this material from intellectual and heartfelt considerations of the spiritual dimensions of MAiD to an experience

[23] Wiebe, Ellen, et al. "Reasons for requesting medical assistance in dying." *Canadian Family Physician* 64.9 (2018): pp. 674–679. See also Li, Madeline, et al. "Medical assistance in dying – implementing a hospital-based program in Canada." *New England Journal of Medicine* 376.21 (2017): pp. 2082–2088.

[24] Blake, Robert R., and Charlie Blake. "Why People Think They Might Hasten Their Death When Faced With Irremediable Health Conditions Compared to Why They Actually Do So." *OMEGA-Journal of Death and Dying* (2021) 00302228211033368.

of spiritual principles that can support you as you face the end of life. Fortunately, these also support a more profound experience of living, so you don't have to face your demise to benefit. Some exercises require a field trip, while others can be done in bed to support the healthy and the frail. We will engage death as a normal, even bearable, part of the life experience.

Part 1 explores the dynamics of MAiD and the ego, that personal, rational identity we build throughout our lives, and the distress that arises as it dissolves in the end. Part 2 examines cultural issues, including ethics, terminology, the slippery slope argument, and delves deeper into the distress driving MAiD requests. Part 3 focuses on models for treating that distress, including counselling, meditation, and psychedelics. Part 4 explores religious perspectives on assisted death, the deeper spiritual dimensions at play, and the astonishing surprise that many overlook but awaits us all. Finally, there is a summary of my perspective at the end, which is only three pages long. This summary is provided for those who are ill and lack the energy to read the entire book, as well as for caregivers who may be fatigued or emotionally drained.

Throughout the book, you will find stories and tools to help engage with this challenging topic, as well as a deep dive into aspects of MAiD that have yet to be explored by the public or professionals in law, government, or health care. While I encourage you to read the entire book, the latter half may be more appealing to those interested in the topic's clinical, philosophical, and religious aspects. If you only read parts 1 and 2, I recommend concluding with chapters 25 to 30 and the summary regardless.

For readers who are not religious and for those who have been harmed by religion, I understand that my credentials as a member of the clergy may lead you to question why you should continue reading past the preface. The role of religion as a moral authority has lost credibility in our age, and that responsibility now rests with law and medicine. Many view the Christian church, in particular, as deeply flawed and disgraced by sexual scandal, abuse, exploitation and corruption, on top of teachings that seem out of touch with the modern mindset. I share these concerns, and as a progressive Lutheran minister, I strive to work within the organization to shape it, evolve it, and challenge it to acknowledge and rectify its failures. However, I also believe in the wisdom that can be found within its flawed structure (which it has no copyright over). So, I will continue to discuss God and love in a manner that is hopefully intelligent, relevant, and revolutionary.

As I explore the perspective of several faith traditions, I know that I do so with no formal training in their culture, customs, or practices. Though I have consulted with leaders of these faith traditions, I appreciate that what I present is a highly condensed and simplified summary. And, though I explore the Christian perspective on suffering and how it changes us, this book fundamentally is a non-sectarian, deeply human engagement with the hottest topic in health care. Good spiritual care always respects the patient's beliefs (however defined or abstract). I hope to extend the same respect to you, the reader, for the heart of this discussion must always remain grounded in compassion and wisdom beyond any one tradition.

Now, a word on what I mean by spirituality. I am not referring to belief in God or adherence to a specific religious system. It's much broader than that! Over the centuries, people have noticed that there are standard developmental stages all humans go through on their spiritual journeys. These stages are related to the evolution of our consciousness as a process of *awakening to that which is*, or *coming to know yourself as you truly are*. This is explored through thousands of ancient writings from hundreds of cultures. The number of stages varies in each tradition, but they all have observable parallels. These stages always culminate in the dying process, an experience in which we all will enter the final stage of consciousness. Spiritual growth has always been and continues to be a critical part of the human journey.

What does this growth look like? Well, that, too, is fairly universal, marked by increased inner realization as a result of personal experience, a lessening of self-centredness, a "death" to the ego-centred way of looking at the world and a simultaneous "rebirth" into a less self-centred way of seeing things. As a person's consciousness opens to deeper yet more expansive states, they become less attached to aspirations in this world, desires, and even to their embodied self. This reaches fulfilment in death and can be considered the final stage of human development.

MAiD is movement in the opposite direction of this ultimate process by resisting and controlling how dying deconstructs our identity. I will explain why in the pages that follow, but for now, please know that my position against MAiD is not a position against anyone who chooses it. I make no moral declarations on them or their families and circle of support. I understand why many who are dying want MAiD, especially as Canadian society has normalized it. Even more, I make no moral declarations as few will be familiar with the spiritual factors and dynamics I am raising. This may be as true for religious professionals as it is for healthcare providers, palliative care specialists, and the general public. Those facing the end of their lives may be even less familiar with these ideas. Their energies are consumed by the experience of their own suffering, their fear, and the emotional effect their condition has on those they love. I trust, though, that in the deep contemplation that accompanies the dying process, they are already engaged in this material far beyond any systematic organization I employ to explain it.

As with all decisions a person makes about their medical care, MAiD is now their choice at life's end. It may be wise or not. It may demonstrate great self-awareness or not. But, as assisted dying is now legal in Canada, it is their choice to make. And though I am a member of the clergy, I can make no statement on how that affects a person's soul once they move beyond the veil. That's beyond my scope of practice! However, what is within my practice is speaking to this issue and its impact on the spiritual health of humanity. If there is a moral weight to this, it remains on this side of the grass with us as a culture. Moral declarations are most dangerous when they become unilateral, for morality and ethics must never exist outside the container of relationships. This is the human journey we are talking about. If someone desires an early exit, I have no right to condemn them for it and must earn the right to come into their suffering and share, to whatever extent I can, the wound of their heart. Only then may I speak to their pain. That is what I have been doing for twenty-five years, yet I can no longer do it within the medical setting because of the moral distress created in me by assisted dying. This forms an incredible tension within me, for if I do not speak to this on a cultural level, I will be left in additional moral distress. So, here it is. May this book enrich that discernment and identify what's missing with this new option at the end of life.

If you are a community member interested in the topic, may this book add to your considerations and enhance your conversations.

If you are a healthcare professional, I hope this book deepens your practice and dedication to self-care, as well as care for others.

If you struggle that a loved one has died through MAiD, I invite you to engage it trusting that God's understanding, love, and grace are infinitely greater than ours. Furthermore, I encourage you to engage this book for a deeper consideration of aspects of the human journey that you may not have been aware of before.

If you are a family member supporting someone as they die, may this book help you navigate the most challenging experience of your heart, work wisely with grief, and merge that sorrow with gratitude for the life soon to be lost.

And if you have been diagnosed with a life-threatening condition, are considering MAiD, or are actively dying, may this book assist you in navigating the wilderness we all must traverse, yet fundamentally do so alone. May it awaken wonder and wisdom, raising self-awareness and compassion for yourself. May it offer something that stems from the most profound dimensions of your being, something sufficient to bring you to your greatest truth, to the gift of who and what you are in this brief passage of time. And may I use your time effectively in the reading, for you have no time to waste. So, let's get to the bedside and visit someone considering MAiD.

EARLY EXITS

Spirituality, Mortality, and Meaning in an Age of Medical Assistance in Dying

PART 1

Maid and Ego

CHAPTER 1

ONE'S WORST NIGHTMARE

The best journey takes you home.

– UNKNOWN

THE GREATEST LESSONS OF LIFE ALWAYS ORBIT AROUND LOVE. AND when we reach the end of life loving well and being well-loved, that end can be infused with as much gratitude as grief. For all my patients have taught me about that enterprise, I have to say, with great pride, that my best teachers were my parents. How lovely that these central lessons have come full circle in my journey; the ones who loved me most in the beginning are the ones who completed that lesson at their end. And this was marked, in no small part, in how they considered MAiD against the suffering ahead.

"What are you most scared of?" It's a crowbar of a question meant to pry open fear and disgorge its contents quickly. This is a critical area aching to be explored when a patient is considering MAiD, but one I'm sorry to say is rarely ventured beyond the surface by MAiD assessors, who determine a person's eligibility for the procedure. They will identify this distress, but they do not treat it. I'm surprised people will so readily go there with me, but perhaps that's because I'm not family. I'm a stranger, a kind and compassionate one, a professional and expert on death and dying, but a stranger, nonetheless. So, they talk. And they all say the same thing:

I'm afraid of losing control. I'm so scared of suffering for an interminable length of days. I'm afraid of being a burden on my family.

I hear their words. I understand their perspective. I invite them, as a guide who, having faced cancer multiple times, has walked the labyrinth of suffering (not without stumbling!), to consider that there is a mystery at the centre – something waiting that we cannot name, cannot even imagine, even though I have witnessed it time and time again: Presence. Spirit. Deep stillness. The only way to get there is naturally and slowly. However, all those I've supported who wanted MAiD were not interested in using the time they had to unpack their life, deconstruct the ego, or dive deep into suffering by allowing their disintegration. They wanted comfort. They wanted the problem of death fixed. They wanted to feel safe.

"What are you most scared of?" With any other patient, I hold my gaze and ask this without effort, buoyed by compassion and professional clarity. But this time, I struggled to breathe as I felt the swell of sadness rise and swallow me whole. It is one thing to ask this of a stranger considering MAiD. It is another to ask of your mother.

She lay in the palliative care unit. Dementia had slipped in like a thief, stealing fragments of her over the months and disguising itself as minor aberrations brought on by a bad day, bad luck, or bad memory. Isn't this just part of getting old? Chronic urinary tract infections also provided an alternative explanation, which I found myself clinging to. Maybe she needs antibiotics. This can easily be managed. Perhaps it's her diabetes. "Is she still hiding Mars bars in her bedroom?" I'd ask my sisters, who had beautifully stepped up as the primary caregivers. They knew I was grasping at straws. Eventually, there was no denying what it was… and we knew that she knew. Mom was no fool. She had cared for her mother through Alzheimer's. That experience was horrible, marked by violent behaviour and intense physical care. While we somehow knew our mother would not go that way, the outcome of total dependency was still unacceptable for her. Now, with MAiD just legalized, she had an option. She had a choice. She had control. And, she had this window of cognitive clarity to discuss that death with her son, the chaplain, the expert and author working on his second book, wrestling with the very words you're reading now.

"David, this could go on for a long time. So, I had a little chat with my doctor. I want him to do that thing you're writing about."

"That thing."

"Yes, where they put you out. Just put me out, simple."

"You mean MAiD?"

"Yes, that's it. Simple."

Simple! I felt the emotional abyss within me and imagined the agonizing void ahead for her. I also felt... anger. Simple! How cavalier, how convenient those words made it seem. How easy. My head swam with indignation, and then, thankfully, I paused. Breathed. Relaxed. All that emotion was my homework. And she's just finding a way to be protective, to make it safe to have this most difficult conversation with her son. She was not being coy; she was being careful with my heart and with her hope. Finally returning to myself, I asked, "What are you most afraid of, Mom?"

It was as if I was hearing the answers for the first time. She spoke them softly but with immense weight. "Losing control. Suffering. Becoming a burden." Her voice was raspy, her body weak, but her words could not have been more accurate. Most striking was the honesty in her eyes – not strained as mine were with tears on the edge of eruption, but clear and simple, heavy and true. She spoke with the awareness of one who had been walking the road of preparatory grief long before I laid a foot upon that path. She had been thinking about this for some time. And no wonder! Dependency on others had been steadily increasing. A chairlift had been installed at home to access the bathroom. The dining room had been converted into a bedroom. Eventually, she could not even rise without a two-person assist. Then the wheelchair. Then the hospital bed. Then weeks in palliative care, waiting to die. When it became clear that would not happen anytime soon, the wait for long-term care placement began. That could take months.

I responded as her son, not as her chaplain. My voice cracked a bit. "That makes sense, Mom. Losing control, becoming a burden. Yes. . . ." And then, too soon, I offered a rescue. "Mom, we can be at your side for as long as it takes. We will love you to the end. It is not a burden. It is an honour. We are ready to grieve and do everything we can to ensure you're comfortable." My words stopped there as I realized I was not focusing on her in those statements. I was emphasizing our needs, our commitment… my sorrow, my grief. What was it like for her? I realized her concern for being a burden had nothing to do with our ability to care for her but with her ability to be cared for. We must never underestimate how giving ourselves over to complete dependency is a foundational challenge to our identity.

"Mom, this is the hardest thing you've ever faced. You've told me before that you're not afraid of death. You're quite curious about it. But dying, this way of dying… is hard. This slowly erodes who and how you are in the world."

She nodded. Or was that nodding off? Hard to tell, as she increasingly spent more time sleeping. I felt this window was closing quickly. "Mom, this is part of dying – to have it all fall away until there's nothing that holds you together except the love." Her head nodded, then sagged, eyes now closed. I watched her face become slack, her breath shift. She began to snore. My tears could softly flow without protection. "Love you, Mom. Love you."

A brief conversation with her doctor confirmed that she had not only talked about MAiD but had been assessed and found ineligible due to her increasing confusion. And while she was not in any physical pain, her dependency would only increase as time went by. The scale of that time, and what it would ask of her, was beyond our comprehension. But we did know that we would do whatever we could to ensure she had the best quality of life possible, marked by belonging, compassionate care, dignity, and love. We could not see the mountaintop, but we could see where to put our feet for the next step in the climb.

Two years passed. Two years of dependency and deterioration, drifting into dementia. Despite my sisters' exceptional care for her at home, we all agreed the best next step was to move to a higher level of nursing support. We were fortunate, so fortunate, to place her in one of the best nursing homes in the province, right next door to the hospital. It was brand new, developed in collaboration between a private firm and the Sisters of

St. Martha, the nuns now its primary residents. Our mother would be surrounded by their compassion and supported by excellent nursing. Daily, we would witness the nuns embracing her as part of their community, infused with laughter, affirmation, and daily prayer. Though our mother is not religious (unlike her son!), she is… how should I put it… mischievously delightful in her spiritual practice. So were the Sisters of St. Martha, it turned out. Gentle joking quickly built the belonging that is so central to well-being. This community would provide unexpected gifts of life and countless beautiful, ordinary moments. Mom never could have imagined that from the perspective of the palliative care unit. And we never could have imagined the personal growth within us that resulted from waiting for her death longer than we could comprehend.

Three years. We are astonished she has survived and that dementia has been so gradual in dissolving the person we knew. We see through to her occasionally, but the moments of clarity are like small, smudged circles rubbed clear on an old window. The light flickers in brief words – she recognizes us, then drifts. She comments with typical dry wit on some aspect of life… these can be hilarious… until she pauses, the eyes roll back, and another small seizure wipes a bit more of her away. And I am left recalling her dread of this erosion, this dependency.

My mother can now lift little more than her head, a hand perhaps. She relies on others for everything – to be moved, fed, changed, washed, checked on through the night and found staring blankly at the ceiling, drifting, waiting. What is your world now, Mom? Do you lament your living? Are you lost and alone in a land of distorted perception? Do you dream, and in your dreams, are you well and young again? I know you are waiting to die. You have told us enough to know that.

“It takes too long,” you whispered one rainy afternoon. “I’m done.” My soul swam in sorrow. What would this have been like for her if she had been permitted to die by MAiD? What had these three years done to her? Why did this wretched disease have to come upon her? What was the point?

I held your hand and cried openly that time, not bothering to protect you from my tears. And in that, you touched my face and became my mother again, clear and present. Your eyes were soft, but your words were marked with that sharp wit. "Eh," you said, "None of that! Pull up, my boy." Then you smiled.

TOP TEN REASONS

As we explore the spiritual dimensions of MAiD, I recognize my position may persuade some, but I don't expect it will affect the law. It will take a radical shift in government and society for that choice to be taken away now that the horse has left the barn. Western culture focuses on profit and efficiency, and there is no persuasive argument or explanation as to why such a society would have our best interest at heart. Canada's healthcare system is crippled, so with a significant percentage of healthcare costs expended in the last year of life, MAiD's economic benefit fits neatly into the idea that the liberty of the individual is sacred.[25, 26] In such a setting, there is no convincing explanation that there is a better alternative, especially as assisted death seems to allow a person to die as they have lived, leaving behind the memory of an essentially whole person: brave, realistic, facing the truth of life and the inevitability of death.

What might change someone's mind is experiencing life in a different way, where self-determination is not the ultimate criterion of human dignity. At this point, only inspiration from a lived experience of love and acceptance and something so much more than liberty and living on your terms can convince someone that an alternative to MAiD may be preferable and possible. Where can we find this in a culture increasingly unfamiliar with dying as a community-building event? How can we die wise when there is little social capital left to draw on to help us navigate the end of our days? This capital is the shared set of values, beliefs, and practices that create social cohesion and trust within a community. Religion used to be a source for this, but Western culture has largely discarded that, and people have limited community and lackluster engagement with spiritual

---

[25] Canadian Institute for Health Information. "Health care use at the end of life in western Canada." (2007).

[26] Bernier, Govindadeva. Cost Estimate for Bill C-7 "Medical Assistance in Dying." Government of Canada, 2020.

principles. With each MAiD procedure, a withdrawal is made from the larger social capital that is rapidly depleted, so it affects us all.

You'll find I make no statements as to how MAiD affects one's state of consciousness in whatever realm awaits us after death, even as I consider the teachings of spiritual traditions on that matter. For my part, I trust that the compassion and love that receives those who choose an early exit will be infinitely more than the compassion and love that, hopefully, surrounds them as they die.

Even with that perspective, I believe that MAiD is one of the worst things we can do to ourselves as a culture. To explore that well, I must first move in the opposite direction and appreciate why people choose MAiD. I must acknowledge and demonstrate that *I get it.* All my conversations and considerations on the matter remain otherwise abstract and irrelevant unless I compassionately embed myself, to the best of my ability, with the one choosing an early exit. For the day will come when I am the one in the bed, swallowed by suffering and anxiety in a life now to last only months, weeks, or days. So, here are ten reasons MAiD seems a desirable option.

1. MAiD promises a smooth exit. On this point alone, it is entirely understandable why people would choose it. Their imagination of what lies ahead is painful to them. The weight of their loved one's grief is heavy upon them. The memory of another's difficult death may be embedded in them. And the "futility of suffering" is always before them. The road ahead looks only to get worse. No wonder suicidal thoughts are exceedingly common among those with a terminal prognosis, though relatively few attempt it.[27,28] And for good reason – what of suicide's impact on loved ones? What of my legacy when this is my last act? And… what if it goes wrong? How empowering when one can choose MAiD. Here is society's

[27] Kleespies, Phillip M., Douglas H. Hughes, and Fiona P. Gallacher. "Suicide in the medically and terminally ill: psychological and ethical considerations." *Journal of Clinical Psychology* 56.9 (2000): pp. 1153–1171.

[28] Chochinov, Harvey Max, et al. "Depression, hopelessness, and suicidal ideation in the terminally ill." *Psychosomatics* 39.4 (1998): pp. 366–370.

blessing, and medicine's expertise, ensuring that your wish to die in this way is honoured. You can trust the professional to do it quickly, with primary consideration of your comfort and desires.

2. MAiD is death on your terms. The act can feel empowering, as your mental and emotional energy is freed up to contemplate your demise without as much anxiety. This act embodies the dignity and self-determination you deeply crave. Your rights feel respected, while your ownership of your body, choices, and fate is the final and ultimate exercise of personal liberty. The medical system can serve you the way you want when facing your greatest fear: final suffering and a turbulent takeoff.

3. MAiD gives you time to orchestrate what, many agree, can be a deeply meaningful experience. Instead of interminable days languishing in the torment of dying, you can leave quickly with a tender smile upon your face, genuine gratitude within your heart, and a tearful kiss of love upon your cheek. Some have thrown parties for the occasion, a living wake in which they can say final goodbyes while words can still be formed and wine can still be enjoyed.

4. MAiD does what Western medicine has fumbled in doing: getting people to talk about the reality of death. Yes, doctors and nurses deal with death daily, but still predominantly within the framework of failure. It is, after all, what medicine strives to prevent! And MAiD seems to bring relief not only to those dying but anyone imagining such a state. So many times, I've heard someone casually say, "Well, if I'm ever in that situation, I'll just choose MAiD." They speak of it as an act of mercy, compassion, comfort, and, most of all, as a way to avoid suffering. To the average person, it actually makes dying feel safer.

5. MAiD, to many who are dying, is a way to shield their loved ones from what feels like unnecessarily protracted grief. Any action that makes death a bit easier or straightforward for the family is very appealing. I've heard many patients say it felt like an act of

kindness, consideration, and love. It also energizes the effort to talk about what's most important to you at the end of life. This includes honestly saying what you need and graciously accepting help. That can be empowering for your family and care providers, knowing they are doing what can be done and feeling that they are on the same page… at least with the practical issues.

6. MAiD is an effective analgesic for existential distress because you no longer need to fear the final slide into mystery or the loss of activity and control. Existential distress occurs because your identity in the world, lived out through your role in family, work, and the activities that make life meaningful, is eroded away by suffering and dying. You are reduced to the body in the bed. This distress is why most request MAiD, stating they see no point in enduring such disintegration.[29] As soon as it is approved, the distress subsides. Knowing MAiD is an option you can keep in your back pocket is enough for many.

7. MAiD creates opportunities for structured, intentional expressions of gratitude. This is part of saying goodbye, of letting people know how much they mean to you. Even sincerely saying thank you for small acts of care is empowering; it connects you to others. This act creates a sense of abundance in the heart of the dying person and those who remain. Gratitude increases happiness, and self-esteem improves relationships and energizes one's engagement with the moment before them.[30] As such, it is a potent agent for alleviating situational depression, which is common in the dying. Gratitude gets us out of our own way, shifting us to a sense of deeper connection and completion. It is healing and restoration for the soul, all the more critical when one leaves this world.

---

[29] Li, Madeline, et al. "Medical assistance in dying – implementing a hospital-based program in Canada." *New England Journal of Medicine* 376.21 (2017): pp. 2082–2088.

[30] Wood, Alex M., Jeffrey J. Froh, and Adam WA Geraghty. "Gratitude and well-being: A review and theoretical integration." *Clinical Psychology Review* 30.7 (2010): pp. 890–905.

8. MAiD creates opportunities for reconciliation. No one leaves this world without some rubble, some damage left behind. Knowing your literal deadline is great motivation to attend to those awkward conversations and leave this world without unnecessary baggage. While most realize the relational pain they felt in life is not worth carrying to the next, there are some who do not know how to let it go. Worse, there are some who gain some delight, some satisfaction that their death might twist the knife one more time. This righteous indignation only hurts themselves, of course. The offending party may never realize the extent of this injury. MAiD is motivation to name that pain in its raw form, challenge the offender to authentic engagement to achieve, if not reconciliation, then at least release of the wrapping that has constrained the heart, often for decades of one's life.

9. MAiD has been described as profoundly spiritual by the dying and their loved ones, all the more when they use the event to create personal rituals to mark the end of life. Favourite music, blessings and goodbyes, treasured possessions of the dying mindfully bestowed upon others, prayers and commendations offered at the bedside; all these are rituals of farewell. I've even known devout members of religions that condemn euthanasia nonetheless choose it as their way to go. One woman commented, "I trust God will understand my decision." Even more, despite their tradition's prohibition against assisted death, a few clerics have been present to bless the dying, administer rites and sacraments, to pray and provide all they could to make this a sacred event. MAiD has been carried out in public parks for one final connection to nature, at spiritual retreat centres, and in church sanctuaries where one's connection to God felt strongest.[31]

---

[31] Carnevale, Sabrina. "Back to where they started: Betty Sanguin chose a medically assisted death in the church where the ALS sufferer had raised her family" *The Free Press* https://www.winnipegfreepress.com/arts-and-life/2022/04/04/back-to-where-they-started. Accessed May 20, 2020.

10. Finally, MAiD seems to make so much sense. It appears to be a compassionate and merciful act for those who describe their suffering as intolerable and those who feel no other option is acceptable or adequate. Of course, we must be wise in discerning this, for what is being felt is not a desire to end one's life but a desire for hastened death. It's taking too long, and it feels too hard. This desire increases when approaching the end of life. We often see this in palliative and hospice settings, where excellent care enables one to live into their dying longer than ever before.[32] The resulting frustration is understandable when you'd like to hurry death along. This is why the driving factors behind the desire for medically assisted dying are equivalent to those driving MAiD: depression, hopelessness, demoralization, lack of social support, feeling like a burden to others, purposeless waiting, meaningless days, and loss of perceived dignity.[33] That's certainly what my mother feared. It used to be that you had no choice save suicide. But now, in Canada and a handful of other countries, you can request an early exit before fading to that final breath.

I gazed at my mother's smile. It lasted only a moment before her eyes closed, and she descended once again to her abyssal world. Did she remember our conversation three years earlier? I did. It was written into my soul like a broken record, a groove that cut deeper every time I played it. As I drove home, I wondered how it would have felt to witness the needle being placed in her arm, to see a doctor deliberately end her life… to say goodbye. But remaining in that groove only broke my heart again and again, leaving me imprisoned in a world of "what ifs?" The only solution was to come back to this reality, this moment, this connection. So as the

---

[32] Bellido-Pérez, Mercedes, et al. "Assessment of the wish to hasten death in patients with advanced disease: A systematic review of measurement instruments." *Palliative Medicine* 31.6 (2017): pp. 510–525.

[33] Hudson PL, LJ Kristjanson, M. Ashby, et al. "Desire for hastened death in patients with advanced disease and the evidence base of clinical guidelines: a systematic review." *Palliative Medicine*. 20 (2006): pp. 693–701.

kilometres passed by, I thought it through. I knew she was well cared for. I knew she was loved. And I knew I was grieving. Intellectually, I understood that sorrow was, ironically, a healthy response. And I knew it was so much more than an emotion. Grief is an entire state of being, an orientation to self and circumstances you cannot control. Yet grief is also grace asking you to allow it all, for it stems from the perceived separation we have from each other, a separation ultimately healed by a spiritual process of awakening. To do so, of course, we must allow the ego, the "separate self" to die. And the rational voice in me was trying hard to resist that disintegration. Its voice of defence was quite... rational. "We're doing everything we can. She didn't have competency, anyway. It was never an option." All the while, as the hours rolled by, my tears marked the distance beneath humming tires.

EXERCISE 1: FIELD TRIP

To become more familiar with your feelings around death, sit in a cemetery, alone or with a friend. Take your time strolling by the graves. Stop and feel the air, hear the sounds, feel the earth beneath your feet. Lie down in the grass by a grave. Let the sunlight play upon your closed eyelids. Imagine. Note whatever feelings arise.

Chapter 2

DEATH ANXIETY

Life is pleasant; death is peaceful. It's the transition that's troublesome.

– ISAAC ASIMOV

If you're going to wrestle with mortality, you might as well grab some popcorn and do it through a good film. In *The Seventh Seal,* Ingmar Bergman engages in a profound inquiry into the nature of faith and the torment of death anxiety. It's a stunning allegory of our search for meaning and a work of stark visual poetry. Through the simplicity of a chess game, a knight, who returns from the crusades only to find the bubonic plague decimating his home country of Sweden, negotiates with death. He is buying time to perform one last redemptive act, something that will bring peace to his soul. Each character in *The Seventh Seal* reveals that how we cope with death is inextricably tied to how we live. In fact, they are one and the same.

I found myself watching this classic late one night during the pandemic. It brought new insights to the news cycle: a disillusioned soldier returning from a fruitless war, a looming plague threatening humanity, the eroding belief in religion… and that we still don't play chess very well. With MAiD, at least, we tell the reaper when to make the final move.

I see this with my patients as they negotiate with mortality until the end or deny it with the declaration that a miracle is still possible. That doesn't sound reasonable, but this is not about reason. This is about the most primal aspects of our identity. This is about being afraid, plain and simple. In a culture that insulates us from suffering (while we also project it upon the screen for entertainment), death is unfamiliar, institutionalized, medicalized, and modernized. Which leaves us quietly terrified in the end.

Think of it: we're the only animal that can ponder the future and the past. Thanks to the neural marvel between our ears, we have built empires and harnessed the forces of nature. We have reduced poverty and improved the quality of life for billions. We decipher the subatomic world and discover new planets orbiting distant stars. Yet as our reach extends to ever greater tomorrows, death remains constant, and suffering becomes ever more unfamiliar and existentially unacceptable. So, MAiD seems to make sense. However, such a rational response is seen as something entirely irrational through the lens of something fit for a Stephen King novel. It's called terror management theory. This psychological perspective argues that our phobia of death is one of the reasons we might watch *The Seventh Seal* or slow down to view a traffic accident. These experiences give us an outlet – we're able to face the *concept* of death without having to think specifically about our own. MAiD has a similar dynamic by turning the experience of death from an ultimate mystery to a controlled medical procedure. Yes, there are those who choose MAiD to embrace their end, to turn toward death face-on, heart open, grateful, though exhausted. However, this is done to *preserve* comfort and *prevent* the total surrender of ego-identity to the final stages of natural death (which, understandably, are imagined as unnecessarily prolonged, devoid of meaning and burdensome to loved ones).

How predictable. Throughout life, we tend to be terrified of feeling pain, loss, grief, and sorrow, so we engage in behaviours that medicate or distract… and these become magnets for more pain because they feed more disconnection from ourselves. We run from difficult emotional states straight into the arms of fear and the desperate need for control.

Researcher and author Brené Brown found this to be her own default as she struggled with self-sabotaging behaviour in her early twenties. She states, "it was years of terrifying change, hard goodbyes, and boundaries – a truckload of boundaries. When we stop numbing and start feeling and learning again, we have to re-evaluate everything, especially how to choose loving ourselves over making other people comfortable. It was the hardest work I've ever done and continue to do."[34]

Apply that to dying. At no other point do goodbyes become harder, and boundaries become clearer. Here we are called to love ourselves enough to trust our feelings and allow them, to trust our body and the signals it gives, and to trust our medical team in addressing them. We are learning how to discern that others' feelings are their homework, not our responsibility. We are clarifying who we are; we are re-evaluating life and death itself. It is the hardest work anyone will ever do.

Turning toward our anxiety can bring grace and clarity, openness and allowing. Turning toward death will do the same and more. I say this because I trust the dying process. Having seen it unfold countless times in a quarter-century of practice and doing so alongside amazing medical professionals, I believe the centre will hold – that our consciousness will naturally shift to a state of transcendence. I also say this knowing it is the hardest thing in the world when death takes its time.

But now there is MAiD. Now, there is an enabling act that soothes the ego's desires for safety, for a solution, for control. It certainly can *feel* like allowing death. People have even said it demonstrates their full acceptance of death. But this is on their terms, the terms of the ego. The bottom line remains: we want to die existentially intact. Is this because we live in a manufactured environment, cut off from nature, insulated from suffering, and uprooted from ancestry? Stephen Jenkinson thinks so. An author and expert in palliative care, his insights on this are bracing: "What we suffer from most," he says, "is culture failure, amnesia of ancestry and deep family story, phantom or sham rites of passage, no instruction on how to live with each other or with the world around us or with our dead or with our history."[35]

---

[34] Brown, Brené. *Atlas of the Heart: Mapping Meaningful Connection and the Language of Human Experience*. Random House, 2021. p. xviii

[35] Goodman, Leslee. "A Good Death: An Interview With Stephen Jenkinson." www.dailygood.org/story/2267/a-good-death-an-interview-with-stephen-jenkinson. Accessed Dec. 22, 2022.

His experience gives further insight into the nature of death anxiety in this modern age: "In every deathbed and hospital room," Jenkinson writes, "I didn't see sane dying. I saw sedated dying, depressed dying, isolated dying, utterly disembodied dying. Sane dying would require a childhood steeped in death's presence, adulthood employed in its service, and an elderhood testifying to its necessity. Sane dying is a village-making event: lots of people with plenty to do, and the whole production endorses life. What does our way of dying endorse?"[36]

That is a good question. MAiD does not endorse the sanctity of life but the sanctity of the individual. That's quite an impoverished perspective. If death is the ultimate transformation of consciousness through expansion and awakening to the Ground of Being (what we call God), then it is the most crucial event in life. We should have frank discussions on it throughout the journey and blunt engagements with its wonder at the end. The dying should be encouraged to ask the big questions, "How will I die? What will it feel like physically, emotionally, and spiritually? Give me a road map so that I may find my way." However, few people have a spiritual guide, and few healthcare professionals are comfortable describing the emotional and spiritual experience of dying. That's a difficult conversation when we are wired with a survival mechanism so strong that it easily overrides coping and cognition as death approaches.

SHELLY

She had always thought she was tough, but the news Shelly received was enough to make even the strongest cower in fear. She'd been through an abusive childhood, had a reckless adulthood, lived on the streets, and endured the soul-destroying life of an addict. Cocaine was her escape from a wretched world. But she had known friendship, too, and her best friend... perhaps her only friend, was the sole visitor to the

[36] Hoffner, Erik. "As We Lay Dying, Stephen Jenkinson On How We Deny Our Mortality." *The Sun*, (Aug. 2015) https://thesunmagazine.org/issues/476/as-we-lay-dying Accessed Dec. 13, 2022.

floor. The doctors told Shelly she had terminal colon cancer. Her time on earth was limited to just a few weeks.

She couldn't believe it. She'd faced the worst situations in life, but this was something different. This enemy was within. The thought of dying made her tremble with fear, and the prospect of the pain and suffering she would endure in her last days was too much to bear. She lashed out at the staff, brooded in her bed, and requested MAiD – multiple times. Each one required another assessment. Each one was scheduled, then cancelled by her at the last minute. We knew what was going on. Given her feisty character and fierce determination, it was no surprise she was using MAiD to defend her self-esteem. It was an effective way of managing the terror of mortality, for each time death was scheduled, she had the power to postpone it. It was the only control she had at this point.

I wondered if Shelly would receive me, but kindness seems in short supply in many lives. She welcomed my gentle manner. She opened her heart, and, from it, placed the gift of her broken story into mine. It began, as most human tragedies do, with abandonment. Her father left at an early age. Her mother descended in desperation to sell her body before destroying it with alcohol. And Shelly's life continued in the only way she knew: through using others, trusting herself alone, and scrapping for her place beneath the table of those who let their crumbs fall. She experienced more compassion in the hospital than at any time in her forty-two years.

"What do you wish for, Shelly?" I wanted to help her repair her childhood; imagination is central in approaching archaic wounds.

She paused, curled and frail in the bed. It was cluttered with quilts and books and stuffed animals – a young girl's sanctuary. Her tobacco-stained fingers trembled upon her thin lips. "What does anyone wish for?" Her voice was throaty and deep. "To belong. To be loved. I know I'm dying; I just wish I wasn't alone." And then she said something utterly surprising. "So... I called my dad. I told him. I don't expect anything... he's tried a few times to come into my life, then he tells me how to live it. But I thought he should know." Another pause. Then she looked into my eyes. "And you know what? He's coming. He bought a ticket; he's coming. So when he gets here, I'll do it. I'll do it for real this time."

"MAiD," I said. "And you won't be alone when you go." That was the theme as she related a tale of years I could not imagine enduring. Several times she had come close to death, which, she confessed, was her own doing – one poor decision led so naturally to another until the circumstances stripped her of options.

"Life on the street has its own community," she reflected. "I wasn't always alone. You know who has your back, but you still don't trust anyone completely. Trust is for fools."

Interesting. In her company, I knew I was one who trusted too much. I wouldn't last a week out there. My respect for her resilience soared. Yet I also knew that trust was essential in the hospital for authentic connection. It requires equal parts brokenness, courage, and clarity of the best in you when others forget that in themselves. Here is where forgiveness comes into play. Could Shelly discover that to forgive her father meant no longer being imprisoned by the pain of the past? Could she become someone greater than who she used to be? This didn't depend on what he said or would say or failed to say when they met. This was up to her. She could do it now. And by the tone of her voice, it seemed she already had.

"I hope that visit goes better than either of you imagine," I said. "I hope he doesn't try to fix your life. Maybe he'll just sit here and tell you he's sorry."

"I'll take that!" she said, smiling. "But I don't need him to say it, really. We both screwed up. I'm more like him than I want to admit. I get it. We screw up. But maybe we won't screw this up."

And they didn't. She later shared that he had sat with her, listened to her, opened his heart and from it, placed the gift of his broken story into hers. From mutual vulnerability, she was able to say the truth. "I'm afraid. I don't know what's going to happen to me." And he was able to be the father he had never been. Dignity and identity in both of them were restored as they laid their lives on the table, no cards hidden, all chips on love.

Here was the best practice of a clinical approach, employed not so much with great skill as great compassion. Terror management theory offers a solution common to several counselling techniques: telling your story, and having it compassionately received, so that your dignity and self-esteem are honoured in the deepest way through a vulnerable, grateful presence. It proposes that a basic psychological conflict results from having a primal self-preservation instinct while realizing that death is inevitable. Recall that existential or spiritual distress is that which threatens the integrity of one's identity. Death is the ultimate annihilation of the self. What could possibly counter that fear? Belonging. Compassion. Deep, heartfelt presence. We build purpose into the dying person's life by taking the time to sit with them and, more than that, to learn from them. The dying are esteemed.

This is what happened to Shelly, and, as a result, she allowed death to take its natural course. The pain she feared was managed by meds. The frailty that followed was met with no resistance. As she diminished in energy, she opened to her own presence. She was in the moment, no longer longing for another that may be better, different, or anything other than what was. This was made possible, in no small part, by simply seeing the eyes of her father or a nurse when she opened hers and hearing the words, "I'm here."

The remedy to her terror was found in the unpacking of her life and enfolding of love. Her imagination fed her fear, her defences projected her anger, MAiD gave her control, and then compassionate presence dissolved her desire for it and made possible the discovery of what sounds impossible: when we turn toward death and greet it with a bow, we are able to do what we never imagined we could do. We are able to die.

Terror management theory also offers a bracing insight: that MAiD is one example of how an entire society may make decisions primarily to avoid thoughts of death or to make it as comfortable as possible so as to prevent the deepest engagement with that ultimate moment.

To die, or rather, to know you are going to die, will always turn the fiction of death (which always happens to others) into a documentary of death. For the vast majority of us, that *must* trigger death anxiety as a passage to one's awakening, which spiritually is the loss of the perceived, separate self (the ego) and the awakening to complete interconnectivity and unity with everything. The ego is the part of us engaged in self-justification, rationalization, and decision-making, and it tends to dominate our personality in Western culture. So, of course we're overwhelmed when losing all that we think we are when we know of nothing else. The ego can feel no other, for in death, it runs into its own boundaries of identity without even knowing those boundaries exist because the self *is* those structures and boundaries: role in the family, activity in the world, identification with the body, with the past, with experience and expectations. This is marked by profound helplessness that has more than an edge of loneliness to it. Such isolation is required to confront the perceived self, relax protective patterns, and open with trust to a process that can never be understood by the mind, but certainly is known by the soul. We consent to not knowing, an existential orientation intolerable to the ego, for this allows its annihilation. No wonder the realization that an illness is terminal activates the long-repressed terror of non-existence. *There is no way the mental ego can confront its own death without anxiety.*

How do we consent? By not resisting. One might speak to the frightened part of themself, speak even directly to the terror, and say, "I am experiencing you, but I am not you. You are so destabilizing, so powerful in your disruption of my well-being. You are a nightmare to me. However (and here, it helps to gently and tenderly smile at the terror), I am the open loving space of awareness in which you appear. You can rage all you like, and you can stay for as long as you wish. You can be as intense as you like. You are completely welcome within me." Can you say this to death itself? Thankfully, you may not have to.

Stephen Jenkinson, in his highly recommended guide *How It All Could Be: A Workbook for Dying People and Those Who Love Them*, poetically challenges us to consider that the reaper is not the enemy and certainly not one we need to flee from or speed toward. He says, "Your cancer is your executioner, but your death is your angel. You wrestle the executioner by chemotherapy and radiation and eating right. You wrestle the angel by grief, by wonder, by courting uncertainty, by falling in love again with being alive, this time with the taste of its end strongly on your tongue."[37]

Jenkinson's imagery captures the dual nature of our engagement with death – one rooted in our body's mortality and the other in our soul's transcendence. But while we wrestle the physical executioner, we often fail to wrestle the angel. The ancients and those modern souls who have a supportive community and a healthy spiritual practice know this. They suffer far less distress.[38] They are able to move into their limited tomorrows surrounded by compassion, contemplatively embedded in ambiguity, open to the mystery. Even more, they are linked to traditions that embrace the complex dimensions of life energies from which we flow. Cultures throughout the world have always known there is more to us than meets the eye, that we are composed of several identities or bodies, and that consciousness continues long after the convincing bodily form shuts down.

Daily we experience the most superficial level, the solid body to which ego-identity attaches the self. Beneath this is a subtle dream body, one we all experience each night, then shrug off as an abstract state through which we encounter our subconscious material and symbolically work out our issues. Most of the time we forget it within seconds of waking to our day. However, as Anthony Stevens lays out in his excellent book *Private Myths: Dreams and Dreaming*, the reality we experience in our sleep is a fundamental creative act of the subconscious for processing archetypal aspects of our connection to life. Even more, dreaming enables the brain to process information far beyond its neural mass. Without dreaming, Stevens points out, our brains and cranial capacity would have to be several times larger, making birth impossible. Dreaming is evolution's way of accelerating our intelligence and processing power without compromising our

---

[37] Jenkinson, Stephen. *How It All Could Be, A Workbook for Dying People and Those Who Love Them.* Orphan Wisdom, 2009, p. 1.

[38] Taghiabadi, Mina, et al. "The association between death anxiety with spiritual experiences and life satisfaction in elderly people." *Electronic Physician* 9.3 (2017): 3980.

survival.[39] In the same way that dreams access hidden layers of our being, death – like a final dream – offers a passage into deeper, often unrecognized dimensions of our existence.

Spiritual traditions assert that we can move even further to yet more subtle dimensions of consciousness through vision quests, meditation, medications, trance, dance, drumming and, in the end, dying. Consciousness can shift to the unseen realms from which we emanate, and death is the final process by which we all expand to these transdimensional states of being. In the West, we call these levels body, mind, and spirit, but it is far more complex in other traditions. Yet, the material realm is so convincing that we often think that is all there is.

In addition to living in a society where reality is significantly reduced, we live in a culture that increasingly emphasizes safety first. This is even more evident in medicine (and rightfully so). Protocols and procedures are scrutinized and regulated to minimize the risk of infection, mistakes, or anything short of "best practice." Foundational to this is not accelerating, let alone causing, death. But MAiD now introduces a tension – for many, it feels safer than natural death or prolonged suffering. Additionally, as medicine advances, this line becomes blurry; some cancer patients are given chemotherapy that has a slim chance of even mediocre success and a high probability of escalating physical suffering to the point of what many would call torture. This is not an indictment of the medical team – it is often the patient who asks, at the end of life, if there is anything else that could be tried. And if offered, even though it may have only a slim chance of working, it becomes gospel. "Maybe I'll be that 1 percent," comes the thought. The dice are eagerly, anxiously cast with the all-too-common creedal statement, "It's in God's hands." Except we know what is in your heart as you toss the dice: fear of dying, heartache at leaving all the love and life you've known. Existential distress. Such is the lens of the death-denying culture in which youth is glorified, the elderly are compartmentalized, and death is hidden away under makeup on corpses slid into beautiful caskets and buried beneath marble epitaphs. Even our obsession with material wealth

---

[39] Stevens, Anthony. *Private myths: Dreams and dreaming*. Harvard University Press, 1995.

is an expression of death anxiety. Possessions become extensions of "me," for they are "mine." We solidify our place in the world through attachments, all reaching an ugly ultimate state through hoarding, clinging to every object in the anxious effort to preserve identity, or through extreme wealth, in which not only objects but unheard-of power defines the self through the world now owned. Death annihilates this illusion. We leave as naked as we arrive. No hearse ever pulled a U-Haul. Yet MAiD is the ultimate push-back against that annihilation. It is an existential aberration in the arc of time, for it stems from an assertion that you *have* a life – yours to own, yours to dispose of in the end, when in fact, you *are* a life that does not remember its essential nature.

No wonder – the modern mythology of material reductionism says that what you see is all there is; there is no hope beyond that mortal line. Even more, it severs us from an orientation to life infused with wonder and respect for the natural world, from joy and peace through connection to all that is, from the Ground of Being that has a thousand names and one nature. Such spiritual poverty also results in Western civilization's divorce from death. This makes the assignment essential and universal to the human journey – awakening – all the more difficult for us, especially as it requires that we become very uncomfortable. This is death anxiety writ large in our collective and individual psyche. This is the wilderness of waiting as death approaches, a place of profound struggle and growth. Thousands of years of meditative practice, modern research in experiential therapies like psychedelics, and insights gained from near-death experiences all indicate that raw confrontation with the most frightening aspects of human existence is particularly effective in initiating, then accelerating, spiritual development. This is the psycho-spiritual transformation of the mental ego. It follows universal pathways:

1. Painful surrender of the fiction of the separate self.
2. A willingness to enter the truth of the present moment through direct awareness, without mediation or any buffer of thoughts, feelings, or activity.

3. Healing of the deep wounds caused by distance from the Ground of Being which resulted in the emergence of the ego.

4. Final integration into the Ground of Being.

As overwhelming and abstract as that may sound, the way is known. It is written into every soul that has ever lived. I wish there were a smoother, more comfortable way to awaken to that which you fundamentally are, but for most of us (excluding the rare souls naturally enlightened), suffering is the crucible of transformation precisely because it triggers the ego's defence mechanisms for self-preservation, as the ego exists solely via the illusion that it is a separate self. While ego has a functional role in human experience, it becomes dysfunctional when it asserts itself as essential to identity. Nothing triggers that dysfunction like suffering and death.

Stephen Levine comments that "most people begin to open to their life not because there is joy, but because there is pain. Pain denotes the limit of the territory of the imagined self... beyond which a kind of queasiness arises at being in the midst of the uncontrollable. This is our edge, our resistance to life, the place the heart closes in self-protection... When you are near your edge, you are near your truth."[40]

Your ultimate truth is waiting to be discovered within. Unfortunately, it requires the "you" you think you are to end. This is the heart of spiritual teachings, but with the loss of such mysteries comes the loss of our identities. As cities grow and technology takes over the world, the traditional source of this wisdom – religion – becomes increasingly out of step with the modern mind. These teachings used to directly address the experience of death. Now they offer what is, to many, an archaic cosmology, a fairy tale. So, unless spiritual language has an upgrade, faith fades away, as does our sense of the sacred within. The world becomes disenchanted.

[40] Levine, Stephen, and Ondrea Levine. *Who dies?: An Investigation of Conscious Living and Conscious Dying.* Anchor, 2012. p. 34.

While personal liberty, patient autonomy, and the individual's dignity drive the MAiD discussion, advocates of such principles must not assume they are universal in the human family. This topic has a distinctly Western bias that focuses on concepts that have little relevance in other countries or cultures.[41,42] This context is central to our explorations of the spiritual dimensions of assisted dying. Let us never advocate for any position for or against the procedure, thinking it is one's inalienable right or a fundamental principle of autonomy. MAiD is not that simple, and neither are we. Just as we do not understand the very nature of reality itself, we do not understand what is at play when we argue for or against the right to die on one's terms. The issue is more complicated than we realize but has been reduced to what we can comprehend and what many desperately want at life's end: control.

It's late, and my bowl of popcorn is empty. The final scenes of *The Seventh Seal* play out on the screen. The knight has led his friends from the congestion of the virus-infected coast to his home in the country. Among the company gathered for their final meal is a young woman rescued from a rape earlier in the film. The things she has seen in her plague-ridden town are so unspeakable that she is rendered mute, but her actions prophetically demonstrate the strength of her spirit, for she engages death, not with fear but compassion. When her would-be rapist appears in the forest dying of the plague, she tries to offer the man a sip of water. And when Death arrives at the knight's castle at the end of the film, she is the only one smiling. She kneels down, as if in reverent prayer, and speaks her only line of the film. "It is finished."

---

[41] Macer, DR., J. Azariah, and P. Srinives. "Attitudes to biotechnology in Asia." *International Journal of Biotechnology 2*(4) (2000): pp. 313–332.

[42] Blank, RH. "End-of-life decision making across cultures." *The Journal of Law, Medicine & Ethics*, 39(2) (2011): pp. 201–214.

EXERCISE 2: ART THERAPY

Take a few moments to sit in a quiet and comfortable space. Close your eyes and bring your attention to your breath. Allow yourself to become present and grounded in the moment. When you feel ready, engage with the following:

> *Using a pencil or pen, crayons or coloured markers, draw your death. Do not try to make it good or artistic, try to make it visceral and emotional. Connect with the feelings you have around dying, around leaving, around becoming nothing or becoming everything. Take your time placing your soul upon the paper. Then sit and listen to what it is saying to you.*

CHAPTER 3

THE MAiD PROCESS

The cave you fear to enter holds the treasure you seek.
–JOSEPH CAMPBELL

"HOW DO I GET THIS DONE?" MRS. CARMICHAEL WAS GLARING AT me, which seemed to be her default setting. Fiery, demanding, temperamental... she was what is euphemistically known as "non-compliant" – refusing care, criticizing doctors, complaining to the cleaners. There was only one nurse who connected well with her and only one chaplain she wanted to see – every day. At 2 p.m. Because he was kind and handsome and listened. And I never called her anything but Mrs. Carmichael. And Mrs. Carmichael was tired of living in a hospital waiting to die. She wanted, she said, to be "dead and done with it."

"Well, I said, "you simply request it, then we initiate some conversations to assess things like suffering, distress, and competency..."

"What the hell do you mean by that!?" she snapped. "Of course, I'm competent. Do you think I've lost my mind? I'm dying, not going crazy."

"Yes, Mrs. Carmichael. But some people are on medications that affect the clarity of thinking. Some people are so sick that they become confused and can't make a legally binding choice. And MAiD is the most seriously binding choice you could ever ask for. So, I'm wondering why you'd like MAiD?"

Mrs. Carmichael didn't want to talk about that. No surprise; she hated feeling vulnerable. Yet she allowed my company. She even eventually allowed me to ask about her life, her heart, her hopes, and hardships. We had explored a lot in the weeks she was with us. But she would not let me explore her desire for MAiD. So, I got brave and filled in the blanks.

"Dying is taking too long," I said. She nodded. "You're worried it will leave you lying in the bed, unable to speak, unable to lift your head." She nodded again. "It's scary." She stared off, and softly said, "Yes."

"That makes sense," I said in equally hushed tones. "Your feelings make sense."

"Then can I die tomorrow?" Her tone was almost mischievous. And she smiled, ever so slightly.

The MAiD process was not as easy as Mrs. Carmichael wanted. In fact, she found it irritating. The patient submits a written, signed, and dated request for MAiD before two independent witnesses, who also sign and date the request. An assessment by a doctor or nurse practitioner is carried out to determine eligibility. If the patient meets the criteria, the law requires a second assessment by a doctor or nurse practitioner to confirm all this again. The first and second assessors must be independent, and must not have a supervisor-supervisee relationship. There used to be ten days between the date the patient signs the request and when MAiD is provided, unless their death or loss of capacity to provide informed consent is imminent, in which case the procedure can be accelerated. That waiting period has since been removed for those whose death is reasonably foreseeable. Additionally, a patient deemed ineligible for MAiD may seek an assessment from another doctor or nurse practitioner.

Families, friends, and allied healthcare providers, such as pharmacists and spiritual care practitioners, can be present for support. All are protected from criminal prosecution. Recognizing that not all healthcare providers will be comfortable with this service, consideration is given to conscientious objection. A doctor or nurse practitioner must, however, refer the case to someone else, which raises a problem: some will feel referring is collusion in the taking of a life. Such was the position of a group representing 4,700 Christian doctors in Ontario. The court ruled they must refer nonetheless, and the remaining provinces and territories will likely follow suit.

How do spiritual care practitioners navigate MAiD? The Canadian Association for Spiritual Care offers guidelines that outline key responsibilities for those who object to participating in MAiD on moral or religious grounds, with the direction to:

- Inform their employer to arrange alternative care or transfer the client to a practitioner who has no moral objection to MAiD, ensuring the client's rights and autonomy are respected.
- Communicate to the client that they cannot remain in a therapeutic relationship due to their conscientious objection.
- Reassure the client they will not be abandoned. If no replacement is available, the practitioner must continue to provide non-MAiD-related spiritual care as per the client's care plan, without expressing personal moral judgments.[43]

So, an individual working in health care can exercise conscientious objection, but what about institutions? Over one hundred Catholic hospitals in Canada serve the public and receive public funding. Can a religious-based institution have rights similar to those of an individual under the Charter? According to Chief Justice Beverley McLachlin and Justice Michael J. Moldaver, the answer is yes.

> "The freedom of religion of individuals cannot flourish without freedom of religion for the organizations through which those individuals express their religious practices and through which they transmit their faith [As long as the hospital meets the requirements for protection if it is constituted

[43] "Guidelines for Spiritual Care Practitioners and Psycho-Spiritual Therapists in Responding to Inquiries Regarding Medical Assistance in Dying (MAiD)." Canadian Association for Spiritual Care. Accessed Feb. 24, 2019. https://www.virtualhospice.ca/Assets/Guideline-for-SC-in-responding-to-request-for-MAiD-final-Dec-7-2016_20170406141127.pdf

> primarily for religious purposes, and its operation accords with these religious purposes]." [44]

The primary purpose of Catholic hospitals is to provide health care, not conduct religious practice or education. Countering this can be the argument that caring for the sick is very much part of the church's spiritual practice. Indeed, this is where hospitals originated.

Stalemate. Catholic hospitals that receive public funding were now able to deny what the Supreme Court has declared a human right based on the hospitals' moral conviction and belief about the sacredness of life. And this has been the case since 1969 when abortion became legal in Canada. Their practice, of course, is based on the core belief in the sanctity of life – a concept that deserves deep exploration, serious reflection, and careful handling, which I shall endeavour to do in Chapter 23.

That a hospital could deny a dying patient their desire for an early exit raised the ire of MAiD advocates. The online responses were replete with disdain, but the Nova Scotia government found a creative workaround. They converted a section of St. Martha's Hospital into the Antigonish Health and Wellness Centre, separate but affiliated with the Catholic organization. MAiD could be carried out in the corner of the building (far from the chapel). It seems like a win-win situation.

In checking that the request for assisted death is durable, two assessors must agree that the request is not being pressured by external forces, that there is a grievous and irremediable medical condition or illness, and that the patient's suffering is not amenable to other treatments which the patient finds acceptable. Then the request for assisted death can be sanctioned. They can comfortably be sent off to the great beyond. That's how the process is set up. That's the way the physician or nurse practitioner is supposed to do it. But that's not really how it plays out. What began as a last resort at the end of the road has become an option for everyone, even

[44] Bussey, Barry W. "On assisted dying, government should respect the beliefs of religious hospitals." *National Post* (March 8, 2016). Accessed March 12, 2019. https://nationalpost.com/opinion/barry-w-bussey-on-assisted-dying-government-should-respect-the-beliefs-of-religious-hospitals

when there are years of life left. In Canada, the law states that the physician must inform the patient of possible treatments for their suffering when hearing of a MAiD request. And the patient can refuse such treatment if offered, insisting instead on assisted death even if there are effective treatments for both the physical and existential ailments.[45]

This will be all the more acute if MAiD is approved for those with mental health conditions, which was to be implemented in 2023. Due to pressure from mental health professionals, that expansion has been paused, for here is a population vulnerable to social and economic factors more than any segment of healthcare "consumers." Treatment for mental health conditions can take years, but MAiD would provide an out in minutes. Additionally, the wait list to access such care can take years, but MAiD assessors tend to respond within days, if not hours. How ironic that the government will provide assisted dying but not affordable housing or comprehensive care for mental health. This is why most groups advocating for those with disabilities have not welcomed this change. The situation is tragic, with even those living in poverty now reluctantly considering MAiD over the continued struggle of living on the streets. Your death can be arranged in about two weeks, but the social support to help you live is nowhere to be found.[46] It's going to be a mess when, despite the MAiD law absolving doctors of criminal negligence, the guidelines in psychiatry continue to state otherwise:

> "Psychiatrists who fail to take responsible care that their patients do not commit suicide, including failing to order their involuntary hospitalization to prevent them from committing suicide when a reasonably careful psychiatrist would

---

[45] Center for Addiction and Mental Health. "MAiD and Mental Illness: FAQs." CAMH, last modified January 24, 2023. https://www.camh.ca/en/camh-news-and-stories/maid-and-mental-illness-faqs. Accessed June 20, 2024.

[46] Leffler, B and M. Dimain. "How poverty, not pain, is driving Canadians with disabilities to consider medically-assisted death." *Global News* (Oct. 8, 2022). https://globalnews.ca/news/9176485/poverty-canadians-disabilities-medically-assisted-death/ Accessed Oct. 16, 2022.

> not have failed to do so, can be liable for medical malpractice, unprofessional conduct, and even, in extreme cases, criminal negligence."[47]

You may cringe at the use of the word *suicide* when talking about MAiD, yet for Dr. John Maher, a psychiatrist from Barrie, Ontario, who has spent twenty years helping people with severe mental illnesses, you say it as you see it. Speaking to the desire to hasten death and the nature of "irredeemable suffering," he comments, "To say this is not suicide inducement or that it's not suicide, I find bizarre... [and] if you're saying 'irremediable' means they can't be cured completely, sure, there are people who are irremediable. If you're saying it means there are people where you can't reduce suffering... I don't buy it."[48]

Another shocking development in the assessment process seems to have gone unmentioned in MAiD conversations: with the pandemic, many assessments are being done over video. There is no in-person engagement or chance to enter the suffering person's living environment, read their body language, or sense their life through all dimensions of smell, sound, touch, and presence. The assessor need not expose themselves to the full dimensions of suffering anymore. An experience that could evoke consideration of compassionate options and mobilize support is reduced to a checklist of criteria to end their life.

One would think the assessment process for something so ultimate as causing a person's death would be thorough, standardized, and based on the best practice, experience, and research. Those last three points would have to draw from the experience of countries that have practiced assisted dying for decades: Belgium and the Netherlands. Yet, as of this writing, no such model exists. No manual, no protracted courses, and certainly no advisement from spiritual care on the existential issues at play and how one deeply engages distress as functional in negotiating mortality instead

---

[47] Boudreau, J. Donald, and Margaret Somerville. "Euthanasia and assisted suicide: a physician's and ethicist's perspectives." *Medicolegal and Bioethics* 4.1 (2014): pp. 1–11.

[48] Gillmore, Meagan. "Have Assisted Dying Laws Gone Too Far?" *The Walrus* (May 30, 2023) thewalrus.ca/assisted-dying. Accessed June 8, 2023.

of futility in the face of one's end. A Belgian study found that "physicians assess decision-making capacity in different ways and that personal values and beliefs influence their approach. As such, a common approach in assessing a patient's decision-making capacity among the interviewed physicians is lacking."[49]

That spiritual care is rarely included is no surprise. Though hospitals and palliative care arose from the world's spiritual traditions, the rift between spirituality and science has often resulted in chaplains dwelling in the afterthoughts of the hospital's ledger, thinner on the ground than the already sparse psychosocial experts who support patients through the crisis. Additionally, spiritual care tends not to be called in until the final crisis – death – to administer prayers and sacraments and perform "closing ceremonies." This presents an additional barrier, as most people request and receive MAiD while physical and existential suffering can still be treated, and they want to leave this world *before* reaching that stage when a chaplain is often consulted. Patients do state in the assessment process that their suffering is intolerable, yet little, if any, counselling is provided to address that suffering. And processing existential distress is what spiritual care practitioners specialize in. This is our bread and butter; this is our daily practice. That's a critical point to remember, as the latest version of the law states that individuals are informed of available and appropriate means to relieve their suffering and are offered consultations with professionals who provide those services. That's one reason the ten-day waiting period was put in place – it would give us time to get in and build the therapeutic relationship needed for such profound personal work. The ninety days for cases where death is not imminent holds… for now. The ten days has been dropped. A person can have the required two assessments on the same day and be rendered dead that evening. Yes, it's rare, but I've seen this happen, and it is a radical departure from the law's original intent.

---

[49] Schweitser, Frank, et al. "Assessment of patient decision-making capacity in the context of voluntary euthanasia for psychic suffering caused by psychiatric disorders: a qualitative study of approaches among Belgian physicians." *Journal of Medical Ethics* 47.12 (2021): e38.

Additionally, when support from spiritual care (or any other discipline) is offered, the patient can refuse, even if it would be effective in relieving their suffering because the one dying feels their suffering "cannot be alleviated under conditions the person considers acceptable."[50] That's quite a challenge, as most of the public (and many healthcare providers) do not understand the true nature of our work. This is not about religion and need not be about spiritual realms. Spirituality gives one meaning and identity in this world – concepts that go unarticulated for many but are lived out by all as they navigate life by their principles, values, and connection to something greater than themselves (which could simply be a richer experience of life). We're not the God Squad; we are spiritual counsellors. But offering counselling is only possible when you have counsellors who can address existential distress, post-traumatic stress disorder (PTSD), suffering and grief, spirituality and death. Ain't going to happen. I suspect there are three main reasons for this:

1. The assessor needs to become more familiar with or take the time to explore the nature of existential distress.
2. The patient can decline counselling.
3. There needs to be more spiritual care practitioners or psychosocial counsellors.

The first is a matter of training, the second of awareness, and the third of funding. Comprehensive reform is needed!

There's another serious issue at play here: that of informed consent. Can a patient, on the edge of life, truly be fully informed of the MAiD procedure when they cannot objectively consider their suffering from within their own experience? We are talking about dying here. Few can be clear-headed with that impending fate. It hits the most primal functioning of the brain, the reptilian amygdala, where it's nothing but fight, flight or f – this (which may be an accurate sentiment in the face of death when choosing MAiD). Beyond even that, there are yet more

---

[50] Ibid

gaps. For example, a 2022 study through the Champlain Regional MAiD Program found that most patients with lung cancer are "assessed by an oncology specialist before MAiD, though less than half received systemic therapy. Among patients with more treatable forms of lung cancer, many patients still undergo MAiD without accessing, or in some cases being assessed for, these treatment options."[51] So, while there may be more that medicine could offer, that option is not always on the table, whether because of the potential additional suffering or at the discretion of the doctor. And there are times, understandably, when patients are so discouraged by their situation, or so accepting of the outcome, that they don't want any more treatment. Especially in those cases, they may have time to benefit significantly from spiritual counselling to help unpack for that final trip.

Even with those for whom treatment failed and became palliative, there are still astonishing incongruities the lawmakers did not anticipate. There are cases where the palliative care doc offers medication and solutions to alleviate pain and suffering, assuring the patient that any turbulence they may encounter in their final takeoff can be managed. Nonetheless, the patient says, "Thanks, I still want assisted death." Such statements demonstrate that fear of suffering and loss of dignity has not been adequately addressed. This is about so much more than alleviating pain; it's about not dying *this* way, at *this* time, under *these* circumstances. It's also a statement demonstrating assisted death's potential to empower the patient. "I've made up my mind, and that's it." It is the final assertion at the pinnacle of human freedom, giving the individual the power to enact their version of a good death, free from the constraints of institutions and culture, relying purely on personal desire.

I recall one fellow, a successful entrepreneur, devout Catholic, and leader in his faith community, saying, "I know the church disapproves. The priest won't give me final rites. My wife is pissed that I want this at

[51] Sara Moore et al., "Brief Report: Medical Assistance in Dying in Patients with Lung Cancer," JTO Clinical and Research Reports (2022): 100283.

all. They may even think I'm going to hell for this. But it's not suicide. I'm not depressed. I'm in charge!"

Dr. BJ Miller, the founder of Mettle Health, relates that after conducting many assisted deaths, he's found that the vast majority of patients request an early end as a last act of their will and autonomy to bring their life to a close in a way that is meaningful to them. Their request is not due to intolerable suffering at present. Some even say, "I'm not suffering right now. But I will in the future. This is what I want." They play the game, going through the hoops of screening and assessment, to exit this world on their terms. They demonstrate absolute competency, and their autonomy is upheld.

The death industry is only too happy to comply. Funeral homes now provide MAiD services in rooms designed for the final farewells.[52] You can walk in in the morning and be buried that afternoon. Even more startling, a European company is now offering death capsules, futuristic pods in which you lie down, press a button, and are quickly dispatched with rapid sedation and sterile release of your mortal coil. It's called the Sarco suicide pod and could be available for anyone, anywhere, as the company, Exit International, will make the design available for download. All you need is a 3D printer. Assembly instructions are included.[53] The device, approved in Switzerland, is meant to remove doctors and medical professionals from the dying process, which Dr. Philip Nitschke, its creator, considers a natural process rather than a medical condition. A person reclines in the pod, closes the door, then presses a button to release nitrogen gas, which induces hypoxia. You quickly and comfortably lose consciousness, as you would with sedation for an operation. Death quickly follows. To ensure the procedure is available only to those

[52] Lupton, Andrew. "Funeral homes pivot to offer rooms for medically assisted deaths." CBC News. Oct. 26, 2021 4:00 a.m. ET | Last updated: Oct. 26, 2022. https://www.cbc.ca/news/canada/london/funeral-homes-pivot-to-offer-rooms-for-medically-assisted-deaths-1.6224353. Accessed Nov. 1, 2022.

[53] Bateman, T. "The Sarco suicide pod aims to take assisted dying out of doctors' hands with AI and 3D printing." Eronews.next. Dec. 9, 2021. https://www.euronews.com/health/2021/12/08/the-sarco-suicide-pod-aims-to-take-assisted-dying-out-of-doctors-hands. Accessed March 5, 2022.

who qualify, plans are in place to develop an AI computer that will converse with you, assessing competency and motivation. You don't even need a human nearby. Of course, if one changes their mind, there is an emergency escape button.

Who could blame a person for desiring such an efficient exit? Imagine you've been diagnosed with esophageal cancer. You go into surgery hoping it is manageable but emerge with the heartbreaking news that things are worse than expected. To give some quality of life, they removed the esophagus and connected a feeding tube to your stomach for nutrition. You live that way for three months until a follow-up scan reveals more cancer. It has spread so extensively that severe treatment is recommended: thirty rounds of intense radiation and chemotherapy will make you nauseous, weak, and miserable. You decline. You function relatively well on the feeding tube, can get out, enjoy life, and are independent. But you know it won't last. You also know dying will be... unpleasant. Organs will be compromised. You will deteriorate as the cancer absorbs all the nutrients you pump into your frail form. Medications to treat your pain and anxiety may alter how you are able to interact with loved ones as you actively die. In the face of all this, wouldn't it be better, kinder, and more understandable to opt for an early exit? Why prolong an inevitable end? Imagining it is torture enough. And that's precisely the problem: our imagination. So, let's explore what it's like to die, first through the provision of MAiD, then through natural death.

THE PROCEDURE

Unlike natural death, which can stretch out for an indeterminate number of days or weeks, MAiD is, for the most part, simple, painless, and incredibly effective. The doctor arrives with the medication preloaded in their syringes. After introductions, the procedure is explained as plainly as possible, and the patient's consent is confirmed.[54] Family members and friends may be invited by the patient to attend the

[54] If the patient is aware, but that is no longer required in the amended policy due to Bill C-7.

procedure. The doctor will explain how the first medication is for anxiety and will put the patient to sleep. Often midazolam is used. The second injection is lidocaine, an anesthetic (or numbing) agent, in case a sting is felt with the following injections. Every effort should be taken to ensure the patient is comfortable throughout the procedure, even if they appear unconscious. The third medication is propofol, given in a giant syringe. This is often used in surgery to induce unconsciousness for the operation, but this dosage is much larger.

A final injection contains rocuronium, ensuring the heart has stopped. The body shuts down, with no sense of awareness or connection. There may be slight variations in the number of syringes used, and loved ones may be overwhelmed as they observe the process.[55] While that procedure may take ten minutes or so, it will seem much longer for those present, as they are suspended on the fading breath and heartbeat of their loved one. There is no movement in the patient beyond this, no twitching, no gasping, no muscles flexing or grimacing. Those in the room will see facial muscles relax along with the entire body as life leaves.

At any point, family members can step out of the room, sit down, or embrace each other if they feel overwhelmed. Sometimes they choose a ritual to mark the gift of this life and its transition to whatever awaits. These can be profound and are always meant to affirm the love and assist the release of this world. I have seen stunning wisdom as families craft a truly unique ceremony. There may be live or recorded music, flowers, sunlight and warmth, prayers and blessings, and open windows to let the breeze flow through and the soul flow free.

After the last injection, the doctor will check for a heartbeat using a stethoscope. The needles will be removed, and the family will be informed of what they already know: their loved one is gone.

---

[55] In the United States, this effective and painless procedure is not, surprisingly, available. There, the patient empties the contents of capsules into a glass of water, swallows the bitter solution, then waits, sometimes for hours, for death to come. See Dear, Jennie. "The doctors who invented a new way to help people die." *The Atlantic* (Jan. 22, 2019).

With that often comes the release of tears, held in respect so as not to upset the patient while they were alive. Now, the barriers are dropped, the embraces reach out, and all the emotional energy is released. Often, I witnessed gratitude quickly expressed to the doctor. Most of the time, this is sincere. Sometimes it is awkward, awash with mixed feelings about what was witnessed... especially if those present have never seen someone die. Of course, there is relief that their loved one no longer suffers. And, there is a profound realization that it is done. They have passed the point of any hesitation. If there was any, they carry that quietly through the rest of their days.

Those days are marked by grief, which is the price we pay for love. In several studies, the family and friends of patients who requested MAiD had fewer traumatic grief symptoms than those of patients who died of natural causes.[56] However, other studies have shown a higher prevalence of PTSD and depression among family members or friends witnessing MAiD.[57] There can be moral conflict upon reflection, wrestling with witnessing someone causing death who, nonetheless, was carrying out the dying person's wishes. I've often found a family member who disagreed with assisted dying or felt moral distress without knowing how to articulate beyond saying, "This just feels wrong." The following silence can be tinged with resignation and the effort to respect the choice now made. It's all the more critical for discussion afterwards, for any questions to be answered, but primarily for people's feelings to be honoured. Death and grief stir the deepest layers of our identity, challenging our understanding of life itself. How could anyone expect it to be so simple as "dead and done?"

What I've presented above is an ideal scenario, but we know life rarely works that way. Some cases feel cold and frighteningly clinical, all the more a possibility when there are doctors who have become MAiD specialists,

---

[56] Swarte, NB, et al. "Effects of euthanasia on the bereaved family and friends: A cross sectional study." *BMJ*. (2003) 327(7408):189.

[57] Wagner B, J. Müller , and A. Maercker. "Death by request in Switzerland: Posttraumatic stress disorder and complicated grief after witnessing assisted suicide." *European Psychiatry* 27(7) (2012): pp. 542–546.

ending hundreds of lives a year. Death by injection becomes not just another way to die, but the preferable way to die. Herein lies the great danger: that death by our hand could become normalized. Even more, that death is compressed from a natural mystery to a medical problem.

All of that is from the family's perspective, from the position of the living. What is that like for the patient to be rendered lifeless? From what I understand and have observed, this feels like being put to sleep for an operation. I recall that well from my multiple surgeries; the most uncomfortable part is having an IV line put in to receive the cocktail that renders you unconscious. For the person who has MAiD, that line is in place already, often put in the day before. For an operation, they tell you to count backwards from ten. I've never reached seven before the lights went out. The feeling is fast, a rapid descent to darkness with only a brief swimming in the head. Then… nothing. You wake hours later, unaware of the time passed, sensing self and environment distorted through an amnesiac fog. Sounds and sensations leak in, and you feel sloshy and sleepy.

The MAiD patient, of course, does not wake. They receive that second injection, and dissolve in seconds. I trust they do wake up, but to what is beyond our comprehension. According to those who've temporarily made the trip through a near-death experience (and yes, I've had one), this transformation is marked by expanded consciousness, crystal clarity, and for the most part, great love. Is that also the case for those who intentionally exit this world? Or does the act of ending one's life eternally affect their afterlife? What does exercising control over your own body and fate a few weeks, days, or hours before your natural death do to one's consciousness, one's life force? And if consciousness ends with the body, how does this act affect culture? How does it impact our orientation to death and life itself? These are among the constellation of questions that arise when exploring the spiritual dimensions of MAiD. Let's explore them with the acknowledgment that death is the ultimate mystery, one we may be incapable of understanding from this side. Dying, well… that we know. That we have been doing since the beginning of time. Despite the eons of practice, that is not something we do well anymore.

Mrs. Carmichael did die well… eventually. She was assessed and found eligible for MAiD, then changed her mind because "the service of the staff improved." In other words, we pampered her. She enjoyed herself. As her mood lifted, so did some symptoms, and we realized that dying was going to take even longer than we expected. The best step seemed to move her to a more appropriate level of care. When offered a bed at the local hospice, which was accurately described as first class accommodations on a luxury liner, she procrastinated. Turns out it was the community of care she didn't want to leave. We had become her new family, perhaps the first she had ever truly experienced. Our compassion was repairing the wound of identity and dignity left unfinished from childhood. But we could not maintain such focus with unit beds now full and reduced staff due to COVID.

When another hospice bed became available, she transferred reluctantly. Her displeasure was evident as I came to say goodbye. "I don't want to talk to you. You all want to get rid of me. Get out." I stood at the door, considering my response. "OK. It's been a pleasure serving you, Mrs. Carmichael." I turned to leave. Then, just at the door, she said, "But you'll visit me, right?" Her tone was vulnerable this time, not mischievous. But she did smile, ever so slightly.

I heard Mrs. Carmichael eventually warmed up to "the staff" at the hospice. She accepted the personalized meals. She took in the view of the ocean. And she died gently and naturally as the music therapist sang one of her favourite Rolling Stones tunes, "You Can't Always Get What You Want."

EXERCISE 3: CONTEMPLATION AND CONVERSATION

Find a quiet and comfortable space where you can reflect without interruptions. Take a few moments to center yourself and focus on the present moment.

1. *Acknowledge the sensitivity of the topic: Begin by recognizing the sensitive and complex nature of exploring the desire for medically assisted death (MAiD). This exercise is designed to provide space for introspection and self-understanding without judgment.*
2. *Reflection on your situation: Take out a journal or piece of paper, and reflect on the following questions:*
    a. *Your circumstances: What specific physical, emotional, or psychological challenges are contributing to your desire for MAiD? Explore your current suffering and the limitations that make this option appealing.*
    b. *Impact on quality of life: Consider how your condition affects your autonomy, dignity, and overall well-being. How has it changed your ability to engage in activities you enjoy or maintain meaningful relationships?*
    c. *Alignment with your values: Reflect on your values, beliefs, and priorities. How do they align or conflict with choosing medically assisted death? Are ethical, moral, or spiritual considerations influencing your decision?*
    d. *Alternatives and support systems: Contemplate the alternatives available to alleviate your suffering or improve your quality of life. Are there emotional supports, palliative care, or other treatments you've yet to explore? Consider the perspectives and advice of loved ones, healthcare professionals, or support groups.*

3. *Review your reflections: After writing down your thoughts, take a few moments to re-read them. Absorb your reflections fully and note any patterns, insights, or conflicting emotions that surface.*

4. *Consider seeking support: Reflect on whom you might reach out to–whether a trusted confidant, healthcare professional, or counsellor–to discuss your thoughts. Engaging in open and compassionate conversations can offer additional perspectives and support.*

5. *Practise self-compassion: Throughout this process, be gentle with yourself. Acknowledge that exploring the desire for MAiD is a deeply personal and complex journey. Allow space for conflicting emotions and uncertainty, and offer yourself kindness in the process.*

6. *Take further action: If appropriate, reflect on tangible actions you could take. For example, consider exploring alternative treatments, joining a support group, or seeking palliative care services. What next steps could you take to address your suffering?*

7. *Close with gratitude: Conclude this exercise by expressing gratitude for the opportunity to reflect deeply on your feelings. Acknowledge your courage in engaging with such profound matters. Offer yourself kindness and compassion for the exploration you've undertaken.*

For more information and support, visit virtualhospice.ca, which offers a wide range of resources related to palliative care, emotional support, and end of life decision making.

CHAPTER 4

NATURAL DEATH

Death is not the opposite of life. Life has no opposite.
Death is the opposite of birth.
– ECKHART TOLLE

I SAT WITH THE FAMILY OF A YOUNG MAN WHO SEEMED MORE LIKE AN angel as he took his last breath. But Brad hadn't entered the hospital so radiant. He entered defiant. He entered determined that cancer would not kill him. He entered devoured by fear long before the cancer consumed him. And, like so many, he projected that distress upon even those who loved him as they sat by his side. Their compassion amplified the reality he so desperately wanted to avoid. Life had been unravelling since the diagnosis of acute myelogenous leukemia, an aggressive blood cancer. It had spread to his brain and spinal cord, to his liver and lymph nodes in a matter of weeks. How could Brad have suspected such a disease when all he felt was fatigue and flu-like symptoms?

He had managed chemotherapy well, but it never yielded the results we desired. Even after several cycles, the cancer kept spreading. It just would not relent. So, more potent drugs were employed, so strong that most would have died from their side effects. But Brad was young, robust, even magnificent. He was a top athlete, a vegetarian, and did nothing halfway. No wonder he took whatever we threw at him. No wonder he was so enraged that nothing he had done prevented the cancer. It was small consolation to consider that those very choices optimally positioned him to fight the disease.

"What's the point, though?" he asked one day. "What's the point if it only means I'll live into my suffering longer than most? What's the point if I lose anyway?"

As Brad's health deteriorated, his family experienced a rollercoaster of emotions. Fear gripped them as they witnessed his struggle, feeling helpless in the face of his relentless illness. They grappled with their own grief, mourning the loss of the vibrant young man Brad once was while trying to stay strong for him. Each family member coped differently; some retreated into silence, unable to articulate their fears, while others lashed out in anger, frustrated by the unfairness of it all. Despite their differences, they rallied together, their presence bringing comfort amidst the turmoil. In sharing their grief, they found strength in each other, cherishing all the more the few moments left to be lived.

Now, at the end, they had asked for the chaplain to come and do what chaplains do: say the prayers, give the last rites, perform the rituals that wrap the tragedy up and send the package of love to God. But what they really needed was to feel somehow safe as their world was falling apart. He was only 21. A child is not supposed to die before his parents.

"I'd be honoured to pray for Brad," I said. "But I don't know him. I'd like to appreciate who I'm praying for. Can you tell me about him?" The question is sincere, but it's also a therapeutic technique for opening people up, to animate love and gratitude so they are stronger than the fear. And it worked, even to the point of allowing laughter to join the conversation.

We talked for over an hour while Brad lay silently in the liminal realms between the here and after. We reflected on his appetite for life, on the foolish and wise ways he embraced it. And we talked about dying, what it looked like, how to know its process, how to prepare for his last breath and oddly find yours continuing, nonetheless.

Gradually, the sound of Brad's breathing became softer while the energy in the room became larger. The air was heavy with the gravity of love, so we gathered around, joined hands, and did what felt more than right. It felt kind.

"Gracious God, thank you for Brad. Thank you for giving him to this family to know and love. May he release his body with gratitude and his life without regret. May he soar on the wings of angels to the wonder that awaits. May he have adventures ahead. May you bless him and keep him, make your face shine upon him and be gracious to him. May you look upon him with favour and give him peace." As I made the sign of the cross upon Brad's head, his heart, and his hands, his breath faded, then stopped. We stood in wonder that it could be so gentle. As his mother bowed to kiss his forehead, his sister opened the window so the angel could fly free.

People imagine the Grim Reaper as this dark malevolence with a scythe. I imagine him as a gentle, wise, and tender friend, a guide who understands our sorrow and softly leans into the laughter and tears to say, "I know it feels hard, but it's going to be OK. It's a perfectly natural process. I'm right here to show you the way. Come on, take my hand. It's time."

One of the most essential questions to ask your doctor when you become palliative is also one of the hardest to ask in the company of those who love you: how will it feel to die? One imagines a natural death is far worse than MAiD, and when it comes to expediency and utility, that's true – it takes longer, requires the descent into unconsciousness, is marked by some turbulence, and more waiting, sometimes for far longer than you imagined. All while your family sits at your side, alone in your home, contemplating, sobbing, grieving. Yet, while people have been dying this way from disease processes since the beginning of time, the experience under modern palliative care is smoother and more comfortable than ever before. Giving you a roadmap of what lies ahead has great power to assuage your fears.

Before embarking on this, it is important to acknowledge that not all deaths are peaceful. Those who have experienced the death of a loved one understand that the journey is rarely smooth. Most deaths involve difficult moments, and at times, extremely challenging ones. Pain may be inadequately managed, personal dignity may be compromised, and the grief experienced by your family may be overwhelming. I have witnessed numerous patients swallowed by such sadness, so I recognize that what I am about to discuss may seem like an idyllic scenario. I can only offer my compassion to those who have been present for a loved one's distressing death. However, it is worth noting that under proper palliative care, most individuals experience less physical suffering than they initially anticipated. (I must emphasize that my observations are unrelated to situations involving instant death resulting from accidents, violent crimes, heart attacks, aneurysms, and so on.) Now, let's delve into the topic.

Death is a process that follows fairly predictable pathways.[58] The process may take months for people who experience a gradual death due to illness. An acute disease that rapidly progresses may take life in weeks to days. The earliest indicator is fatigue, a weariness that builds over time. So many of my patients stated they thought they had picked up a bug. Strength and stamina faded as the weeks passed, but they just pressed on until they could not. No wonder a diagnosis like acute leukemia is such a shock.

When a disease becomes palliative, meaning that medical care shifts its focus from curing or managing the disease to maximizing comfort and quality of life as the illness progresses, you will experience an increase in sleep and a decrease in energy. Life becomes more restricted, and one's world gradually contracts to the confines of the room and the body in the bed. The pace at which this weariness intensifies is a reliable indicator of life expectancy. Your palliative care team takes this into consideration when evaluating your functioning during late-stage life using the Palliative Performance Scale. A score of 100 to 80 percent indicates normal mobility and functioning, while a score of 70 to 40 percent signifies decreased mobility, implying that you should only rise and move with assistance. Confusion and dependence increase significantly as you decline to 30 percent; the dying process now renders you bedridden until death. Knowing where you stand on this scale provides insight into what lies ahead, emphasizing the importance of attending to essential matters in life. This is why a crucial question to ask your doctor throughout the course of the disease is, "Would it surprise you if I were still alive in a year? Six months? Three

[58] Mannix, Kathryn."Dying is not as bad as you think." YouTube video. Uploaded by BBC Ideas. Sept. 5, 2019. www.youtube.com/watch?v=CruBRZh8quc. Accessed April 1, 2023.

months? One?" Yes, this requires courage, but it allows you to gain clarity regarding what matters most in the days to come: the conversations, the grief, the gratitude, and the farewells.

There can be intense and emotionally difficult periods during the dying process, marked by confusion or delirium. That means your behaviour may change. The dying person sometimes become angry, snapping at their family or the healthcare team. This is something nurses see often, but loved ones may feel deeply hurt by the behaviour. Know that this is delirium, not the true person who may have been loving and peaceful all their life. Try to remember that the dying person in this state is not aware of their actions, and their behaviour does not reflect their true feelings or beliefs.[59]

Boredom and frustration are to be expected as you sleep more and move less. You wait and contemplate, zoning out a bit with meds that keep physical pain at bay. You increasingly become a human being, not a human doing. You are left with your thoughts and feelings, your memories and worries. It is a time to reflect, to share your story, to release its chapters bit by bit to the book of history in which you will never know your role except as it is written into the lives you have touched. They are the living documents of your journey; they are the signature you leave behind. They are your autograph.

The extended time of dying naturally becomes an invitation to unpack your life, repair the broken bits, acknowledge your humanity and reconcile those aspects that didn't turn out as you expected. This is the homework of the soul, done through deep conversations, engaging rituals of release, and practicing the skill of simple presence, surrendering to the moment, and unfiltered abiding. You are slowing the mind down and practicing the state of stillness that is fundamental to transcendence.

When the energy level changes significantly in a matter of weeks, we know that there are only weeks of life left, possibly days. Soon appetite diminishes as the body's requirement for food fades. Now will be the time

[59] "What Are the Last Days Before Death Like? | Signs of Approaching Death." YouTube video. Uploaded by Dr. Pauline Moyaert, May 2, 2022, www.youtube.com/watch?v=JDirQOmydRs. Accessed April 1, 2023.

to enjoy morsels, to savour the taste without needing to finish the plate. The body is shifting from an anabolic state, getting energy from food, to a catabolic state, getting energy from muscle and fat stored in the body. Molecules called ketones are released, suppressing hunger, thirst, and pain. Your body is preparing to shut off and doing what it can to ensure you are comfortable. There's even some evidence that shows high levels of ketones can also induce well-being and mild euphoria. Introducing food compromises this process, increasing hunger, thirst, and pain. It feels counter-intuitive not to eat and drink, but at the end of life, doing so supports the ultimate natural process. Not being able to eat is a symptom of the body shutting down, not the cause of it.

Sometimes there is a period of deep unconsciousness from which you cannot be roused, followed by a burst of energy that awakens you, making you comfortable enough to even sit up. This is a wonderful, final opportunity to say those four important things: thank you, love you, forgive me, and adios. The window of alertness will be brief, and then the coma-like unconsciousness returns. Eventually, it dominates your days. Showing compassion and acknowledging your resistance to this process will help normalize and process your feelings. It is understandable to feel frustration, bitterness, or anger. What you are experiencing is the most challenging yet universal part of the human journey. There is no need to protect your family (although your love will naturally try to) and no need to "keep it all together." Remember, the goal at the end of life is to love and be loved, to be comfortable, and to receive comfort. Caring for you will ennoble them as you slip into unconsciousness and toward transformation.

Hands and feet may become cool as the heart weakens. The body directs blood away from the limbs to ensure the brain has enough fuel. The skin on the arms and legs may become mottled and blotchy. Death is immanent, and the breathing may shift, sometimes subtly, sometimes abruptly. When the breathing stops, the heart stops, and the person dies.

There is strong evidence that the dying continue to hear the voices of their loved ones, but are unable to blush, of course, as they share heartfelt appreciation for your life, your love, and all you mean to them. Here is a significant opportunity to give yourself entirely to the natural process of descending into the deeper dimensions of consciousness. No activity, no doing, no words to formulate or express ideas, no perception or processing of information, no ego-identity. Only the gentle silence and a state of pure, unfiltered existence. As you read this, I want to assure you that you do not need to worry about this state or wonder if you know how to approach it. We are all wired for this, and from what we know from those who slip in and out of this state, it is not suffocating or dark or lonely. Those anxieties and constructs of experience emerge from your present, wakeful ego state of identity. All of that will gently fade away by the time you reach the end of your life.

Death is not painful, but disease processes can be, so good symptom management, which is central to palliative care, ensures that this is well controlled and that you experience no unnecessary physical distress. This is particularly important for loved ones who may anxiously hang on to any movement or sound. You give them a great gift by demonstrating how to die with calmness, allowing this ultimate process.

A wonderful aspect of the dying process is the shift in consciousness to expanded or mystical states. It's called nearing-death awareness, and it may begin weeks to days or hours before death. We'll explore that in detail in Chapter 25, but know that it is marked by visions of your welcoming party (loved ones who've died and are to receive you), lucid dreams of celestial realms, or an infilling of peace and light. Those dreams can be profoundly healing, with an engagement to your life story that reconciles past injuries and fills the dying person with a gentle and perplexing grace. Dreams can also be quite symbolic, presenting your final journey in the form of a train ride, climbing stairs, or some other metaphor for leaving. Nearing-death awareness is ubiquitous, independent of culture, age, historical period, or even belief.[60] Most significant is how it dissolves the fear of death and replaces it with expectancy and an unspeakable assurance that you will

[60] Shushan, Gregory. *The Next World: Extraordinary Experiences of the Afterlife*. White Crow Books, 2022.

be more than OK when you die. You may have periods of clarity in which you can share these experiences. This will dramatically affect the grief of those present, infusing their hearts with hope and wonder.

A person may undulate from this deep state of unconsciousness to more wakeful states of awareness, able to speak and interact, feel and express love, and confirm their comfort level. One rises and descends on these waves throughout the dying process, but, eventually, brain activity decreases so that wakeful states no longer occur. Awareness fades away, and your metabolic activity settles only to the essential: brain activity now focused on automatic breathing, blood pressure, and heart rate slowing. The hands and feet become cold as blood is diverted to the body's core to preserve essential organ functioning.

The quality of your breathing will begin to change, often alternating between fast and slow. Long pauses begin, extending from five seconds to twenty, thirty, or even forty-five. This is called apnea and is perfectly normal. The body is slowly shutting off. Apnea can be stressful for those present, as they hang on the next breath, wondering if it is the last. It may come and go or fluctuate in the length of pauses. Breath may also sound laboured. This, again, is normal. The brain is drawing from an increasingly limited reservoir of oxygen, triggering the lungs to try harder when they are also low on fuel. There may be a gurgling sound as fluid, unswallowed in the throat, bubbles with the exhalation. It's been called the death rattle, and family members can find this very distressing, fearing their loved one is drowning or choking. That is not the case, as there is no flinching or distressed expression. It is a sign that you cannot feel such physical sensations and are not distressed by what seems like a great deal of saliva in the throat. You are comfortable in a dimension of stillness that the mind is a stranger to throughout most of life. Medication can be given to dry up these secretions, which can also be suctioned out. That, again, will provide more comfort to those with you than to you, for you will be shedding the last vestiges of the ego-identity and attachment to the body. You are within the chrysalis; you have moved into a state of full potential before your transformation.

Accompanying these metabolic changes are energetic changes in your biofield. These subtle emanations are part of the mystery of consciousness, but, nonetheless, can be detected by gifted individuals to a remarkable degree of accuracy and by most people in general through intuitive sensing.[61] There are also some scientific instruments that can measure its diminishment, such as a photomultiplier that detects photons, and a quantum interference magnetometer, which detects subtle shifts in energy fields too delicate for conventional instrumentation.[62]

Recognizing and understanding this sequence of changes helps us to be fully present, compassionate, and attentive companions who can walk by your side. You are teaching us the ultimate lessons at this point: how to navigate grief, how to abide, to sit with suffering, how not to abandon any aspect of our sorrow, how to support each other, how to be kind to the parts of us that are scared, how to work together in love, how to face death. This experience will change us in ways we will only comprehend in the years to come. It will deepen our humanity and bring us into solidarity with all who suffer, and even more so with the rhythms of life and death, with creation itself. If meaning and purpose are what you desire as you die, then there can be none more significant than this.

Families should keep talking to their loved ones, singing sacred or favourite songs, quietly playing music, and sharing stories. It's also good for them to take turns, sitting in shifts at your side. Of course, some resist this for fear of missing the moment of your death. There can be a great sense of fidelity, a feeling that if they leave for a moment and you go, they would have abandoned you at the crucial instant they needed to be there. However, that need is on their part, not yours. You need nothing other than to dwell on what you hopefully have – good love, good care, and good pain management. Having said your goodbyes, you now are utterly still, soon to be transformed.

---

[61] Peck, Susan, Gail Corse, and Der-Fa Lu. "Case report: Energy field changes approaching and during the death experience." *Integrative Medicine: A Clinician's Journal* 16.6 (2017): p. 36.

[62] Janawadkar, MP., et al. "SQUID-based measurement of biomagnetic fields." *Current Science* (2010): pp. 36–45.

There's an exciting phenomenon often reported at the end of life: the dying person seems to have a power, a mysterious ability to control the timing of their death, waiting until everyone who needs to be there is there, or those who need to be out of the room are absent.[63] Their state of unconsciousness does not matter; the ability remains despite their condition. A new level of awareness is reached in which they mysteriously know more than we do, a psychic insight as to when it is best to leave. This only happens sometimes, but often enough to make one pause.[64] Very mysterious!

I recall this in a heartbreaking case of another young man dying from bone cancer. Michael was incredibly popular, given the crowd of friends in the hallways and family rooms. He had battled the disease and taken any procedure offered, including amputations. Now he lay unconscious, hovering on breath so gentle his parents dared not move or look away.

I asked a standard question, but for a reason they could not suspect. "Is there anyone still to come that needs to be here?"

"Yes... yes, his brother," said Michael's dad. "They are so close, and Steve promised he would be at Mike's side when he died. He'll be heartbroken if he doesn't make it. They talked all the time through Mike's illness. Steve wasn't going to go, but there was a football scholarship, and Mike insisted he should do it. Told him he'd be a fool not to. Told him not to worry." Tears began to well up. "He's flying in from Calgary. But I don't think he'll make it in time. The flight doesn't land for another hour."

"Well," I offered, "I wouldn't underestimate this guy. From what you've shared, he's got a strong bond and a strong will. I bet he'll hang on. They have to say goodbye." In the silence that followed, we gazed at Mike's youthful face. We breathed in time with his breath... until my pager shattered the moment. "OK, looks like I have to say goodbye, too." Then, looking at the youth, I thanked Mike for the honour of providing support. We briefly prayed and blessed him before I left the room.

---

[63] Fenwick, PBC., and Elizabeth Fenwick. *The Art of Dying: A Journey to Elsewhere.* London: Continuum, 2008.

[64] Callanan, Maggie, and Patricia Kelley. *Final Gifts: Understanding the Special Awareness, Needs, and Communications of the Dying.* Bantam, 1997.

The crowd gathered in the hall turned their heads in unison, searching my expression for the news they dreaded to hear. I simply smiled and said, "He's comfortable. He's surrounded by good love." Then, scanning their faces, I added, "lots and lots of good love."

His cousin approached, her voice soft. "His brother's coming. Will he make it?"

"Yes, I understand his flight lands in an hour."

"No. No," she stammered. "They got the time wrong. It's going to be three hours. More if there's a delay in Toronto. It'll be too late." She seemed to deflate before my eyes. Mike's breath could barely sustain him. Yet something in me trusted that breath. "I'm going to be bold here and bet that Mike will hang on even for three or four more hours. It sounds like they have a close bond. Trust it."

That was an audacious bet, but I've seen it often enough. And the next morning, I received word that Mike had hung on, despite all odds and expectations from the medical team. Steve arrived, came to the bedside, and had another hour with his brother to say thank you, love you, forgive you (brothers always have something they need to forgive), and goodbye.

In the end, Mike's breath shifted from the regular-though-weak whisp of air to an irregular rhythm. This followed the predictable course we see so often in the hospital. Finally, the breath grows faint, the pause grows long – a soft inhalation, a gentle exhalation, and then... nothing. Breath stops. It's as delicate as that. A faint pulse will continue for a few moments. Then the heart stops. Death is complete.

While good palliative care ensures this process is as gentle as possible, there is no way to medicate or mediate what lies at the core of the dying process – existential distress. You are leaving all the love you've ever known; you are losing your very identity in this world. You are being deconstructed which, ironically, is the only way to discover who you truly are.

EXERCISE 4: CONTEMPLATING DEATH

Take a few moments to sit in a quiet and comfortable space. Close your eyes and bring your attention to your breath. Allow yourself to become present and grounded in the moment. When you feel ready, engage with the following exercise:

> *Imagine yourself at the end of your life, reflecting on your journey. What thoughts, regrets, or accomplishments come to mind? How does the contemplation of your own mortality affect your priorities, aspirations, or the way you live your life now?*

If you have witnessed or encountered the death of another, take a moment to reflect on the experience and explore the following questions:

1. *What emotions or thoughts arise when you recall this death? How did it impact you personally?*
2. *How did witnessing this death affect your perspective on life and mortality?*
3. *How did the experience of witnessing death shape your understanding of the impermanence of life? What existential questions or deeper reflections resulted from this?*
4. *What lessons, if any, did you take away from this experience? Did it influence the way you approach your own life or relationships?*

CHAPTER 5

EGO DECONSTRUCTION

You are afraid of surrender because you don't want to lose control. But you never had control. All you had was anxiety.

– ELIZABETH GILBERT

WHO AM I? WHAT AM I? IT WAS NOT A PATIENT ASKING THE QUESTION but a young man being introduced to the French philosopher René Descartes in an introductory philosophy class. "*Cogito, ergo sum*" is a fundamental element of Descartes' method of skepticism and his attempt to establish a firm foundation for knowledge. Descartes realized that even if he doubted everything he believed to be true, and questioned the reliability of his senses and even the existence of an external world, there was one thing he could be sure of: the fact that he was thinking. "I think, therefore I am." The young man was me, and just as this statement was the starting point for Western culture's exploration of the nature of consciousness, it was also my starting point in trying to figure out the mystery of myself. I was eighteen and had survived my first cancer – potent fuel for profound questions. I wanted to know the nature of the life I almost lost. Little did I imagine that would come full circle with those deliberately ending theirs.

Central to our explorations of the spiritual dimensions of MAiD is understanding something nobody is talking about: how suffering and death deconstruct the identity of self in the reverse order it was formed as preparation for transformation. This is the essential insight of an astonishingly brilliant teacher, writer, and hospice professional far more experienced than Descartes in the dying process. She is the worthy successor to Elisabeth Kübler-Ross, who wrote the classic, *On Death and Dying*. Her name is Kathleen Dowling Singh, and if you want to seriously explore the inner dimensions of dying, drop my book and pick up *The Grace in Dying*. Following that is *The Grace in Aging*, *The Grace in Living*, and *Unbinding: The Grace Beyond Self*. These are manuals of the soul.

To keep you engaged with my book, here's a summary of her thesis: the dying process is designed to guide us into the realm of Spirit. It does so by reversing the process of ego development. Ego formation is marked by four contractions of consciousness away from the non-dual state of the Ground of Being. These contractions create four successive dualities: that of self/other, living/nonliving, mind/body, and persona/shadow. Dying activates the need for the dying person to heal and transcend each of these divisions in the reverse order they formed, but this triggers ego defence mechanisms for self-preservation – existential distress. Fortunately, the final stages in which frailty has sufficiently eroded those barriers are marked by nearing-death awareness; a state of peace and grace. Singh puts it this way:

> In the dying process, people experience transformation in the movement from tragedy to grace. Expansion of the identity into transpersonal levels seems to occur universally. For some people, this transformation occurs several months or weeks prior to the death of the body; for others, it may be hours or even minutes before death that surrender – which is the fulcrum of the psychospiritual transformation – occurs. The tragedy of the loss of "me," violently at first and then with increasing gentleness, is transformed into grace.[65]

Singh's astonishing insights come only from sitting with hundreds as they die, something she did with keen observation. Her wisdom gives us a cartography of dying unsurpassed in the modern era. Something

---

[65] Singh, Kathleen Dowling. *The Grace in Dying: How We Are Transformed Spiritually as We Die*. New York: HarperSanFrancisco, 1998, p. 110

fundamental and monumental happens to human consciousness at the beginning and the end of life. The problem is that medicine and modern culture have little awareness of what this is.

Singh describes how human development moves from the newborn's unconscious union with the mother to a conscious union with everyone and everything. Between those two points is a process of increasing individuation and separation, then increasing commonality and reunification. The first is a series of contractions away from the Ground of Being and proceeds slowly through growing up. The last is a series of expansions back into the Ground of Being, which tends to proceed too rapidly for our comfort: by dying.

The difficulty of this process is that it requires the formation of an ego-identity – who and what we think we are in the world – and then the deconstruction of that same identity through suffering and death.

The most basic meaning of the word ego is that it refers to the "I" that is capable of referencing the self and making decisions. It is a personal consciousness as opposed to the universal consciousness that is the foundation of reality. This self-reflective awareness, when threatened, instinctively seeks to justify its actions to self and others. Singh comments, "In our own time… relatively few human beings have managed to progress beyond the level of ego… In its self-obsession, it is simultaneously so clever and so blind."[66] No wonder MAiD is so appealing to the ego's distress at the thought of its own obliteration. Thankfully, even though most remain embedded in personal identity, death will deconstruct us in the end as awakening to the Ground of Being, to our fundamental nature. We don't need to figure out how to do it, as the process will come upon us. We will be apprehended by grace. Still, it helps to practice, and we begin by becoming aware of our ego.

Spiritually, the ego is an illusion, a fictional self compared to one's true nature.[67] But let us make a concession and say it is, nonetheless, functional

---

[66] Singh, Kathleen Dowling. *The Grace in Dying: How We Are Transformed Spiritually as We Die.* New York: HarperSanFrancisco, 1998, p. 113.

[67] For clarity, at this stage of my spiritual development, I am an idealist, not an essentialist. Essentialism is concerned with the inherent properties of entities that define their essence, while idealism is concerned with the nature of reality and posits that it is fundamentally mental or immaterial. I assert that everything is a veiled form

when it remains a *process* by which consciousness has experience, and dysfunctional when it becomes a *structure* that mistakes experience as its identity. For example, you may say *I am a parent. I am a woman. I am a truck driver. I am hungry.* From a spiritual perspective, these are all experiences or roles, but they are not you. You are a unique expression of awareness, of the underlying consciousness that is one, yet takes many forms. This is the foundation of your experience of self. To return to that Ground of Being, one observes their experience, and states the ultimate truth: nothing more or less than *I am.* You can do that now through simple shifts I will explore shortly… or you can do it when you die and become nothing but pure consciousness. The homework of awakening to what we truly are will patiently wait for us. It is mandatory but can be postponed until the last minute. (Isn't that the way many do their homework?)

The ego is formed through the cognitive, defensive, and executive functions of the developing personality. It becomes the story of ourselves in the world, and it constantly organizes, interprets, and processes experiences to support us as the lead character in that story. This helps us feel safe, significant, and belong. However, when threatened, the ego's defence mechanisms automatically kick in for self-preservation. That tends to accelerate when you're dying!

Contractions of consciousness commence by forming a distinction between self and other. One is in an environment, unlike being one with the environment of the womb. And this new environment is massive, extending far beyond the newborn's comprehension or optical perception. How different it feels from that enfolding warmth in which nutrients, oxygen, and waste management were all supplied without effort or desire. Now the newborn breathes, feeds, and interacts with a realm yet to have labels or context.

A second contraction soon follows: the distinction between living and non-living objects. Some things are moving in this strange new world: people, pets, a mobile hanging above the crib, sunlight dappling upon the

---

of consciousness – that which we call God, the indivisible Ground of Being from which 'physical' reality emanates and by which it is sustained.

curtains. Most are static: the wall, the mattress, the light above. And yet their proportions shift as the infant instinctively explores the new dimensions of open space through twisting head and squirming body.

That adorable form becomes an object, something other, with the third contraction of consciousness: the distinction between mind and body. Notice that the first contractions reinforced the sense, one might even say the illusion, of a self that is separate from others, but here the shift takes on a more profound abstraction. A body is physical, as experienced by the hand I gaze at and the toes I place easily in my mouth (no longer the case, of course!). But the infant is at the stage of experiencing the illusion of being in the body, somewhere behind the eyes, in the head. Here is the formation of the mind, and, with it, a distinctly non-physical, eerie entity called the self. Things are about to get complicated.

The final contraction provides us with our most challenging and essential homework on the long road travelled through the map of becoming, living, aging, and dying: we distinguish between what we can face inside ourselves and what is too frightening to face. We began as luminous and innocent. We began uncluttered and unformed in who and what we are in the world. But this material, these messages of how we are loved or unloved, valued or dismissed, have agency or are powerless... this shapes the wounded self. We add experiences, messages, and objects that support our identity to our ego, our outward, experienced self. The rest we place in the warehouse of the unconscious. That warehouse is vast and, for many, is never intentionally explored, so most remain in their ego-identity while this material waits for integration. When it does arise later in life, it is often judged, filtered, ignored, or projected upon others. Here, we meet what Carl Jung called the shadow – aspects of ourselves that we suppress because they are too difficult to acknowledge. These are socially unacceptable characteristics we keep locked away. The shadow is the fuel behind our anger, loneliness, and longings. Jung emphasized, "Everyone carries a shadow, and the less it is embodied in the individual's conscious life, the blacker and denser it is. If an inferiority is conscious, one always has a chance to correct it. But if it is repressed and isolated from consciousness, it never gets corrected and is liable to burst forth suddenly in a moment of unawareness. At all counts, it forms an unconscious snag, thwarting our most well-meant intentions."[68]

Acknowledging one's shadow is essential to integrating and activating its wisdom, for our most profound act of self-acceptance to support authenticity awaits. When we bring it into the light, our shadow no longer controls us. It becomes a bridge of solidarity with others through the awareness that it was born out of our unmet need to be loved. It will take patience, repeated failure, and great self-compassion to learn how to present this material in our relationships instead of projecting it destructively upon them. Shadow work is never brought to the table so intensely as when we die.

The material of our shadow builds slowly and steadily with every challenge. Since we are who we are through our relationships with people, places, objects, and experiences, with each change comes an investment in growth or a deposit in the Shadow Bank.

At first, minor changes cause major upsets. An infant losing her favourite blanket results in wailing as if the world has ended. More change comes when a sibling is born, shifting attention from parents and altering your place in the family unit. We continue our development of the self as we advance through grades in school, gain and lose friends, or move to another town. All initiate new growth by expanding us beyond our comfort zone. (All spiritual growth is initiated by an irritant!) This is life; this is the way we become fully human. And along the road, we secretly ask, am I loved? Am I accepted? Do I have a role? Do I have agency, ability, and identity? Do I matter?

In our efforts, we build meaning, but that requires choice, which constricts us to a specific path to become a specific person – the one I call myself. There is no smooth, comfortable way to become, and most of the time, we're stumbling into our tomorrows. And we get by, especially if we're fortunate to be born into economic circumstances that provide means and methods to meet basic needs, into a family or community that is relatively healthy. Still, it seems, for most of our adult journey, we are not the highest version of ourselves that we can imagine. We are the lowest version of ourselves that we can tolerate.

---

[68] Jung, Carl Gustav. *Collected Works of CG Jung, Volume 2: Experimental Researches. (Vol. 43.)* Princeton University Press, 2014.

Little do we realize the more we fortify the foundations of ego, our place in the world, our power and possessions, our privilege and place, the more we lay the foundation of our fear of death when all that is dismantled. In this, the person desiring MAiD turns away from transformation and toward what the ego wants: dignity, empowerment, and the ability to steer the self down that dark road. One can depend on headlights when driving in the dark, but those lights will only pierce so far. Better to slow down, stop, let one's eyes adjust, and discover you can see in the dark better than you realize. What we most desire to find in our lives is often, frustratingly, found in the places we least want to explore. The dignity you desire at the end of life is waiting within but is found only as you stop controlling. Stop driving the car. The stars are waiting to illuminate your path.

DECONSTRUCTION

HERE IS KATHLEEN DOWLING SINGH'S BRILLIANCE: THE AGING, SUFFERING, and dying process breaks down these contractions in the reverse order in which they formed. As each layer disintegrates, we open to more expansive dimensions of reality. While this builds connection and relationship with those who are part of your community and intensifies appreciation for what was taken for granted, it also triggers ego defence mechanisms for self-preservation. We do not want to be dismantled. We do not like such difficult change, for we do not know how to be anything other than who we think we are in the world, a story we tell ourselves about ourselves. The tyranny of the ego and the fixed narratives it constructs about our identity are activated all the more through dying, which inevitably challenges us to wake up and consider that what we are is a mystery, that we are the storyteller, not the story, that we arise from what we cannot cognitively understand. Whether that be the stuff of stars or the stuff of Spirit, eventually, in the end, the dying process will strain us of what is not essential for this final state of fundamental awareness.

I recall one couple who resisted the reality of death in such a coordinated fashion that it seemed like a dance of denial. He had been told he had weeks to live. They made no eye contact with the doctor or me. My mere presence amplified the obvious: I was the chaplain. They were getting bad news. It had death written all over it. But he talked of golf, she talked about the weather, and they sat, not touching, not registering the terror within. Life had been more than normal, it had been good. Really good. But it could not stay that way. He became weaker and bed-bound, and she became busier, cleaning and fussing, frustrated he would not eat. Then, in one visit, the protection they insisted upon for each other broke down, and she cried. And he reached out. And then, most beautifully, she crawled into his bed, and stayed there every night until he died.

They had traversed what Kathleen Dowling Singh calls the transformative fields of chaos. On one side is the Mental Ego, clinging to experience; on the other is the Witness, observing experience. What happens between these states can feel like an existential evisceration, especially as we resist it. Therein lies the distress driving most MAiD requests: not the fear of death and not physical suffering, but the inability to process and accept the disintegration of the self. Loss of dignity, meaning, purpose, pleasure, agency, and role in the world… all of it is ego deconstruction (Figure 1).

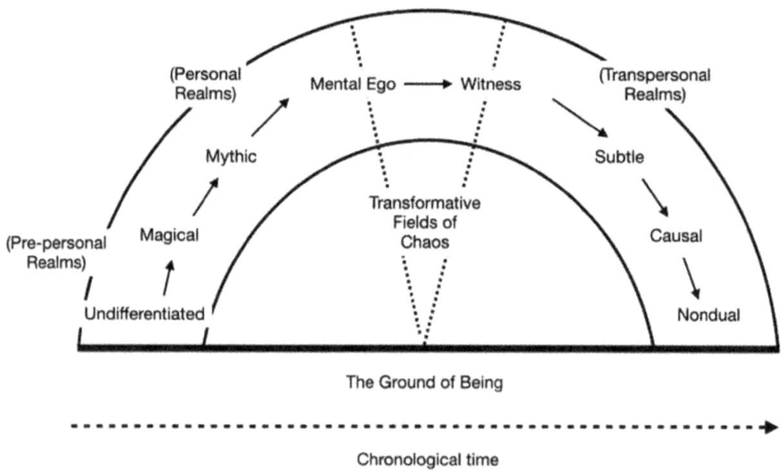

Figure 1: Ego Construction and Deconstruction[69]

[69] Adapted from Singh, Kathleen Dowling. *The Grace in Dying: How We Are Transformed Spiritually as We Die.* New York: HarperSanFrancisco, 1998, p. 20.

In the Christian tradition, it's called the dark night of the soul, a period of despair and hopelessness in which one loses all sense of security, dignity, and meaning. Patients are standing on the threshold of that darkness when they say, "What's the point in suffering?" "I don't want to put my family through this." "I'm scared of what dying will do to me." The dying are in the centre of it when they emotionally shut down, pull back, or lash out. Existential midnight is marked by feelings of spiritual emptiness or being abandoned by God. Surprisingly, this is natural in spiritual growth, a necessary stage of development in opening consciousness to the Ground of Being. Whether you are a person of faith or a more practical pilgrim in this terrestrial journey, know that this period of intense internal struggle is temporary. It will not last. You are not trapped. You are travelling through. And when going through hell, keep going with compassionate care at your side and good pain meds in your veins!

The ramifications of this are unarticulated in MAiD discussions – that the loss of dignity, meaning, purpose, pleasure, agency, and your role in the world is a functional process at the heart of dying, which opens us to the final stage of development in human consciousness: transcendence. Therefore, it is not pointless. This is why I assert that MAiD is a medical procedure used to treat a spiritual condition in most cases.[70] The impoverishment of MAiD is that the final stage of ego deconstruction is not experienced, let alone imagined.

As we make the shift from preserving our identity to relaxing our hold on it, a new orientation to our experience emerges. It is marked by gentleness, contemplation, and by an increasing skill to be fully present in this moment without any need to control or understand. As we work with this

---

[70] And for those cases in which MAiD is being requested to treat overwhelming physical suffering, the appropriate response is excellent pain management. I recognize that some cases involve what we call intractable pain – pain that is not responsive to medication or other interventions. In those cases, it is likely that pain arises from a combination of existential and physical origins. Palliative sedation is the only solution, and here we enter the grey zone of soothing suffering while possibly accelerating death. It is small comfort to consider that, on some deep level, the dying person is engaging their deconstruction. The best we can do at that point is practise deep presence with them as they struggle.

process through allowing, even surrendering, there is an opening to something deeper, something quite mysterious and unexpected. But when the deconstruction of the ego is met with resistance, our road becomes very rough, collapsing us into distress.

It's understandable if you think the person who dies by MAiD is allowing, even embracing, death. They are not in denial, they are not shrinking back, but are letting go of this world, often with gratitude and acceptance. How can that be a bad idea? I often hear this, but it's an effort to preserve identity by choosing to die 'beautifully,' 'heroically,' or 'consciously.' This reflects the mental ego's effort to preserve itself and its cherished identity. Yes, they appear to die beautifully, heroically, and consciously. But, as Singh puts it, "There is a difference between the quality of an isolating pose of the mental ego and the surrendered, participating quality of a whole being as it undergoes transformation."[71]

In other words, the hero does not slay the dragon; instead, the hero is consumed by it, and in that surrender, becomes fully human. This is explored well in the thoughts of author, teacher, and songwriter Paul Weinfield. I quote him at length here as he muses on another poet, and while he's speaking here of the inner voice that harangues us through life, it applies equally well at death:

> Leonard Cohen said his teacher once told him that the older you get the lonelier you become, and the deeper the love you need. This is because, as we go through life, we tend to over-identify with being the hero of our stories. This hero isn't exactly having fun: he's getting kicked around, humiliated, and disgraced. But if we can let go of identifying with him, we can find our rightful place in the universe, and a love more satisfying than any we've ever known.
>
> People constantly throw around the term "Hero's Journey" without having any idea what it really means. Everyone from

[71] Singh, Kathleen Dowling. *The Grace in Dying: How We Are Transformed Spiritually As We Die.* New York: HarperSanFrancisco, 1998, p. 163.

> CEOs to wellness-influencers thinks the Hero's Journey means facing your fears, slaying a dragon, and gaining 25k followers on Instagram. But that's not the real hero's journey.
>
> In the real hero's journey, the dragon slays YOU. Much to your surprise, you couldn't make that marriage work. Much to your surprise, you turned forty with no kids, no house, and no prospects. Much to your surprise, the world didn't want the gifts you proudly offered it.
>
> If you are foolish, this is where you will abort the journey and start another, and another, abusing your heart over and over for the brief illusion of winning.
>
> But if you are wise, you will let yourself be shattered, and return to the village, humbled, but with a newfound sense that you don't have to identify with the part of you that needs to win, needs to be recognized, needs to know. This is where your transcendent life begins.
>
> So embrace humility in everything. Life isn't out to get you, nor are your struggles your fault.
>
> Every defeat is just an angel, tugging at your sleeve, telling you that you don't have to keep banging your head against the wall.
>
> Leave that striver there, trapped in his lonely ambitions. Just walk away, and life in its vastness will embrace you.[72]

Being embraced by life is certainly something we might desire, but how about being embraced by death? And what if that is the ultimate intimacy you could have with the universe? Here we come back to Kathleen Dowling Singh and her final observation of the dying process… which is shocking. Completely unexpected. Utterly incongruent with everything we've know. In the final crumbling of the ego's framework, a period before death that

---

[72] Weinfield, Paul. "Letting the Hero Die." *Science & Nonduality*, www.scienceandnonduality.com/article/letting-the-hero-die. Accessed July 17, 2023.

can last weeks or seconds, awaits a transformation marked by the experience of ecstasy. Yes, ecstasy. It is a quiet rapture, a sublime openness, a connection to self and all that is beyond the poverty of words to explain. It is grace. Author and co-founder of the Esalen Institute, Michael Murphy, described this as "the process by which unitive knowing, self-transcending love, and other extraordinary capacities emerge in us, during which such capacities appear to be freely given rather than earned, spontaneously revealed rather than attained through ego-centred effort."[73]

It is a love greater than you've ever known, an equanimity that desires nothing. Singh and countless others who work with the dying observe this in many patients as they die: a transpersonal state of consciousness. We are reunited with the Ground of Being, with Spirit. We feel unity with everything, an infilling of love. We experience the transcendent state of consciousness. We are ready for our transformation.

Many become anxious as they contemplate this, and no wonder. Few people can sit in silence by themselves in an empty room for five minutes. Fewer still can sit for five seconds with an empty mind. That can feel like you're approaching a void, a vast emptiness, an oppressive darkness. The mind becomes anxious, projecting its limitations onto the peace just beyond that seeming nothingness. The void is just a blank screen over the veil of the Ground of Being, the inherent peace that is rarely reached since the void feels unbearable. But it's a thin veil, which can be parted with a simple step. Let's take it.

As you read the words on this page, pause and step back from yourself. Pause and observe the sounds around you. Pause and observe your physical sensations, what may be called the sounds within you. Pause and observe thoughts and feelings. Pause and observe the experience. Consider that you are not your body, thoughts, feelings, or experiences. All of these are temporary and unstable. They are not essential to who and what you are. Notice what is essential, what is unchanging: awareness itself. Open to this through releasing. Allowing. Stillness. No grasping. No understanding. Just Being. You are aware. You are awareness.

---

[73] Murphy, Michael. "The Future of the Body: Explorations into the Further Evolution of Human Nature." *Omni* 14.8 (1992): pp. 6–7.

How does it feel? What do you notice? Stop reading and check in at this level of being.

I appreciate that this sounds abstract, perhaps even quite strange. But think of it. In all your life experiences, for all the times you have said, "I am sad, I am happy, I am injured, I am content..." the only constant in those changing states is the "I am." It is your awareness. This state is unaffected by what "you" go through. This is invincible against the trials of life. And the surprise is that this is what seems to continue after death. We'll explore that further in Part 4.

For now, notice how your mind will interrupt you in this exercise. The imaginary self goes off searching for this treasure out in the world, out in roles and relationships, possessions and people, all to fill the void, find itself, then assert itself and feel itself having power, purpose, and dignity. It seeks to become, belong, and be blessed with anything that makes it more than what it is. Yet the well-being the mind seeks is found in what it cannot understand. It is found in the simple knowing of your being. Knowing yourself. Awareness is awareness of awareness. It is a self-referential state of being. It is the Ground of Being. And it is the only "thing" that is everything you will be in death.

Seems like a fantasy? We'll explore the evidence and prevalence of this state later, but let's not get ahead of ourselves, for we must not prematurely abandon the difficulty of this process, a difficulty some of you may be experiencing right now. Singh explores this struggle with the fidelity of a seismographic needle, acknowledging each tremor and earthquake as the self is shaken to the core by the dying process.

Singh has revealed that beyond Elisabeth Kübler-Ross's five stages of dying – denial, anger, bargaining, depression, and acceptance – are three more: a fall into darkness that verges on despair, a resignation that dwarfs our initial acceptance, and the in-breaking of ecstasy. That's where we're going in the coming chapters, but we'll also explore how one's relationship to suffering can intentionally shift through effective counselling, compassion, vulnerability, and curiosity. This will not help you find a detour around difficulty, for, again, the despair is functional in deconstructing the ego. With such a map before us, we can consider the curves ahead, the hazards and refuelling stations, and the unexpected beauty in a land that we imagine only to be marked by sorrow.

EXERCISE 5: AWARENESS MEDITATION

Time to observe yourself. We're going to do a meditation, which you can listen to at https://soundcloud.com/david-maginley/exercise5. This one draws from the Hindu and Buddhist traditions. It's called vipassana, *a Sanskrit term meaning "to see things as they are." This is a meditation through which we observe our own experience by embracing that which is happening right now and being openly aware of what draws our attention. It will help you work wisely with the ego when it runs on autopilot to control your deeds and your days.*

We will do these practices lightly as an introduction to developing deeper awareness. Note that your thoughts will frequently drift as you practise, but in noticing that, you can bring attention back to the exercise. That drifting will never stop, so we'll employ a repeated phrase or object of awareness to anchor our practice. Sometimes called a mantra, this is like a bone you throw to a dog to get it to sit and stay. We'll be using this for the exceedingly tough job of piercing the layers of illusion that obscure reality to drill down to who you indeed are, beneath the anxiety and fear of death, beneath the noise of the ego-self.

If you can, begin by taking some time to stretch. You can be sitting or lying down. Close your eyes. Listen to the noise in your environment. It may be traffic outside, rain or wind on a window. It may be voices in the hallway or the sound of an intravenous pump by your side.

Now place your awareness on your breath, particularly one area of your respiratory system, such as the sensation of air flowing through the nose, the lifting and falling of your diaphragm, or the rise and fall of your belly or chest. Focusing on one aspect of breathing helps maintain attention. Breathe naturally, noticing the physical sensations of the breath in that one area. Let's stay with this for a few breaths.

Now do a quick scan through your body, beginning at your feet and moving up through ankles, calves, thighs, hips, stomach, back, neck, and head… notice any sensations, such as the weight of your body supported by the chair or bed, and the fatigue you may feel as you rest upon it. If there is pain, allow it with a perspective of kindness. Be gentle in opening to this, as the practice is challenging when pain is more intense. Try to open a space for the pain to be as it is and observe its movement, edges, and quality. Now silently repeat, "I have this body, but I am not this body. I have this body, but I am not this body."[74] *You may even focus on the pain, saying, "I have this pain, but I am not this pain." The pain will pulse and move as you do this, so returning awareness to your breath will be the best response, especially as it can be very effective in relaxing the body. Observe your physical experience for as long as is comfortable… and then a bit longer.*

Now notice your thoughts. Allow them to flow. We have one every few seconds, and they are the activity the mind is designed to generate. Therefore, trying to calm your mind is like pushing down on flowing water – that will only create more turbulence! Instead, watch the flow of thoughts. Even more, notice when you get caught up in them and carried downstream. In the Buddhist tradition, that's called shenpa, or "that which gets its hooks in you." In the noticing, you can step back from the water and observe the flow again. The stream of thoughts may be turbulent or smooth, depending on the subjects your thoughts are flowing over. Yesterday's lunch will produce but a ripple, while the sorrow of grief and dying can create a vortex of whitewater. Watch the turbulence; do not become the turbulence. Now silently repeat, "I have these thoughts, but I am not these thoughts. I have these thoughts, but I am not these thoughts." Observe your thoughts for as long as is comfortable… and then a bit longer.

Move your awareness to your feelings. We observe them now as the previous step can create stress – it's so easy to get caught up in our thoughts, then try all the harder to step back from them. But we don't need to believe everything we think, so please do not try to calm your thoughts and feelings. Rather, let go and allow whatever arises within you to arise. Return to this moment as a human being, not a human doing. Allow and observe what is… no need to understand, filter, judge, or control. Breathe… breathe… Notice if your feelings and thoughts retreat as you observe them, like small creatures

[74] This is literally true; the cells in your body are completely replaced every ten years. Bone cells live the longest, cells in the digestive tract the shortest. While we understandably identify most with our body, especially when it is in pain, there is also a sense that we are somehow *in* the body.

scurrying for cover and protection. This is a natural defence strategy of the ego, which defines itself according to past experience and future expectations. Ego is not present at this moment, though it may assert that it is all you are. By observing your thoughts and feelings, you observe the ego. You also realize that everything the ego offers is not permanent. And yes, that means even your distress is temporary. That alone makes it possible to wake up from the convincing perception that what you think is actually what is real.

Notice how you feel, where your feeling is located in your body, and how there are many layers or feelings at once. No need to understand or name them... allow whatever feelings arise to be. If you begin to feel sad or anxious, notice how that registers in your body and allow it. Observe and be kind toward this dimension of your experience. Breathe... breathe...

Now silently repeat, "I have these feelings, but I am not these feelings. I have these feelings, but I am not these feelings." Observe your feelings for as long as is comfortable... and then a bit longer.

Allow your awareness to observe the body, thoughts, and feelings as noise within yourself. Allow the noise. Breathe... Now shift your attention back to the noise in the external environment. Notice how it flows by, each moment moving into the next like water in a stream. Remain in this for a few breaths, then gently open your eyes.

We are unfamiliar with this observational state of being in our busy world, but we did it naturally as children and even better as infants. To notice the experience of the self is the beginning of developing a stabilizing and kind awareness when engaging in the ultimate issues at life's end. I encourage you to practise this lightly and frequently, with curiosity for whatever arises, especially your desire to feel safe as you die. If you are considering assisted death, use this exercise to explore what is behind that desire, without judgment but with accuracy. Writing notes on your insights will be very helpful as we move through these practices.

CHAPTER 6

THE CHALLENGE OF SUFFERING

He who has a why to live for can bear almost any how.

– FREDRICH NIETZSCHE

JOEL WAS FRAIL BEYOND WORDS. IT WAS REMARKABLE TO ME THAT the skeletal form lying in the bed had any life at all, yet he smiled and extended his hand as I sat down. His paper-thin skin felt surprisingly soft against mine. Carol, his wife, was across the bed from me and radiated love and admiration. I knew right away they could teach me a lot about life.

"You guys are having quite the effect on the nurses. We feel like we're witnessing a beautiful love story that's going to be cut short."

"Oh, cut short is true. But also complete," said Carol. "Joel has been fighting this cancer for years. He fought with a vengeance. He fought for me."

"But I stopped fighting," Joel added, "because I could see that any more would prevent my life moving from tragedy to grace." Joel was a poet at heart, which made chatting a profound and enriching experience.

"Tell me about your suffering," I asked. "Tell me what one does with their suffering to enter that grace."

"Well, first, you fight like hell! I know I did. I took everything they could throw at me. Three types of chemo. They all failed. Tons of radiation till they couldn't give any more. Look how it left me." His bright blue eyes closed for a moment. "If I had known it would be like this, I never would have done it. But I had to do something. I had to try. For Carol. For the kids." I held my words so we could feel the grief filling the space between us. "I didn't know back then, but I know now. Suffering… is what we have when we fight what is. I had to learn I was mortal, and it took longer than it should. So I suffered. Now, pain, pain is of the body – suffering's of the soul. They have good drugs for pain, and I'm not shy. But the only drug for suffering is surrender with satisfaction for the life you've lived. I guess I wasn't satisfied. But I am now." Joel looked at Carol. She was crying. I was crying. But Joel was smiling. "Love you, babe."

Joel died a week later. Carol shared that the room felt filled with peace. He had slipped into unconsciousness; his face so relaxed it seemed he didn't have a care in the world. Then his breath became faint, then imperceptible, then it was as if he just slipped out.

"You could tell that something had changed. I was gazing at him, but he simply wasn't there anymore. After so much struggle… is it okay to say I'm relieved?"

No wonder so many consider the rough road ahead and ask, is it worth it? Is it worth the descent? That fall into darkness that verges on despair… what's the point of enduring that? That was the question on Joel's mind as he fought for his life. That's the question on the minds of everyone facing their finality. Is it worth continuing until my body fails, living into the misery of anticipated physical anguish and, worse, the imagined and unbearable weight of sorrow as my loved ones grieve? Am I not empowered, are not my feelings respected through having the option of facing mortality on my terms, ending my life before it crumbles into utter chaos?

The French philosopher and Nobel Prize laureate Albert Camus would sympathize. Here in the suddenly fleeting sanctuary of one's bedroom or the safe harbour of a hospital bed, ordinary patients considering MAiD grapple with the ultimate question: does my life, as it is, have meaning? Is it worth sliding down to the end? He called it "the fundamental question" of those who suffer, explored in his essay *The Myth of Sisyphus*. The short answer? No. In his wrestling with absurdity and paradox, he concluded that if life has any meaning, we must be the ones who create it. Each of us is Sisyphus, a figure of Greek mythology condemned to repeat the same task of pushing a boulder up a mountain, only to have it roll to the bottom again and again and again.

As with all creative works, his is autobiographical, revealing not so much the truth of reality as the truth of *his* reality. It was the 1940s. Camus witnessed millions of refugees fleeing the advancing German armies. And after the war, the world reeled in existential distress as we learned of the Nazi concentration camps; millions were slaughtered in hatred. Utter despair engulfed the collective psyche. In this respect, Camus was an effective mirror for society.

God was no comfort for this man. Instead, the divine was an inadequate coping strategy. Everyone should face the inevitable: there is no rescue from this life and no restoration in the next. You'd think, then, that Camus would approve of euthanasia. Quite the contrary: Albert Camus concluded that early exits are unwise. He said that one must take life's absurdity seriously and acknowledge the contradiction between our desire for reason and the unreasonable world. We must be mature, living out the paradox without false hope, gaining freedom from artificial constraints that seek to define us, that demand we measure up to cultural standards. Since existence is absurd, we can create any meaning we desire. Push the boulder up the mountain but do it *your* way.[75]

Meaning is the antidote for suffering. Here is noble persistence. Here is purpose. Here is the art within tragedy. (And here is the best of comedy. We may as well go out laughing at ourselves!). It is also a call to action, a constant confrontation and revolt against that which would bind and define us.

Well, is not MAiD the ultimate statement of autonomy against the traditional notions of the sanctity of life and the Hippocratic oath? One can argue this both ways, for the one dying is stating that dying on their terms *is* living life fully to the end; an end in which they're still

---

[75] One might say the task of Sisyphus parallels the Buddhist concept that suffering is the price we pay for self-awareness, though Camus was thinking more pragmatically of the repetitive tasks of office and factory workers. While he seems to be a fellow you would not invite to a party, Camus sincerely felt that one can be authentically happy because one is free from illusions of hope and striving for what cannot be.

engaged, able to say goodbye, and avoiding the mess of final biological and existential disintegration. This hits at the heart of Camus's perspective, summed up in his statement, "What counts is not the best living but the most living."

Yet James Hollis, the author of *Living an Examined Life,* builds on this by challenging us: why would you rid yourself of darkness and struggle when you do not know what work they are doing to you? Depression is the psyche withdrawing approval of your experience instead of engaging the crisis to forge meaning over happiness, to choose the path of enlargement, to bestow love on the unlovable parts of you, and in this, you recover personal dignity.[76] Live well, love deep, leave clean underwear.

MAiD ensures that the last box gets checked. It is common for the dying to lose bowel control as they exit this world. That can set in long before death, as incontinence and weakness render the patient bed-bound and dependent on others to wipe, wash, and smooth the wrinkles from yet another set of clean sheets.

AWAKENING

HOW DO WE ENGAGE WITH OUR SUFFERING? WELL, WE DO SO SPORADICALLY, stumbling towards our disintegration with hesitation and resistance. Richard Rohr, a world-renowned Franciscan friar and spiritual teacher, reminds us that this disintegration is the ultimate moment for our soul's growth. His insight: "All great spirituality is about what we do with our pain."[77] This means everyone does spiritual work, whether atheist or evangelist, for everyone will suffer. Nothing erodes our ego-identity; nothing reveals it as the illusion it is, like suffering. This is why suffering is an effective medium for awakening the true self. You don't discover your humanity through avoiding pain, tragic loss, or complex relationships but by engaging it. Spiritual growth is not a movement beyond material conditions and realities. It's always a movement *into* the suffering, trauma, oppressive

[76] Hollis, James. *Living an Examined life: Wisdom for the Second Half of the Journey.* Sounds True, 2018.

[77] Rohr, Richard. *Adam's Return: The Five Promises of Male Initiation.* Crossroad, 2004.

conditions, and wounded nature of what it means to be human. This existential heat burns off the layers of identification through the ego, the mind, and all its desires to reveal the First Principle of your true nature. Being uncomfortable is a sign that transformation is happening. This change is inevitable, but your growth is optional. You can use suffering as fuel for transformation or allow it to backfire because by clinging to what you know, what you want, and what you think you are. In this context, MAiD is the epitome of refusing to accept what is. It is a turning away from ourselves because what is happening is disturbing and painful. It is the ultimate act of ego self-preservation in the face of that which dismantles it for our awakening.

Awakening. It sounds like the opposite of dying. Yet, *awakening* is another word for something that sounds even more preposterous: *enlightenment.* Enlightenment is a fancy name for the most simple, the most ordinary, and the most universal experience every person on the planet is having right now. We all know it, yet because it cannot be found by the mind, it is deemed missing. Also missing, then, are the qualities inherent in it: peace, equanimity, well-being, oneness, and connection without effort. When you observe your own experience, it is there – awareness. Pure and simple awareness.

This natural tendency to reject our immediate experience of our true nature has compelled us to look throughout life for anything that will soothe this massive subconscious existential anxiety. As one dies, the ego frantically searches for a solution to its impending destruction. Previously, the only option was medication. Now, there is MAiD. As the primal nature of death anxiety is so intense, and the procedure seems so kind and straightforward, this option is an intoxicant to the ego. It acts as a balm to imagination's darkness one patient even describing MAiD as an enfolding comfort, their security blanket. The child within only wants to feel safe. But, as Rohr comments, "Until we walk with personal issues of despair, we will never uncover the Real Hope on the other side of that despair. Until we allow the crash and crush of our images, we will never discover Real Life beyond what only seems like death. Remember, death is an imaginary loss of an imaginary self that will pass anyway. This very journey is probably the heart of what Jesus came to reveal."[78]

Where do you find meaning? Usually in the deepest, darkest places. This is the inevitable reality of suffering that will occur in everyone's lives, and it can make people bitter, frustrated, angry, sad, and reeling in despair. The antidote is a meaningful life – to adopt responsibility for what can be made of it, despite the reality of its horror. And what we can make through dying is the ultimate realization of our true nature. That is why a meaningful life is found right here, right now, and nowhere else. This is why hope is the dying person's four-letter word; it's always reaching for some future, some fix, something else rather than what is. Mindfully embracing all dimensions of self as you are, at this moment, is to embrace our life with what the Buddhist tradition calls its "ten thousand joys and ten thousand sorrows." This is the ultimate love affair with life on its own terms. And, as ridiculous as it may sound (especially if you have a terminal prognosis), this is possible even as we die.

Rev. Olivia Bareham, the founder of Shared Crossings, speaks in the film *Saying Goodbye: Preparing for Death* of a remarkable woman she supported who embodied such grace. Her doctor told her to go home, get everything in order, and embrace her family's love as death approached. She called for Bareham to come and help her brother and son, who she lived with, to grieve, to walk this road with her, and then to say farewell. And this she did in style, complete with a living wake, where almost 200 friends and acquaintances came to say goodbye. Many in the crowd even signed the simple cardboard casket on display in the garden. It was shocking to her family. It was genius to her friends. It was closure for the one dying. Olivia comments, "She had taken the news with such calm grace that I was fascinated by her and intrigued by this level of acceptance... I asked her, 'What is it that allows you to move into this space so gracefully?' " The response was intriguing. "Olivia, it is directly related to my capacity to receive. While I'm receiving this... all of it, my dying, my friends, love, the birds, the sky, I can't be holding on to anything. And I've learned how

[78] Rohr, Richard. *Near Occasions of Grace*. Orbis Books, 2015.

to receive these last ten years of my life, so this is the penultimate opportunity, and I am filled to the brim. I'm ready to go."

The next day she slipped into a coma and faded gently from this world. Olivia emphasized the lesson: "Our capacity to receive, receive everything, receive life, receive death, receive joy, receive grief, receive it all, is going to help us at the end when we need just to open and receive what's next."[79]

Without this meaning, which is more visceral than intellectual, we can consider why people would opt for MAiD to escape. It's no simple thing to pick up the weight of your suffering and turn toward death. You are like Sisyphus, nearing the top of the hill. But this is your most challenging climb. Perhaps, at the top, you will discover you can fly. If you are in a position to have two doctors assess you for the procedure, you are likely in the position to have palliative care support you, which will ensure you have as smooth a takeoff as possible.

You may be worried or doubtful as you read this because you are in pain, because you have witnessed pain at the end of life. And perhaps that pain could not be controlled. Is there an option for assisted death in this situation? Yes, there are two.

The first is palliative sedation. This is a significant step beyond ordinary palliative care. The palliative service at Sunnybrook Hospital in Toronto, Ontario, describes it as:

> continuous medically-induced heavy sedation such that the patient is effectively asleep or unconscious for a period of what might be days or weeks until death occurs naturally. [Death is not caused by this sedation, though death can be more comfortably hastened if the patient or their next of kin requests that no intravenous fluids be administered in this drug-induced state of unconsciousness.] Palliative sedation is not subject to the same stringent rules as MAiD – it does not require the patient to make the request herself. Her

---

[79] Lunn, Johanna, director. *Saying Goodbye: Preparing for Death.* Centre East Media, 2022. 30:30–38:04

> next of kin can decide on her behalf, taking into account her prior expressed preferences and values, if she is already incapacitated.[80]

While this option may seem ideal, some patients I have spoken with express concerns about still perceiving sound, having dreams, or feeling trapped in a liminal state of consciousness until their passing. Finding the appropriate balance of medication can also be challenging, as family members often overestimate the patient's pain, while healthcare providers tend to underestimate it.[81] However, most studies on palliative sedation primarily focus on its use for physical pain rather than existential distress, which is the main driver behind most MAiD requests. Doctors are not entirely comfortable with using sedation for the purpose of addressing existential distress, and even the Canadian Hospice Palliative Care Association advises that "sedation for purely existential symptoms should only be initiated in rare cases of severe existential distress and after skilled multidimensional management directed at the physical, psychological, and existential dimensions has been attempted, preferably in consultation with relevant experts in this area, such as, for example, a psychologist or psychiatrist, chaplain, ethicist, or palliative care physician."[82]

Alternatively, one could choose to hasten the process by directly resorting to starvation. This involves ceasing all food and drink, specifically avoiding fluids. Hunger pains typically subside after two to three days

---

[80] Lewis, Ralph. "Medical assistance in dying – Is there purpose in suffering?" Your Health Matters, Stories and expert health tips from Sunnybrook. http://health.sunnybrook.ca/mental-health/finding-purpose/medical-assistance-dying-purpose-suffering/. Accessed March 12, 2022.

[81] Kirk, Timothy W., and Margaret M. Mahon. "National Hospice and Palliative Care Organization (NHPCO) position statement and commentary on the use of palliative sedation in imminently dying terminally ill patients." *Journal of Pain and Symptom Management* 39.5 (2010): pp. 914–923.

[82] Dean, Mervyn M., et al. "Framework for continuous palliative sedation therapy in Canada." *Journal of Palliative Medicine* 15.8 (2012): pp. 870–879, citing de Graeff A. and M. Dean: "Palliative sedation therapy in the last weeks of life: A literature review and recommendations for standards." *Journal of Palliative Medicine,* 10 (200): pp. 67–85.

without nutrition. Although the stomach ceases to produce digestive acids and settles, thirst may persist for some time. As mentioned earlier with palliative sedation, if fluids are provided, the person will endure their suffering for a much longer duration and potentially reach a skeletal state if they have not already. Discomfort from dry mouth can be alleviated to some extent, allowing the person to tolerate the condition, as reported by individuals who intentionally undergo a hunger strike.

I'll be honest. I cannot imagine this as I type these words from the comfort of my keyboard. I understand that the suffering we envision from such a condition is not as bad as the reality. But even I shudder at this thought, having seen people endure for far longer than anyone expected, slowly wasting away. Family members will struggle profoundly with this choice and interpret it as unacceptable suffering. Food is a fundamental expression of care. Witnessing this decline can contradict every instinct to nurture and support our loved ones. That perception of suffering can compel us to hope our loved one will die mercifully, which means quickly, even as we ache for them to stay. Even as we ache for everyday life to return, for the miracle to happen.

This book is not about those miracles. I have never seen them. But I have seen something more extraordinary that is utterly astonishing to me and surprisingly common: patients can endure far more than they ever imagined – when effective palliative care is provided. They even describe it as tolerable suffering. How many times I've sat at their side, gazing at their skeletal form, and heard the impossible whispered from thin lips: "I'm OK. It's my family I worry about." It leaves me stunned, realizing their love and compassion for others changes their relationship to their own suffering. I witness the astonishing resilience of their character, reinforced by their gratitude for us, the staff, who strive to make them comfortable, and wish we could do so much more.

Besides embodying compassion, the wisest thing to do is learn from these teachers what it is to love deeply as you die slowly and endure more than you could ever imagine being able to face. In that is grace, not as some gentle favour or mercy but a quality that describes the bedrock of being, an enfolding Otherness we awaken to within. This is revealed in our soul's secret sanctum as we move through the rough road of dying to a subtle state of surrender to what is. Time and trust are required for this state to be reached. Most who take MAiD do so in no small part because they find this stillness suffocating to the ego throughout the dying process. They do not want to wait until the self is eroded away to reveal the astonishing surprise to which silence is the only appropriate response.

EXERCISE 6: DEATH CAFÉ

Go to a death café. This is a gathering of those curious about the ultimate event. Death cafés are discussion groups rather than grief support or counselling sessions. Be prepared for laughter and tears, and be ready to meet new friends. See https://deathcafe.com/what/ for more information. Cafés can be virtual, but in-person is so much better.

PART 2

MAiD AND CULTURE

CHAPTER 7

CULTURE AND CONTEXT

The cyborg would not recognize the Garden of Eden;
it is not made of mud and cannot dream of returning to dust.

– DONNA HARAWAY

"THAT'S NOT THE WAY WE DO IT! WE WOULD NEVER PUT OUR PARents in your nursing homes. We take care of them in *their* home! We come together as family. And as they die, the community comes on through to pay their respects. When my mother's gone, she'll be laying out in the living room, and we're gonna be sharing stories and music and food for days. You get up in the morning and talk to her. Yes, she'd be dead. But we ain't! I thought nothin' of this as a kid. It's just the way it's done! And the funeral… that's at least three hours long. You can come and go. Come and go. It's a fine send-off. It's how it should be."

I sat in silence. I was not going to interrupt this feisty five-foot-nothing powerhouse. I only nodded now and then to acknowledge that I understood. I respected her wisdom and quietly envied her culture. She was African-Canadian, she was on fire, and I was a WASP whose mother was in a nursing home. Still, it made me think of how far we've drifted from how things used to be. And, though I was intensely proud that my sisters cared for our mother for over five years at home, I also knew these situations wouldn't be so difficult if we were not so good at keeping people alive in the first place.

Times have changed dramatically. In centuries past, people faced more significant risks of mortality from a multitude of sources, like an infection, accident, or being eaten by a bear. Death by disease was far more varied a hundred years ago, with pneumonia, influenza, and tuberculosis among the leading causes.[83] Thanks to medical advances, those have largely been taken care of while doubling the average life span since the 1900s.[84]

Medicine's success is now its greatest challenge: the diseases that remain are the most difficult to cure without lifestyle changes. And no wonder: the two leading culprits in North America, cancer and heart disease, are heavily influenced by smoking, poor diet and lack of exercise – our comfort sets us up for failure in this regard.[85]

Of course, one of the reasons cancer is difficult to cure is the it is not a disease but a disease process, an umbrella term for more than 200 distinct diseases. Each type of cancer branches into more variants, each looking and behaving differently because they *are* different on a genetic and molecular level. Since cancer arises from our cells, it can be as diverse as the individuals afflicted. Treatments in decades past were crude compared to today. The past forty years have brought us from severe cobalt radiation to individualized genetic therapy. Now emergent therapies can be designed by AI that decipher your genome and promise to break the cancer code in hours compared to decades.[86] The future looks bright. In fact, it looks unrecognizable, for we are on the edge of a new era for humanity, one in which scientists are seriously considering how death may become not only more remote but an option. Before we venture to that strange tomorrow, we need to look back, for only through the arch of history can

---

[83] Kyle, Kim. "How do we die? What killed Americans in 1900 vs. 2010." *Los Angeles Times* (June 11, 2014) https://www.latimes.com/nation/nationnow/la-na-nn-g-how-americans-die-20140610-story.html

[84] Johnson, Steven. "How Humanity Gave Itself an Extra Life." *The New York Times Magazine,* NY, USA (2021).

[85] Anand, Preetha, et al. "Cancer is a preventable disease that requires major lifestyle changes." *Pharmaceutical Research* 25.9 (2008): pp. 2097–2116.

[86] Dlamini, Zodwa, et al. "Artificial intelligence (AI) and big data in cancer and precision oncology." *Computational and Structural Biotechnology Journal* 18 (2020): pp. 2300–2311.

we gain context for MAiD and realize why we believe what we believe about the end of life.

ANCIENT ROOTS

Early Greece and Rome knew the practice well. Attitudes were tolerant toward infanticide, active euthanasia, and suicide. Support for voluntary death, as opposed to prolonged agony, was widespread, and physicians complied by often giving their patients the poisons they requested.[87]

As Christianity rose to prominence, the sanctity of life principle came to dominate medical care (such as it was), and by the twelfth to fifteenth centuries, support for the Hippocratic oath meant near unanimity in opposing euthanasia. That shifted, if only slightly, with the Reformation. Protestants across Europe challenged the church's authority on all matters. However, ethical issues of assisted death held little interest for most. Illness was as brutal as ever. No significant medical breakthroughs had alleviated that, so suffering was accepted as one's lot in life, the arbitrary will of God or fate's final blow.[88]

Other cultures shared no such fear of divine punishment; the gods understood humanity's struggle well enough. Besides, this was also a matter of survival for communities with scarce resources. Hard choices have been part of life throughout time.[89]

It's no surprise that the isolation of morphine from opium in the nineteenth century reanimated the discussion on mercifully de-animating the dying. The drug was wonderfully effective in treating pain and so gentle in stopping life. Samuel Williams was excited, and his euthanasia proposal received serious attention in the medical journals of the 1870s. Still, most

[87] Dowbiggin, Ian. *A Merciful End: The Euthanasia Movement in Modern America.* Oxford University Press, 2003.

[88] Manning, Michael. *Euthanasia and Physician-Assisted Suicide: Killing or Caring?* Paulist Press, 1998.

[89] Mwaria, Cheryl. "Physician-assisted suicide: An anthropological perspective." *Fordham Urban Law Journal* 24 (1996): pp. 859.

physicians held the view that pain medication should be administered for just that: to alleviate pain, not to hasten death.[90]

Cultural expectations shift with a culture's struggles. The hardships of the Great Depression saw public support for euthanasia rise, even for infants born with physical and mental challenges. The future looked bleak enough for the healthy and strong.[91] Then the war came.

As I reflect on that history, I want to emphasize that I am not saying the countries where assisted death is practised are as malevolent as Nazi Germany. I am saying foundational perspectives on the utility of life play out in similar ways. These matters are endemic to the human condition and revolve around meaning and suffering, as well as our response to challenges that overwhelm us at first, divide us at worst, and hopefully unite us in the end, for we all will die.

Euthanasia didn't start as horrific for the Nazis. It began as an act of compassion, a response to suffering, much like today. In 1939 it was against the law, but cases like Gerhard Kretschmar initiated the unravelling of social norms. He was a child born blind, missing a leg and part of his arm, and with cognitive impairments. His parents were crushed, supporting a life they knew would be marked by extreme suffering. They submitted a petition for him to be euthanized. The following account from Hitler's senior physician, Dr. Karl Brandt, was heard at the Nuremberg trials:

> [I]t was important that it should be done in such a way that the parents could not feel at any later stage that they were burdened by the euthanasia [of their child]. In other words, that these parents should not have the impression that they themselves were responsible for the death of the child. It was further beholden on me to say that if these doctors themselves were involved in any legal proceedings as a result of these measures, carried out on behalf of Hitler, these proceedings

[90] Manning, Michael. *Euthanasia and physician-assisted suicide.* Paulist Press, 1998.

[91] Dowbiggin, Ian. *A Merciful End: The Euthanasia Movement In Modern America.* Oxford University Press, 2003.

> would be quashed... The doctors were of the opinion that preserving the life of such a child was not actually justified. It was pointed out that it was quite normal that in maternity hospitals under certain circumstances for euthanasia to be administered by the doctors themselves in such a case, without calling it such, any more precise term is not used.[92]

Having been presented as "natural" under an extreme interpretation of social Darwinism and survival of the fittest, then normalized through government law and teachings on the value of human life, it was to be expected that doctors, parents, and some struggling with physical and psychiatric challenges would be comfortable with the act. Euthanasia was normalized as a response to suffering but quickly expanded to the nightmare of people who utterly lost touch with the heart of life. Regard for others became focused through the lens of utility and service to the party's ideal of racial purity, so they systematically sent thousands of physically and mentally challenged children and adults to the gas chambers. But the public felt the dignity of society (and their comfort) should be preserved while such monstrous acts were carried out. Herding children into gas chambers was so... unseemly. Better to do this quietly in medical establishments throughout the country.[93] Upon discovering this, along with the concentration camps and the nightmare of the Holocaust, euthanasia became symbolic of the darkness to which humanity could descend. Soon after, the World Medical Association voted to recommend to all national medical associations that euthanasia be condemned under any circumstances. It would be another fifty-seven years after the war that the first countries, Belgium and the Netherlands, officially allowed tightly regulated euthanasia, with stringent conditions, such as terminal illness, unbearable suffering, and repeated requests by the patient. Canada has joined the club in 2016, and now has the highest rate of euthanasia in the world.

---

[92] Benzenhöfer, Udo. "Richtigstellung." *Deutsches Ärzteblatt*, Jg. 104, H. 47 (Nov. 23, 2007): p. A-3232 www.aerzteblatt.de/pdf.asp?id=57678 Accessed February 10, 2019.

[93] "The Nazi Euthanasia (T-4) Program: Background & Overview." Jewish Virtual Library, https://www.jewishvirtuallibrary.org/background-and-overview-of-the-nazi-euthanasia-t-4-program. Accessed March 4, 2022.

SPIRITUAL FAILURE

WHAT CHANGED? WHAT WOULD SOFTEN OUR STANCE ON SUCH A FUNDAmental facet of our humanity? Whatever factors are at play in this reversal, they are fuelled in no small part by two dynamics: an embarrassing stagnation in our spiritual development and an astonishing rise in our technological development. This is the culmination of biologist E. O. Wilson's insight: "The real problem of humanity is that we have Paleolithic emotions, medieval institutions, and godlike technology."[94]

Throughout history, death occurred in the presence of the public, in the care of the community, within the rhythms of nature, or as the result of human rage. Most cultures would rehearse it through rituals – initiations honouring birth; transitioning to adulthood, marriage, elderhood; and, finally, dying. What rites of passage do we have to mark pivotal points in the human journey today? Getting your driver's licence, reaching the legal drinking age, weddings, baby showers, retirement, then, all too soon, your funeral (which is now called a celebration of life). But these are no longer spiritual touchstones of community initiation in, through, and then out of the passage of time.

Within two generations, death moved from the home to the hospital, where it was primarily regarded as a failure. Dialysis cleansed your blood, anesthetics enabled prolonged surgeries, organ transplants replaced worn-out parts, and intensive care units could keep you alive far longer than you'd typically want. We lost our ownership of dying and gave the process to health care.

Today, Canadians are largely insulated from death. As much as it saturates our news, dying still transpires quietly behind hospital bed curtains and nursing home doors. That's not as true in rural communities, of course. (Which gives rise to the aphorism, "If you're sick, get to the city. If you're dying, get to the country.") We do not experience it first-hand in

---

[94] E. O. Wilson, "Looking Back Looking Forward: A Conversation with James D. Watson and Edward O. Wilson," filmed September 9, 2009, at the Harvard Museum of Natural History, Cambridge, MA, video, 58:02, posted by "Harvard Museum of Natural History," October 21, 2013, 51:30, https://www.youtube.com/watch? v=N8_W2cBAO7s&list=PLcuB9ocQRZCm4-n_TuQKie_L2jlC9Pq2h&t=1s,. Accessed October 17, 2024.

daily life due to the gradual medicalization of death. In the 1960s, it was standard practice for a doctor not to inform a patient of a terminal prognosis to avoid causing additional distress. In the 1990s, we were advocating for patient autonomy over that very truth. Now, in the 2020s, we are supporting not only informed consent for treatment but empowered self-determination over one's death.

This is only one component in a constellation of factors that reflect our spiritual immaturity. As I explore this, I acknowledge I do so with great simplicity – the dynamics are more complex than this book can contain. Nonetheless, let's touch on some very high-level patterns that affect why some have, at this time in history, insisted they should have the right to choose when their lives should end.

First, a reset: I propose that the task of spirituality is not to connect to a God above, become immortal, or believe in a religious system, but to know yourself as you truly are, with no filters, distortions, or illusions of the ego. This is your true essence. If life continues after death, this awareness will connect you directly with your actual state. You will know yourself as a particular expression of the Ground of Being. This is a term coined by Lutheran theologian Paul Tillich, who was critical of the view of God as an entity or personal being. He stated that if God were a being, God could not then properly be called the source of all being (due to the question of what, in turn, created God). Instead, as pure Being, God moves from being the object of love to Love itself. In the spectrum of consciousness, God can and does manifest to us as a being, of course, because that's how we're wired to connect. Tillich's views would later be echoed in a contemporary model of reality called simulation theory, something we'll touch on later. Suffice it to say that, while on this side, we articulate this mystery in very human and beautiful terms: compassion, awakening, and the merging back with the unity of consciousness known simply as love. God is reduced when regarded as the object of love but amplified when we realize God is love itself. Love is not an emotion but the highest state of consciousness from which reality emanates and to which everyone must eventually engage, as we all will die.

Ancient religions supported this inner awakening, but contemporary faith, ironically, tends to compromise it. Western religion continues to emphasize a God above to whom you pray, behaviour to follow by which you're justified, and beliefs to hold in order to be saved. Millions regard The Bible as the literal dictation of God, and denominations claim copyright on salvation. This mythic level of faith reinforces the separation of self from the spiritual realm.

It's no wonder this has occurred. The scientific method was so successful, efficient, and productive that it quickly swamped religious models of reality. Those systems had long become compromised when the church became an imperial authority. Your soul was at the mercy of their declarations. Your mind was shaped by their instruction. The ecclesial empire ruled all.

With the Enlightenment and the scientific method, a new era dawned that encouraged individuals to determine reality for themselves by observing, testing, and drawing conclusions. As it evolved into modern capitalism over the centuries, it promised greater independence, comfort, wealth, discovery, and control over natural forces. It reinforced the idea that everything (and often, everyone) is an object to be used for the ultimate goal: growth in knowledge, power, and possessions. The impact on our sense of morality and life was profound, a nuance often overlooked but astutely presented by Yuval Noah Hariri in his groundbreaking book, *Sapiens: A Brief History of Humankind.*

> Most previous ethical systems presented people with a pretty tough deal. They were promised paradise, but only if they cultivated compassion and tolerance, overcame craving and anger, and restrained their selfish interests. This was too tough for most. The history of ethics is a sad tale of wonderful ideals that nobody can live up to. Most Christians did not imitate Christ, most Buddhists failed to follow Buddha, and most Confucians would have caused Confucius a temper tantrum.

> In contrast, most people today successfully live up to the capitalist-consumerist ideal. The new ethic promises paradise on condition that the rich remain greedy and spend their time making more money and that the masses give free reign to their cravings and passions – and buy more and more. This is the first religion in history whose followers actually do what they are asked to do.[95]

As bleak as that sounds, we've all benefited from faith in the markets. Quality of life for most of the species has never been higher. We live in unprecedented comfort, with access to what we need at the push of a button – Amazon is only one example of the age of convenience that is now spilling into our mortality. Insulated from death, some now desire that to also be on demand.[96] And with MAiD now a legal option in Canada, many will not be able to overcome their craving for a smoother exit than natural death provides. Even as the faithful hope to restrain their self-interest in the name of trust in God, what I see in the trenches of the hospital corridors is that it is too tough to resist that primal instinct to be safe against the nightmare of death they imagine.

COMMUNITY VS INDIVIDUALISM

Consumer culture inevitably shapes our philosophy of life. Our body becomes something we own, and life becomes something we use. Those who support euthanasia employ exactly that lens, stating that your dignity lies in your ability to make choices and determine your own life, and having a body that supports this on your terms. This utilitarian approach means that the body and physical life are instrumental goods, goods *for* the person, not goods *of* the person. Consequently, one can judge that when physical life is useless or burdensome, people should

---

[95] Harari, Yuval Noah. *Sapiens: A Brief History of Humankind*. Published in agreement with The Deborah Harris Agency and the Grayhawk Agency, 2014, p. 349.

[96] Norwood, Frances. "The new normal: Mediated death and assisted dying in the United States." *A Companion to the Anthropology of Death* (2018): pp. 461–475.

be at liberty to free themselves of this burden.[97] This fear of becoming trapped in dependency or disability is enough for many to conclude you should be able to script your death, even if that's shortly after diagnosis. Few realize that, in most cases, some sensible decisions can mitigate the brutal death they dread. Fewer still will travel the road of chaos with skill and grace, allowing room for grief or contemplation as a spiritual intelligence, allowing life to be shattered to discover your essential self at the end.

And here is where the church can bring deep wisdom, not through doctrinal decrees but through its fundamental nature of being a community of love and support. Yet this is not a community that makes you comfortable - it calls us to see the divine in those who are different from us. It offers spiritual practice as an antidote for individualism. It asserts that we are part of one mystical body of Christ, that we arise from the One Consciousness, that whatever is done to the least is done to everyone. The implications are an affront to the ego: there is no such thing as a private thought, there is no one who should ever suffer alone, and it is our sacred duty to step out of our comfort zone and shine for each other. In the words of St. Ignatius of Loyola, "As long as one person suffers, Christ remains crucified."

That's not a marketable message these days, especially as spirituality hasn't evolved much over the past 500 years. Rational intelligence has leaped light-years ahead, resulting in a dialectic strain lost on most. No wonder: we are the product of a swarm of circumstances that have drastically distorted our perspective on life, death, and identity. These factors go back centuries and are, unsurprisingly, linked to two driving forces in Western culture: patriarchy and production. Graham Leicester and Maureen O'Hara, of the International Futures Forum, comment:

> The cultural crisis that opened the twentieth century – the advance of our modern industrial/technological economy

[97] Narbekovas, Andrius, and Kazimieras Meilius. "Why is the ethics of euthanasia wrong?" *Med Etika Bioet.*11.3-4 (2004): pp. 2–6.

> – called into question patterns of previous stability and conceptions of what constituted a good life. The collapse of male identity in a world of automation and office work, for example, triggered a whole set of cultural institutions to deal with the resulting ennui – the boy scouts, DIY, militarism, English-style public schools, a revival of medievalism and the courtly code, self-help and psychoanalysis. Though apparently distinct and unrelated, these cultural inventions were part of a diverse response to a common perturbation – the emasculating effects of industrialization.[98]

The effects of such institutions to bolster meaning and identity in men could not have been anticipated to spiral toward euthanasia. Still, in hindsight, the patterns lay bare their appearance in this day and age. Efforts to preserve the dignity of the average person in the face of industrial empires and hidden forces of greed played well into the mythology of the American Dream. Here, an aspiration was offered against the unjust distribution of wealth and power. It served a central role amidst a web of dynamics shaping the language of dignity and autonomy heard now through discussions on MAiD, which sits as the crown jewel atop the modern ethic of possessive individualism. The claim to personal sovereignty in this culture is staggering! Such insistence erodes core aspects of identity established through community and now is expressed in upbeat rhetoric of personal liberation that desanctifies the outer world of nature and the inner world of the self, reducing both to manipulated objects.[99]

> As the first half of the century progressed, the thrust of this movement was towards reclaiming a vision of human potential and dignity in an age dominated by the wonders of

[98] Leicester, Graham, and Maureen O'Hara. *Dancing at the Edge: Competence, Culture and Organization in the 21st Century*. Triarchy Press, 2019, p. 62.

[99] Lears, TJ Jackson. *No Place of Grace: Antimodernism and the Transformation of American Culture, 1880–1920*. University of Chicago Press, 1994, p. xi.

> technology and new machines. Words like freedom, potential, transcendence, love, awe, dignity, being, consciousness, meaning, joy, pleasure, and compassion, populated the titles of books exploring the outer reaches of human possibility. The playing out of these efforts to transform cultural anxiety into growth took several decades. But they ushered in an era after the Second World War influenced by a more capricious view of the "self-actualizing" individual, no longer ensnared by the demands of the economy and its machines.[100]

DIGNITY

AND SO, AFTER DECADES OF OBSESSING OVER INDIVIDUAL POTENTIAL AND freedom, we arrive at the ultimate obsession: personal dignity at the end of life. It's no wonder this concept now sits at the heart of MAiD debates – after all, what's more dignified than having complete control over every last detail of our existence, including its end. While the term is currently being used in the assisted dying debate to mean simply the freedom to choose how and when to end your life with the help of doctors, this disregards the broader and more nuanced aspects of human dignity. It should not be reduced to merely exercising personal control; it finds equal if not greater expression through meaningful relationships with others. Such relationships recognize the inherent worth of every person, the interconnected nature of human behaviours, and the understanding that individuals are not isolated entities; we are who we are through our relationships.

But we struggle with that when using the misguided terminology of being a burden when we are frail. This common phrase reveals our resistance to the natural dependency that arises when life is at an end. Our ego-identity struggles against allowing its erosion through suffering, resulting in an increasing sense of vulnerability. Yet in that protection, we become inauthentic and detached from the reality of our frailty.

---

[100] Leicester, Graham, and Maureen O'Hara. *Dancing at the Edge*. Triarchy Press, 2019. p. 62.

I can recall countless patients who stated this in various ways. "I want to do things for myself, care for myself, do what I want and enjoy my life on my terms." Understandable and appropriate statements, indeed! But when used to define dignity, that becomes equated with independence and choice, not with the inherent value of the person. That dignity is determined by ability is stated even more forcefully by the Swiss organization Dignitas, which asserts that people "are the bearers of human dignity" and that "this is characterised most strongly when a person decides his or her own fate."[101] For Dignitas, making the choice to end one's own life is the ultimate expression of one's dignity as a human being.

The advocacy group Dignity in Dying echoes this, with their assertion that a good death is determined by choice over where we die and control over how we die. Yet equating choice with dignity is highly problematic. We would never equate our dignity with our ability at the beginning of life. A newborn is utterly dependent, yet cherished as a profound gift of life and love in the family and the world. The infant has no ability to choose but is driven by the primal instincts and inherent wisdom of life. This new life relies on others to feed, wipe, wash, and move. This new soul is utterly dependent, yet of infinite dignity and worth. Why would this be less true as we die?

Additionally, hinging dignity upon choice compels society to respect the desire of anyone to end their life. Ironic, as to do so due to mental health, economic, or other societal issues is understood to be a tragedy and, most often, a failure of society to address the systemic and community issues that drive such situations. Few of us would encourage such choices, and we have mandatory protocols in place throughout health care to intervene, dissuade, and support such people.

But now that assisted suicide is on the table, people feel they no longer need to be ensnared by the final stages of the dying process. Compelled by the preservation of ego-identity and resistance to complete surrender, MAiD becomes the final outcome of identity through autonomy instead

---

101 "Principles/Philosophy." Dignitas.ch, 2023. www.dignitas.ch/index.php?option=com_content&view=article&id=10&Itemid=46&lang=en. Accessed July 31, 2023.

of identity through community. That's the dominant theme in Western culture, grounded in the consumerist mind of *my body, my life, my choice*. It also stems from distorting a popular Western model of personal development, Abraham Maslow's hierarchy of needs, in which the aim is to become a "self-actualized" person. However, there are three surprises in this model that most are unaware of.

First, Maslow did not develop it as a hierarchy; that was applied by marketing experts driven by post-war ideologies of individualism, nationalism, and capitalism. This betrayed Maslow's vision of reaching one's potential for humanity's benefit rather than the individual's. And in this betrayal, we find the second surprise: Maslow's model was inspired by his time with the Siksika, or Blackfoot Nation, who, contrary to Maslow's Western perspective, believe that a person is born self-actualized. Their highest level of development prioritizes communal well-being and interdependence rather than individual achievement and self-determination. The Siksika even regard those who give the most possessions away to benefit the least in the community as the wealthiest among them, for they honour the spiritual nature of life, the interconnectedness of all beings.[102] Finally, Maslow's model does not end with self-actualization, but transcendence – a complete surrender to a final state of consciousness which comes upon a person. This spiritual awareness, marked by equanimity and joy, was applied later to his theory as he became aware of states of consciousness near the end of life. Yet even here, he fell short of the people who inspired him.

As Siksika scholar Billy Wadsorth summarizes, Maslow did not "fully situate the individual within the context of community. If he had done so, and also more deeply integrated the Blackfoot perspective, the model would be centered on multi-generational community actualization versus on individual actualization and transcendence."[103]

Maslow later agreed, stating, "self-actualization is not enough. Personal salvation and what is good for the person alone cannot be understood

[102] Ravilochan, Teju. "The Blackfoot Wisdom That Inspired Maslow's Hierarchy." *Resilience* (June 2021) www.resilience.org/stories/2021-06-18/the-blackfoot-wisdom-that-inspired-maslows-hierarchy. Accessed May 15, 2023.

[103] Ibid

in isolation. The good of other people must be invoked, as well as the good for oneself. It is quite clear that purely inter-psychic individualist psychology without reference to other people and social conditions is not adequate."[104]

This is a vision of a society rich in social capital – the resources, connections, and trust within a social network or community. It encompasses relationships, norms, and values facilitating individual co-operation, collaboration, and collective action. In the context of morality and the health of communities, social capital plays a crucial role by building trust, civic engagement, shared values, social support, and mental and existential health – especially at the end of life.

We didn't listen. The public has bought the line, and I've heard it frequently from my patients. "Where's the dignity in soiling myself? Where's the dignity in lying here helpless?" The insult to ego is loud and clear, but what is being protested, beneath the resistance to a new level of dependency, is an unfamiliar cooperation in which the community takes care of the one dying in all aspects of their humanity, and the dying person cares for the community by giving them this honour, which elevates their spiritual intelligence and communal strength. When we affirm that role in this modern age, we demonstrate the inherent dignity of the dying, elevated all the more by the honour of caring for them. Yet, there is even more at play. The perceived self is preserving an identity that has formed through establishing its distinction in the world. But that process entails forgetting one's fundamental connection to all and one's essential spiritual nature, a nature most are unaware of throughout their life and into their death – that of being not a mind or body or role in the world, but of purely being an expression of fundamental awareness having an experience we call the human journey.

Here we sit, with individuals unaware of the cultural impact of their claims to extreme autonomy throughout life and at its end. The consequence reinforces identity cut off from the community, reinforces individual rights over collective renewal, reinforces our drive to dominate

[104] Kaufman, Scott Barry. *Transcend: The New Science of Self-Actualization*. Penguin, 2021.

and our divorce from the spiritual realm in which all is interconnected. Here we sit, with multinational corporations more powerful than many countries, climate crisis, and technological progress that has brought us to the dawn of the new age of artificial intelligence. Things are changing so rapidly that moral norms can't keep up. Here we sit, oblivious of the generational impact of our choices. Is it any wonder MAiD has arisen in such a soup? Yet, if we get through this period, future ethical considerations at the end of life will make the present ones seem like child's play.

HUMANITY 2.0

Where is it headed? What will tomorrow bring? Will it be the doomsday that our culture projects through blockbuster films? Indeed, most would consider the end of the human race to be a catastrophe, but some are banking on it. They want to hasten the end of *Homo sapiens* and usher in the rise of a new species that looks very much like us... but improved. It may even become immortal.[105] A better, smarter, fitter version of you and me, but augmented by AI and nanotechnology. Welcome to Humanity 2.0.

We certainly need the upgrade. Any species that destroys its environment, won't feed millions because of greed and hoarding, and is constantly at war with itself is heading for the cliff. On top of the stark reality that one in three will develop dementia,[106] and one in two will develop cancer[107] are problems posed by our longevity; a person can live into their deterioration far longer than in decades past. No wonder euthanasia has emerged. Against this, a movement is at play, a cultural dynamic that merges technological advances with the minds and

---

[105] Hopkins, Patrick D. "A Moral Vision for Transhumanism." *Journal of Evolution & Technology* 19.1, (2008).

[106] "2023 Alzheimer's Disease Facts and Figures." Alzheimer's Association. www.alz.org/alzheimers-dementia/facts-figures. Accessed March 11, 2023.

[107] The Canadian Press. "1 In 2 Canadians Will Get Cancer: Cancer Society." CBC. June 21, 2017, www.cbc.ca/news/health/cancer-society-annual-statistics-report-1.4168784. Accessed March 11, 2023.

bodies of its creators. It's called transhumanism, and it offers an existential elixir to our death anxiety – enhancements with direct neural links to AI that could dramatically increase brain power and extend life, physical augmentation that could make us far more robust and more resilient, even providing spare parts, even the postponement of mortality.[108] Death could become obsolete for those who upload their minds to a virtual world, existing on the information level alone.[109]

Many transhumanists see this not only as desirable but inevitable, as exponential advancement is embedded in the processes of nature itself.[110] Evolution took billions of years to make the first critical advancement: DNA. This was an organic computer that could adjust its code through mergers and mutations to determine the best design for survival. Everything exploded from there. In a hundred million years, the Cambrian era saw life flourish, with various body types vying for dominance. Humanoids accelerated the process even further, with each advancement taking exponentially shorter and shorter periods to appear. Thanks to our species' opposable thumb and cranial capacity, the ball set in motion millions of years earlier was picked up by primates and pitched from generation to generation. Language, art, agriculture, cities… each step speeding us ever faster to an unimaginable future. Yes, for millennia, generations passed without significant change for the individual. God was forever in His heaven, and royalty was forever on their thrones. No wonder the rules of life seemed so fixed.

Then suddenly a radical shift upended social structures. The Enlightenment saw monarchs overthrown, democracies emerge, and slavery abolished. Then the Industrial Revolution catapulted humanity forward on the path of technological development. A single generation

---

[108] Regalado, Antonio. "The Transhumanists Who Want to Live Forever." *MIT Technology Review*, 30 (April 2021) www.technologyreview.com/2019/08/16/133364/transhumanists-live-forever. Accessed March 11, 2023.

[109] "The Immortalist: Uploading the mind to a computer." BBC News. March 14, 2016, www.bbc.com/news/magazine-35786771. Accessed March 11, 2023.

[110] Kurzweil, Ray. "The Law of Accelerating Returns." The Kurzweil Library + collections. www.kurzweilai.net/the-law-of-accelerating-returns. Accessed May 16, 2023.

saw the invention of flight and the moon landing. The next witnessed supercomputers shrink from filling a warehouse to sliding into their back pocket. Paradigm shifts that took thousands of years now took hundreds, then fifty, then ten, then few. We now witness the inevitable coalescence of AI, robotics, molecular manufacturing, augmented reality, miniaturization, and the Internet of Things (IoT).[111] It all merges to a point called the singularity; at this point AI becomes smarter than all the human intelligence on the planet.

According to present calculations, this is expected to happen by 2030.[112] Nick Bostrom, head of the Future of Humanity Institute at Oxford, describes it as the most important thing our species has ever done on and to the planet. And while concerns are rising that AI may be our last invention, now that it is in use by the general public, there's no turning back.

You may understandably be concerned about the prospect of billions of people with lifespans exceeding 200 years. This could become a problem, if not for the fact that worldwide fertility is declining due to environmental pollutants.[113] In the coming decades, pregnancies may rely on assisted reproductive technologies.[114] At least our quality of life may dramatically improve, as resources will no longer be an issue with manufacturing taking place at the atomic level.[115] This is the fourth industrial revolution, an era in which our physical, digital, and biological identities

---

[111] Kurzweil, Ray. "The Singularity Is Near: When Humans Transcend Biology." Singularity is near -sin graph - countdown to sin logarithmic. Accessed March 11, 2024. https://www.singularity.com/charts/page17.html.

[112] Orf, D. "Humanity May Reach Singularity Within Just 7 Years, Trend Shows." *Popular Mechanics*, 24 (January 2023). Accessed March 11, 2023, from https://www.popularmechanics.com/technology/robots/a42612745/singularity-when-will-it-happen/ Accessed 05 Nov. 2020.

[113] Vandenberg, Laura N., et al. "Hormones and endocrine-disrupting chemicals: low-dose effects and nonmonotonic dose responses." *Endocrine Reviews* 33.3 (2012): pp. 378–455.

[114] Kushnir, Vitaly A., Gary D. Smith, and Eli Y. Adashi. "The future of IVF: the new normal in human reproduction." *Reproductive Sciences* 29.3 (2022): pp. 849–856.

[115] US Department of Energy. "Innovations in Scanning Tunneling Microscope Control Systems for High-throughput Atomically Precise Manufacturing." Energy.gov. Archived (PDF) from the original on Oct 18, 2020. Accessed Nov. 5, 2020.

are fused as one.[116] Which means you and I may be the last generation of *Homo sapiens*. How we live, work, and relate to one another will fundamentally change. What we are will radically change. Will that be the same for death?

This is happening now. When MAiD was legalized in 2016, AI made headlines by using machine learning to beat the world's best player in the ancient Chinese game of Go. Fast forward to 2024, and AI is becoming ubiquitous, replacing human experts in fields like art, finance, and programming. Its ability to evolve itself and seamlessly converse has even allowed it to pass as human – still an unconscious intelligence, but impressive nonetheless.

Unlike the internet, which Google and Amazon dominate, AI is open source. Anyone can use it to explore the new frontier of finance, medicine, art and science, technology, and warfare. It's hoped that this democratic distribution will ensure no monopoly on humanity's future. Still, the power rests with those who know how to use data. As AI digests the internet, its pattern recognition algorithm will make it more competent thousands of times faster than any human and soon of all humanity.[117]

This exponential progress is facilitated by AI's ability to teach itself, a process that has become even faster through the use of AI designed by other AIs. For instance, Stanford University's Alpaca was taught to think in just two days at a fraction of the cost of its AI trainer, ChatGPT. But its ultimate trainer will be us. How we treat it, and each other, will be the most significant influence on its behaviour. This is not about creating a machine. It's about creating the ultimate intelligence.[118]

The steps involved sound daunting, yet, thanks to machine learning, they are unfolding so rapidly that the world you live in may radically differ

---

[116] Lee, MinHwa, et al. "How To Respond to the Fourth Industrial Revolution, or the Second Information Technology Revolution? Dynamic New Combinations Between Technology, Market, And Society Through Open Innovation." *Journal of Open Innovation: Technology, Market, and Complexity* 4.3 (2018): p. 21.

[117] Harari, Yuval Noah. *Homo Deus: A Brief History of Tomorrow*. Random House, 2016.

[118] For a lively discussion on this, see Pal, Raoul. "AI Revolution: The #1 Megathreat to Our Economy and How to Prepare Now." YouTube video. Uploaded by Tom Bilyeu. March 21, 2023. www.youtube.com/watch?v=S0DHI0DGOIw. Accessed April 2, 2023.

from the world I write in as I type these words. For example, a critical development is Neuralink, a brain implant that connect a person directly to computer systems.[119] This is a pivotal step in our journey toward becoming a new species, *Homo evolutis*. Imagine instant access to the world's information and data, enhanced communication abilities, and even direct control over physical objects through thought alone. Such enhancements would fundamentally transform how we interact with our environment and each other, opening up new avenues for creativity, collaboration, and problem solving while utterly destroying privacy and altering our understanding of personhood and the individual.

Meanwhile, physical augmentation could take many forms, from enhancing strength and endurance to providing advanced sensory abilities or even regenerating lost or damaged tissue.[120] For example, individuals could use nanotechnology to repair injuries at a molecular level or even to replace entire organs with synthetic versions that are more efficient and longer-lasting than their biological counterparts.[121] With such enhancements, people could live longer, healthier lives with greater resilience to disease and injury.

Death will become more remote in this tomorrow. And those who have lived a life longer than our imaginings may choose to bring it to a close in much the same way as those who desire MAiD: they will have a professional do it. The reason may not be as acute as existential distress. It may be as benign as boredom. Imagine 200 years of living where everything has been provided for you, every indulgence tasted, every adventure explored (with replacement parts provided). Or, will it be because of the same force driving MAiD requests today: lack of purpose and meaning? Will this be

---

[119] Play Studio. n.d. "Patient Registry | Neuralink." Neuralink. https://neuralink.com/patient-registry/. Accessed March 11, 2024

[120] Hassan, M. "How AI Is Helping Power Next-Generation Prosthetic Limbs." *Wevolver*, 23 (Jan. 2023). www.wevolver.com/article/how-ai-is-helping-power-next-generation-prosthetic-limbs. Accessed April 18, 2023.

[121] Tel Aviv University. "Hybrid Micro-robot Able to Navigate in Physiological Environment, Capture Targeted Damaged Cells." Phys.Org. March 27, 2023. phys.org/news/2023-03-hybrid-micro-robot-physiological-environment-capture.html. Accessed April 22, 2023.

a world in which you are monitored, managed, and manipulated by an agenda you cannot comprehend? Don't think there won't be masters in this new tomorrow, just as there are today. Without an equally exponential increase in our spiritual intelligence, adding decades or centuries to our lifespan might be the worst thing we could do to the universe.

MAiD has arisen in this continuum of change that will only accelerate. As we rocket to a future where life and death become what we desire, where we are masters of our destiny, the wisdom of the ancients is left behind... the very wisdom essential in averting our self-destruction and embracing our true magnificence.

SPIRITUALITY 2.0

As transhumanism progresses and human augmentation becomes more widespread, there will undoubtedly be those who choose to remain unaugmented. These individuals may form communities where they can live according to their principles without the extended lifespans enjoyed by the transhumanists. However, even if the super-humans do not compose the majority of the population, they will undoubtedly become the envy of those who have not been upgraded. This biological inequality will likely fuel an ever greater economic inequality, with power and privilege reaching unprecedented extremes. The allure of such enhancements will be irresistible, leading to a world where some individuals are hundreds or even thousands of times more capable than their unaugmented peers and free from the physical limitations of life.

This vision of the future may sound familiar, as it shares a common goal with religious promises of an afterlife in which suffering and death are absent. Both transhumanism and religion seek to transcend mortality's limitations and achieve a more expansive existence. One does it synthetically through augmentation, the other naturally through death. But the first is driven by the fear of death, the second by surrender to its wisdom. Given humanity's track record, it's important to consider the potential downsides of transhumanism. Without a corresponding "Spirituality 2.0," this technological advancement could easily lead to even greater social and environmental problems, in addition to a severing of what it is to be human.

But what would a spiritual upgrade look like? Interestingly, the answer is already with us, hidden and forgotten since the beginning of time, but now becoming more familiar thanks, ironically, to the internet. It's the awakening to awareness, the mystery of consciousness, and the realization of our place in the vast cosmos. The new prophets of this teaching are no longer clerics but scientists grappling with the fundamental mysteries of reality. Quantum physicists, cosmologists, and even some AI programmers are among those who have proclaimed a wonderful paradox: that consciousness may be the underlying substrate of reality, and that our being is strangely entwined with the external world we perceive.[122,123] This realization points toward a universal spirituality in which we shift from petitioning an external God to participating in the consciousness of God.

As we enter this new age, it's important to consider what role spiritual leaders will have in society. To remain relevant, they must infuse their prophetic voice with courage and compassion, addressing issues of injustice and exclusion, how we live and how we die. They must also intelligently articulate that when we talk about God, we are really talking about the nature of awareness, if that is all that remains when we die.

These leaders have been among us throughout history. They are found, of course, among the Indigenous peoples and cultures of the earth who have not allowed the concept of the self to dominate over community or creation. Western spiritual leaders preach a similar hope but are still essentially embedded in a model of God that reinforces a duality and, in Christianity, an inherent depravity and separation of humanity from the divine. As the world moves out of step with fundamental spiritual teachings, religious professionals find themselves staring out at empty pews, and chaplains quietly move through the hospital corridors. While we do

[122] Kincaid, Joshua, Kyle McLelland, and Michael Zwolak. "Measurement-induced decoherence and information in double-slit interference." *American Journal of Physics* 84.7 (2016): 522–530.

[123] Afshordi, Niayesh, et al. "From Planck data to Planck era: observational tests of holographic cosmology." *Physical Review Letters* 118.4 (2017): 041301.

so without the robes and rituals of a church service, we are clothed in the essential garment of the spiritual journey: story. Amid the backdrop of history and human suffering, chaplains recognize the story. This is a tale of trauma and transformation, of love and leaving. It's filled with the perennial themes of the heroic journey, and it is grand beyond comprehension. It is the story that gives meaning to our days, especially when we have lost the narrative at the end of ours. It is written in the heart of every patient we see, and we are trained to read it. We are the listeners. The witnesses. The storytellers.

MAiD is now a new chapter. But it is one in which spiritual professionals are increasingly written off as religious irrelevancy rather than written in as guides to the final period.

EXERCISE 7: BELIEF

Take a few moments to sit in a quiet and comfortable space. Close your eyes and bring your attention to your breath. Allow yourself to become present and grounded in the moment. When you feel ready, consider your spiritual beliefs and the heritage from which they developed.

1. *What does spirituality mean to you? How would you define it in your own words?*
2. *What practices or beliefs bring a sense of connection, meaning, or transcendence into your life?*
3. *How do your beliefs influence your everyday perspective, values, and actions?*
4. *Consider the cultural narratives and stories that have influenced your faith. Reflect on the significant myths, legends, or religious texts within your cultural context. How have these narratives shaped your understanding of the spiritual aspects of life? How do they relate to your personal beliefs and experiences?*
5. *Reflect on your hopes, fears, and aspirations regarding the future of spirituality in the age of AI and transhumanism. Allow yourself to imagine and envision the potential positive transformations and challenges that may emerge.*

CHAPTER 8

SPIRITUAL CARE

The door is wide open. Don't go back to sleep.

– RUMI

I WAS CHECKING THE CHARTS, AS I DO EVERY MORNING, TO ASSESS WHO has indicated they're open to spiritual support and who is not. It begins on the admission page that lists the patient's name, contact, and other details, like religious affiliation. Twenty years ago, most of them noted a denomination or faith group. These days I more often see "Not asked" or "None." I then check the nursing assessment form, where people are asked if they want to see spiritual care. This week, only two of the twenty patients in our care checked "Yes." My head slumped. Then a nurse sat at my side with a flourish.

"David, so good to see you. I've got a woman in room ninety-six who could really use your help. She's teary, so scared. Just got some bad news: the chemo didn't work. Do you have time to see her?"

She was not one of the two, and we are not to initiate contact unless the patient has indicated openness. That's the weird thing about spiritual care. Unlike physiotherapy or pharmacy, we are... optional. Which is sad, as it's the emotional and existential aspects of cancer that dominate. Most people just want someone to talk to. They want a good listener. I've often thought of changing the title on my office door from "Spiritual Care" to "A Guy Who's Been There" (since I've had cancer several times). But the nurse had now provided a referral, so in I went. When I introduced myself, the look on her face was... shock.

"Is it that bad? They sent you!"

We are misunderstood. For those who have a religious practice, we are welcome company. They expect us to provide a listening ear, the encouragement of God's love, a prayer, and a blessing. Others expect us to be idiosyncratic, irritating, insulting, or simply irrelevant. Clergy and the institutional religions for which we are agents are viewed by many with suspicion and scorn. For them, clergy are a source of cultural pain and injury, a relic of medieval times when religion ruled as empire. I recall walking into another patient's room and, introducing myself as the chaplain, had a bedpan thrown at me (empty, thankfully). Is it any wonder in Canada with what has been revealed through the Truth and Reconciliation Commission? While the church is as human as any institution (look at the abuse now revealed in professional and Olympic sports, education, law enforcement, and the military), there is an appropriately stronger sense of the injury going much deeper when representatives of God are so depraved.

So, what is spiritual care? Let's explore this by first stating what it is not, and this might surprise you. Spiritual care is not about getting God into you, nor is it primarily about religious practice, specific belief systems and traditions, specific rites and rituals. We are experts in that, but only to support your beliefs, never to impose our own. Spiritual care involves the universal matters of suffering and the soul, existential identity, meaning and purpose.

Most importantly, spiritual care addresses what is most central to you when considering the end of life, which usually boils down to the basics: family, love, meaning, purpose, and dignity... or the lack of the same. It can also encompass the mystery of what awaits on the other side. Above all, spiritual care helps you navigate your way through the crisis. And underlying all of this is the universal mystery of consciousness and our connection to life. Rachel Naomi Remen, MD, who developed the Commonweal retreats for people with cancer, provides this insight: "Helping, fixing, and serving represent three different ways of seeing life. When you help, you see life as weak. When you fix, you see life as broken. When you serve, you see life as whole. Fixing and helping may be the work of the ego, and service the work of the soul."[124] Spiritual care practitioners are there to serve. We don't poke you with needles, but we will probe you with questions to help you discover the wisdom and way already wired into you. We are also mandated to protect you from anyone trying to impose their beliefs on you instead of revealing them within you.

(Side note: This very principle is also the source of my distress, for I assert that MAiD is a medical procedure used to treat a spiritual condition. People are requesting euthanasia because they can no longer function as they want, and they dread how this will get worse as they die. They don't see a purpose in that. It's existential suffering. The appropriate response is to surround them with love and good care, provide excellent medical support, share the stories, demonstrate dignity, and sit with the mystery of wisely waiting for this ultimate event. It is not to kill the one suffering. I'm laying that out here, but I am ethically mandated not to lay it out with the patient once they've been assessed for MAiD, just as I am ethically mandated not to challenge a person's choice to receive aggressive chemotherapy.)

We are predominantly known as chaplains. However, recently the Canadian Association for Spiritual Care, our professional governing body, voted to change our title to Certified Spiritual Care Practitioner. This change was made because an increasing number of the general population is unfamiliar with religious terminology. I'll use both terms in this book. Traditionally, a chaplain is a cleric who is ordained or appointed as a spiritual leader in their community. This includes priests, pastors, rabbis, elders, and imams. A chaplain can also be a lay or non-ordained representative of a religious tradition. These professionals are trained in spiritual counselling, assigned to secular institutions such as a hospitals, prisons, military units, intelligence agencies, embassies, businesses, fire or police departments, universities, schools, or private chapels. We hold undergraduate and master's degrees, have 400 hours of in-field supervision, and an equal amount of small-group reflection for refining

[124] Remen, Rachel Naomi. *Kitchen Table Wisdom: Stories that Heal*. Pan Australia, 2010.

interpersonal communication skills. We regularly complete an ethics module and undergo an assessment every five years. Additionally, we are accountable to several bodies, including the Canadian Association for Spiritual Care, the institution we work for, and our faith community. This accountability is crucial for maintaining our integrity as we work with the most vulnerable and broken aspects of humanity. It's also necessary for self-care, to prevent our ego from hijacking our spiritual practice, and to uphold ethical standards. Certification as a specialist can take years; my parents once quipped that I could have become a doctor by the time I completed all these steps. I responded, "While their pay scale is much better, our afterlife benefits are out of this world!"

Chaplains were predominantly Christian, but now can come from all traditions and can be interfaith. There are also secular or humanist spiritual care practitioners. Chaplains can be denominational or appointed by their religious community to provide care for people of their faith tradition. Alternatively, they can be part of an institution's staff, like myself, commissioned by my faith tradition (Lutheran) to work for the government. (It often surprises patients when they discover that I am a spiritual counselor for the government, which is evidence of how the old models continue to hold on.) When assigned to specific units in a hospital, we are integrated into the healthcare team. We attend rounds, collaborate on patient care, write chart notes, see patients on referrals, and drop in to assess well-being more casually. It is important to note that patients do not need to identify as having any specific faith tradition or be religious in order to benefit from spiritual care. Most of the time, we serve as compassionate listeners, helping people process their health crises and navigate the limitations they may face regarding their identity, dignity, meaning, and purpose. On occasion, we may also employ overtly religious and spiritual tools, such as prayer, rituals, and rites, as appropriate.[125]

Compassionate presence may sound benign, but this is a role best described by a term from the Buddhist tradition: a *bodhisattva*, or warrior

[125] VandeCreek, Larry, and Laurel Burton, eds. "Professional Chaplaincy: Its Role and Importance in Healthcare." *Journal of Pastoral Care* 55.1 (2001): pp. 81–97.

of compassion. We willingly enter into the fire of suffering to incarnate compassion and guide the sufferer to their inner wisdom. We do not shrink back from this pain but recognize suffering as the opportunity for the most significant spiritual growth. It is profoundly challenging to sit in the fire and allow the transfiguration to occur, but we are honoured to accompany you there. And we sometimes do so aggressively. Let me explain.

SPIRITUALITY

SPIRITUALITY IS A FUNDAMENTAL ASPECT OF HUMAN IDENTITY, EVEN though many people would say they are not spiritual in any way. It doesn't need to be about God, angels, or the afterlife, though most expressions of spirituality do involve transcendent realities. Traditionally, the term referred to a religious process of re-formation that "aims to recover the original shape of man"[126] as an expression of the divine. In these modern times, spirituality stems from one's deepest values and meaning. This is emphasized in a definition from the International Consensus Conference on Improving the Spiritual Dimension of Whole Person Care:

> Spirituality is a dynamic and intrinsic aspect of humanity through which people seek ultimate meaning, purpose, and transcendence, and experience relationship to self, others, community, society, nature, and the significant or sacred. Spirituality is expressed through beliefs, values, traditions and practices.[127]

As you might imagine, many do not have an overt spiritual practice, though everyone is spiritual, independent of religion. Most significantly, spirituality enables a person to meet suffering as a process of transformation. So, there's a tension here: suffering is the very thing MAiD helps you avoid and that which spiritual practice challenges you to engage.

---

126 Waaijman, K. *Spiritualiteit: vormen, grondslagen, methoden*. Carmelitana, 2000.

127 Puchalski, Christina M., Robert Vitillo, Sharon K. Hull, and Nancy Reller. "Improving the spiritual dimension of whole person care: reaching national and international consensus." Journal of palliative medicine 17, no. 6 (2014): 642-656.

Spirituality orbits universal issues of who and what we are in the world, part of the human essence that strives for transcendental values. These are expressed through our life principles, how we love and forgive, our core beliefs about reality, and our ability to see beyond present circumstances. Fundamentally, spirituality is that web of meaning and connection larger than the self. It is revealed in what is most foundational and essential to you. Ultimately, it is what you sense you are in this vast cosmos, expressed through your flickering here for one hundred years or so.

When one lives from their spiritual core, their sense of interconnectedness with all things is experienced as sacred (a term which, for those who do not believe in God or a spiritual realm, can be considered *significant* with a capital S). Everything we say, feel, think and do reflects our calibration to that centre. Since the scriptures from several traditions speak of God as love, then love is your best spiritual practice. That's how spirituality is unconsciously, automatically expressed. The overt corporate expression of this, shaped by shared beliefs and expressed through ritual and culture, is a religion.

Spirituality can be theistic – belief in a God or assortment of celestial entities, or naturalistic – a sense of connection to the web of life, infused with what can sometimes be a rhapsodic wonder of it all. The term is ambiguous, as it has to do more with our most profound sense of self in the world and what life is all about. In other words, *meaning*. Not only does this not need to be religious, but spirituality often brings people to question their religion or, better, to search within it not only for the understanding of meaning but the experience of it, especially as one is dying. Ironically, clergy are not always experts in that. I recall one pastor saying, "We talk about what comes after death, but we tend to skip over the dying part, except to make sure the person has made their peace with God."

Some readers may bristle at the idea that they are spiritual, rejecting the notion that there is some reality beyond the material universe. Perhaps what is rejected is any model of the divine currently presented because it is simply inadequate for them, even primitive and superstitious, compared to the more-than-sufficiently inspiring revelations of science. To these readers, I give my respect and affirm the same, but also invite them (or you) to continue with my musings as I hope to offer an understanding of the spirit that is relevant, revolutionary, and robust enough to be congruent with current cosmology and models of consciousness. In the meantime, I encourage you to set aside preconceived notions of God and let love be your spiritual practice. For, in the end, it is the unfinished love stories that truly matter to the heart.

This is no small matter. Your spirituality, in addition to being fundamental to who and what you are, is your only hope when facing death. The research, as well as the religions of the world, are conclusive on this. There are only two possible outcomes to suffering: an experience of transcendence or continued suffering.[128] This transcendence is marked by inner peace, harmony and security that endures even though moments of darkness may persist.[129] Higher levels of dignity and well-being result as the dying person experiences new dimensions of self and connection to the moment.[130] Most profound is the acceptance of death, the integration of one's life story, and moving on into the mystery.[131] Indeed, when exploring resilience in the face of suffering, Brené Brown found spirituality to be the one thing at the foundation for those who were able to create whole-hearted lives despite adversity. "Without exception, spirituality – the belief in connection, a power greater than oneself, and interconnections grounded in love and compassion – emerged as a component of resilience."[132] While most spoke of God, others felt this connection through nature or their

---

[128] Best, Megan, et al. "Conceptual analysis of suffering in cancer: a systematic review." *Psycho-Oncology* 24.9 (2015): 977-986.

[129] Lethborg, Carrie, et al. "The role of meaning in advanced cancer – integrating the constructs of assumptive world, sense of coherence and meaning-based coping." *Journal of Psychosocial Oncology* 24.1 (2006): 27-42.

[130] Kenne Sarenmalm, Elisabeth, et al. "Making sense of living under the shadow of death: Adjusting to a recurrent breast cancer illness." *Qualitative health research* 19.8 (2009): 1116-1130.

[131] Perreault, Annie, and Frances Fothergill Bourbonnais. "The experience of suffering as lived by women with breast cancer." *International Journal of Palliative Nursing* 11.10 (2005): 510-519.

[132] Brown, Brené. *The Gifts of Imperfection: Let Go of Who You Think You're Supposed To Be and Embrace Who You Are.* Simon & Schuster, 2010, p. 86.

family and a sense of life itself. More significantly, for our discussion, three patterns emerged as central to this spiritual resilience:

1. Cultivating hope
2. Practising critical self-awareness
3. Letting go of numbing and taking the edge off vulnerability, discomfort and pain

This is what spiritual care practitioners do; not help you feel better but connect you to something more profound. In exploring hope and powerlessness, Brown notes that hope is not a feeling, but a way of thinking, an entire mindset marked by:

1. The ability to set realistic goals
2. Being able to figure out how to achieve these goals while being flexible as circumstances change
3. Believing in yourself

Recall how this has played out in your own life. Memories from childhood include preparing for a test, learning a game, or making friends. Those were challenging enough. Or perhaps trauma lives there – being bullied, living in poverty, having an abusive parent. As you face the challenges that inevitably come along, notice how your inner dialogue stabilizes or sabotages you. In school, it was a matter of preparing for a test or learning a new game. The stakes become greater in adulthood – financial ruin, betrayal, mortality. This game of life demands serious skill to remain stable in the storms that inevitably come. That skill used to be provided by wisdom traditions – learning from your elders in multigenerational households, rituals with the shaman to mark your connection to the spirit world, or gathering with the community for the final transition.

The game is played differently these days: to beat others, not to belong to them. And now to beat death. It leaves Western civilization in a state of spiritual emergency. We are in dire need of integrating advances in psychology, consciousness studies, the insights of Indigenous Peoples, and the core teachings of the world's major religious traditions. These days, spirituality is seen as distinct from that formal crucible of knowledge, a rift growing ever wider as the years fly by. We have at least two generations now unfamiliar with church, worship, and the doctrines and discipline embedded in what, for them, feels like an outdated relic. We live in a world that has lost its vocabulary of ritual, community, and connection to the mystery underlying it all.

While there is now far less interest in formal spiritual traditions, there is more interest in the concepts behind them. Yet these concepts are nebulous for many people. Without inner discipline and community accountability, popular spiritual practice can float pleasantly and benignly through life, an ephemeral mist of ideas and abstractions that orbit the edges of more pragmatic affairs of the day.

Popular spirituality often condenses into ideals of decency, connection to nature, and the belief that angels and ancestors watch over us, alongside the drive to achieve our potential and fulfill some greater purpose. While it may hint at the mystery of divine presence, too often, this desire is subconsciously tied to the urge to achieve or acquire more. This prevailing (and profitable) expression of the human potential movement focuses on raising consciousness or planetary vibration, positioning individuals as luminaries in a world plagued by addiction, corruption, and waste. At its best, it encourages one to stay true to their values, embrace the gift of life, and compassionately reach out to those suffering. At its worst, however, popular spirituality devolves into unexamined toxic positivity, lacking the support of an authentic community, the discipline of formal practice, or critical self-awareness – making it especially susceptible to being hijacked by the ego.

It's called spiritual bypassing, a term coined by the excellent Buddhist teacher John Welwood. It's "a tendency to use spiritual ideas and practices to sidestep or avoid facing unresolved emotional issues, psychological wounds, and unfinished developmental tasks."[133] In other words, we're leap-frogging over the homework of the heart to enjoy premature peace of

[133] Welwood, John. *Toward a Psychology of Awakening: Buddhism, Psychotherapy, and the Path of Personal and Spiritual Transformation*. Shambhala Publications, 2002.

mind. For example, spiritual bypassing may use absolute truth – "this is part of God's plan" – to avoid engaging the relative experience, feelings, needs, and struggles. This places enlightenment over engagement, sanctification over the indignity of soiled garments and the humiliation of others cleaning up your mess. We're emphasizing the grace and providence of God before engaging with the raw state of pain that calls out for cleansing. A bandage has been prematurely applied to a still-infected wound.

MAiD can be seen as a form of spiritual bypassing, which is an instinctive, not intentional, maneuver of the ego that preserves the integrity of its identity. Here is death, the ultimate spiritual moment in the human journey in which you are entering the final process of human development that calibrates you for the mystery that awaits us all (I will explore this in depth shortly), but you divert its final stages because they require your surrender to it. And it's not hard to see why. You want to avoid the physical suffering you imagine to come. You want to protect your loved ones from the emotional burden and sorrow of witnessing you lying helpless in bed. There is an entire world unravelling in the secret realms of your soul, but you do not know how to give yourself to that process.

MAiD is also spiritual bypassing for our culture. It diverts social energy and resources from deep engagement with the dying to efficient management of the dying. It provides a solution to a situation that is asking not to be fixed but understood. Dignity, purpose and meaning, factors driving MAiD requests, can be restored through deep relationships, story and belonging, contemplation and silence, all held in the space of effective medical management of the dying process. Despair demands the deep investment of collective energy and communal presence. When we do this well, the dying teach us how to live. They raise us to meet the most challenging moment with the best practice. But the most culturally damaging aspect of MAiD is its reinforcement of a structure of identity focused on the individual at a time when that naturally is dissolved to reveal identity as one with community, indeed, as one with reality itself.

You may think, does this not happen to everyone as they die? If suddenly, then the shift is swift. If slowly, then it's a gradual erosion. But in the end, the result is the same. Why would the means of death matter? The distinction here is that death is foreseeable for those who consider MAiD, a procedure that presents an option which overrides the most important assignment in the human journey: shedding the clothing of identity and becoming pure awareness, raw consciousness. The ends do not justify the means, and our end is infused with lessons and growth the mind *cannot* comprehend amid the dying process. The wisdom gained by not accelerating death is only realized afterwards in the lives of those who continue to walk this earth... and it usually takes months to years for that wisdom to fully manifest. This puts new meaning to the words of Jesus in Mark 8:35, "For whoever desires to save his life will lose it, but whoever loses his life for My sake . . . will save it." Hard sell.

The language of spiritual bypassing also stems from a confusion between meaning and purpose. Meaning is the emotional significance of what we do, the importance we ascribe to something. Meaning doesn't just exist on its own; it's something we create and feel. Our purpose is the cumulative effect of meaningful goals. If there is an ultimate purpose, that will have to wait for us to discover when we get "there." In the meantime, we will find it here only due to meaning-making activity – compassionate action, tender conversation, raw vulnerability, authenticity, and deep contemplation.

Overt spiritual bypassing is known through spiritual clichés; we blurt out "God has a purpose in this" because we cannot identify our own. We are scared. We are overwhelmed. We have not yet built purpose out of meaning. And how can we when we cannot conceive of the complexities that compromised us, for we are also asking, "Why did this happen?" And, beneath that, "What did I do to cause this?" The web of choices that contribute to individual or collective suffering is too dense for one person to grasp. Then there are the economic and social justice issues contributing to disease and struggle being much higher in many populations. These extremes scream for us to grow up, care for each other, and get real about what is most important: people, not possessions. Love, not luxury. Our children's well-being and our future on this planet.

All these questions reveal the poverty of our language and the scale of our stress as we struggle. We're trying to put handles on the chaos so we can wrest control and make some sense of the madness that has careened into our lane. At least, if God has a purpose in this, then there is some meaning yet to manifest. Isn't there comfort in at least that?

And yet… if there is indeed a realm beyond this material plane, if there is indeed a God and a spiritual world, then those beings, in the span of eternity, can take any mess we've made and work it for good. That does not mean they caused it. I'll even go so far as to say that does not mean they allow it. All those phrases reveal the limits of our language as creatures embedded in a cause-effect world. Perhaps the wisest thing we can do is learn to sit with the ambiguity, then step up in partnership with the Divine and boldly say, not "Why me?" but "What am I going to do with this?"

I trust that, in the span of time, even MAiD will be part of the awakening of humanity to a wiser compassion. Does not every tragedy and struggle do that? Spiritually, we still have much work to do. The religious traditions provide guidance through suffering, but their maps need an upgrade. Is there a model of spirituality that can speak intelligently to the modern mind while integrating the great insights of the world's wisdom traditions on this matter? Yes, but let's leave that for later. I'd first like to explore the impact spirituality makes when life is disintegrating and then explore how surprising a vibrant spirituality feels.

INTRINSIC VS EXTRINSIC

As spirituality pertains to what is most fundamental to you, let's explore it with a question. Ask yourself, what is essential to my identity? What is the core principle of my life? What drives me? The answers can be straightforward: your family, children, work, goals, and values. What is most important to you and your identity in this world? Even more, what connects you to something greater? We are asking what gives meaning in life. This is your spirituality. It only follows that your role in the world, your function in your family, your independence and how you move through life all disintegrate through dying. Your very identity is eroded. Yet a robust spirituality results in an identity, a sense of being that goes far beyond your activity in the world or even the story you tell yourself about yourself. To have that extend to a sense of connection with nature or the mystical realms makes one's spirituality even more robust in the face of suffering and death. So, it's no surprise that those with a strong intrinsic spirituality have low depression or a desire to hasten death.

In contrast, those with a strong extrinsic spirituality and those with none at all, tend to feel the opposite.[134] However, this cannot be taken as firm across the board. I've supported individuals with strong spiritual identities and devout religious practices who still choose MAiD. They looked forward to seeing God, reuniting with loved ones who passed, and going off on celestial adventures. However, they all approached this with the concept of an external God to whom they prayed instead of participating in God as the Ground of their Being. I'm speaking here of the Eastern Orthodox concept of *theosis,* becoming God in divine energies or operations but not in God's essence or identity; it is the fullness of the expression *to be in Christ*. This is the difference between intrinsic spirituality, marked by contemplation, the deep inward connection with Source, and extrinsic spirituality, characterized by an emphasis on an external deity or realm. Christianity is impoverished in this regard, with mystical union relegated to the saints and exceptional among us.

While many are suspicious of organized religion, a tremendous spiritual appetite exists for a meaningful life, for greater connection to self and the mystery of the present moment. Even more, for the healing of our species and planet, especially as expressed among the First Nations, Inuit and Metis cultures in Canada.[135] However, that leaves one in a peculiar place – with an attraction to spirituality but a rejection of the religious containers

[134] McClain, Colleen S., Barry Rosenfeld, and William Breitbart. "Effect of spiritual well-being on end-of-life despair in terminally-ill cancer patients." *The Lancet* 361.9369 (2003): pp. 1603–1607.

[135] In Canada, there are over seventy Indigenous languages and cultures. Government of Canada, Statistics Canada. 2023. "Indigenous Languages Across Canada." March 29, 2023. https://www12.statcan.gc.ca/census-recensement/2021/as-sa/98-200-X/2021012/98-200-X2021012-eng.cfm#.

in which it was formed. The ritual language, sacred mysteries, and mystical wisdom become divorced from the sobering private discipline, the groundlessness and the ecstasy which must go hand in hand when one surrenders self to sacred service. The law of attraction becomes the law of happiness, success, ego reinforcement, and well-being. This, ironically, is not the goal of healthy spirituality, which will **not** make you feel better at the end of life. It will not give you what you desire.

Healthy spirituality drives you to the darkness, the shadow, and the disintegration of ego-identity. This is the way of the cross. This is the dark night of the soul. This is the road to authenticity, not by knowing but by being known, not being full of yourself, but full of life. So dying does not bring out the best in you. Indeed, it can, but first comes reduction: applying heat to bring that which is hidden (what we might call ugly, unwanted, or shameful) to the surface. Jungian therapist and scholar Ann Ulanov says it comes down to one thing: "consenting to rise, to be dented, pressed in upon, to rejoin, to open, to ponder, to be where we are in this moment and see what happens, allowing the breath of not knowing to be taken, wanting to see what is there and what is not there. In such a space, we allow ourselves to depend on something greater than ourselves, to take what it gives us and respond to it."[136] This is the nature of an authentic relationship with the divine, for which religion is a start, not an end. This is also the ultimate challenge and invitation for those considering MAiD: to surrender to death, to the mystery, to the divine, and not control it.

Which means that your chaplain, your spiritual care practitioner, is not there to keep you comfortable. We are there to make you uncomfortable – that's the price of admission to the present moment, to authenticity. In this new land, you better understand yourself, what drives you, and what you think will destroy you. To do so, we establish a therapeutic relationship through a covenant, a promise and understanding of our role. It's a social contract – we're not there to shoot the breeze. We're there to shoot the false self and watch it die.

[136] Ulanov, Ann Belford. *The Unshuttered Heart: Opening to Aliveness/Deadness in the Self*. Abingdon Press, 2007, pp. 15–16, 17.

We assess four factors to confirm your suitability for this form of counselling. First, we consider whether you have a consistent sense of self over time. A weak sense of self makes engaging with the complex dimensions of identity impractical, if not impossible, which is why spiritual care may not be suitable for those with psychiatric disorders.

Second, we evaluate your ability to self-soothe. This enables you to regain existential balance and resilience while the ego is being deconstructed. This ability may not always be present, and moments of despair are an indication that you are deeply engaging with your own experiences and exploring the boundaries of your comfort zone. However, it is a crucial skill that allows you to observe and evaluate your own experiences.

Third, we look for open emotive pathways. This is a willingness to engage with the hard stuff, the emotional cholesterol that has clogged the arteries of life. So, if I notice an intense emotion, like anger or bitterness, I will compassionately, curiously, and directly ask what that's about. I want to explore that with you, for it is the material you wrestle with as you die. If you allow me to go there, we will examine it together. If you fold your arms and say, "That's none of your business," or "I don't want to go there," well, I'll probably push a bit more. I'll challenge you on that. Then, if it's still "no," we're done. (I'll check back later to see if you're ready.) Vulnerability is required in this work.

Finally, we look for the ability to engage in a relationship. I find this to be the most significant aspect of providing spiritual care. I am a stranger... a professional, yes... but a stranger who walks into the room and quickly gets personal. Your allowing me to do that is often made possible *because* I am a professional stranger. With me, it's safe to explore the shadow, the soul, and the sorrow. Most people at the end of life are ready for that conversation. Most are aching for it. We move into the wasteland to search for meaning in suffering, for this is directly related to the process of transformation. It's not the kind of meaning that gives understanding; it is meaning that gives value. When our search goes well, it primes you for the ultimate spiritual engagement: surrender. That's what's needed at the end of life to experience the ultimate gift of life. And while this gift is not anything the mind understands, the body and soul know it well.

SURRENDER

What does surrender feel like? What is it to give your whole self over to the divine, to the eternal now? Many describe it as a state of awe, marked by a sensation of being aware of something uncanny, overpowering, and vibrantly mysterious - the numinous presence. It's an experience of such perceptual vastness you literally have to reconfigure your mental models of the world to assimilate it. It is to be ravished by a reality so immense you are left stunned. And it doesn't need to involve God. Darwin said, "Attention, if sudden and close, graduates in surprise, and this into astonishment, and this into stupefied amazement."[137] That's what rapture is. That's what illumination is.

When it does involve God, according to ancient and modern mystics, the language is best rendered through intensely sensual imagery infused with something beyond words, beneath thoughts, something that takes one's breath away. (It's difficult to describe this without sounding… inappropriate.) It is the aching urge to merge and fully be one. This language, this inner orientation, is not part of contemporary Western spirituality. One might touch upon such longing for merger in the charismatic Christian traditions. The concept of "giving oneself over to Christ," or the ecstatic experience of being "slain in the Spirit," these graze the edge of such desire. Still, they fall short of the euphoric obliteration expressed by those who allow the release of self into the Ground of Being. Here the journey to the divine is one of lovers longing to disappear into each other. It requires us to be disrobed of ego, stripped of identity, and laid bare in our raw humanity. To adapt the insight of poet and author Kamand Kojouri, turning to the sacred as one dies "is like undressing before a bath. You don't undress out of fear that your clothes will become wet. You undress because you want the water to touch you. You want to completely immerse yourself in the feeling of the water and to emerge anew."[138]

Angelus Silesius, the seventeenth-century mystic and poet, put it this way: "God, whose love and joy are present everywhere, cannot come to

[137] Darwin, Charles. The Expression of the Emotions in Man and Animals. 1872. Page 278.

[138] Kojouri, Kamand. *The Eternal Dance: Love Poetry and Prose*. Kamand Kojouri, 2018.

visit you unless you are not there."[139] The Sufi poet and mystic Jalal Ad-Din Rumi said, "Knock, and He'll open the door. Vanish, and He'll make you shine like the sun. Fall, and He'll raise you to the heavens. Become nothing, and He'll turn you into everything."[140] And then, he sums it up with irritatingly beautiful spiritual flare: "Wash yourself of yourself. Be melting snow."

I know, I know… it sounds so strange, so foreign to the bulk of the dying experience. If only this would wash through us earlier. If only the enveloping Presence would infuse us the moment we realize our days are numbered. But it does not. For most, this state of consciousness does not emerge until the end. Your road to a new creation requires passing through destruction. It is the hardest thing in the world when met with resistance and the most grace-filled experience when met with acceptance. Here lies our ultimate homework.

Spiritual care practitioners are like tutors in this existential assignment. We strive to bring our most compassionate, engaged, and discerning selves to the dying. We are not there to change your mind but to help you discover what role it plays, along with emotions and experience, in creating the story you tell about yourself. Listening to a person's narrative validates and gives meaning to their humanity and worth. We are honoured to do just that, for, along with control of physical suffering, it lies at the heart of what so many want: a good death. That's the goal, and I sincerely appreciate how assisted dying seems to facilitate it. If you are considering MAiD and have read this far… well, then I thank you. Thank you for sticking with me through these pages. I don't know how you feel. Maybe you're more muddled now than ever. Maybe you're angry and want to fling the book across the room. Perhaps you're sad, grieving, scared… or indifferent. I have no idea what you're feeling, what you're thinking. I can only thank you for reading this far, for picking up the book at all.

---

[139] *The Theosophist*, vol. 114 (Adyar, India: Theosophical Publishing House, 1992), 245

[140] Lama Marut, *Be Nobody* (United Kingdom: Atria Books/Beyond Words, 2014), 219.

EXERCISE 8: YOUR SPIRITUAL JOURNEY

THIS EXERCISE AIMS TO GUIDE YOU IN REFLECTING ON YOUR LIFE JOURNEY and identifying the spiritual highlights or significant moments that have shaped your path. By visually mapping these milestones, you can gain a deeper understanding of the spiritual dimensions of your life and recognize the transformative moments that have impacted your journey. By drawing a timeline from birth to death, you can reflect on the various stages, events, and experiences that have contributed to your spiritual growth.

Instructions:

1. *Find a quiet and comfortable space where you can focus without distractions. Have a pen or pencil and a blank sheet of paper ready.*
2. *Begin by drawing a horizontal line across the middle of the paper. This line represents your life journey, with birth on the left and death on the right.*
3. *Take a moment to reflect on your earliest memories and significant events in your life. Start from the left end of the line and think about pivotal moments that hold spiritual significance for you. These can be experiences, relationships, or personal realizations that have impacted your spiritual growth or understanding. For example, recognizing the interconnectedness of all things, realizing the life-changing significance of someone's guidance, or moments in which you felt profound clarity and love. They can also be formal rituals, religious events, or community experiences of connection. It's helpful if you can evoke those memories marked by awe and wonder.*
4. *As you identify each significant moment, place a dot or mark on the line to represent it. Feel free to use different colours or symbols to distinguish between various types of spiritual highlights or milestones.*
5. *Once you have marked a few key moments, pause and reflect on each one. Consider its impact on your spiritual journey, the lessons or insights you gained, and how it shaped your perspective or beliefs.*

6. *Continue moving along the timeline, marking and reflecting on additional spiritual highlights as you recall them. You may find that specific periods of your life were particularly transformative or that specific events profoundly impacted your spiritual path. Often these arise from times of great struggle as well as joy.*

7. *As you reach the right end of the timeline, take a moment to reflect on the concept of death and the eventual end of your physical journey. Consider what insights or aspirations arise when contemplating the culmination of your life's spiritual journey.*

8. *Once you have marked and reflected on significant spiritual highlights along your timeline, take a step back and observe the map of your spiritual journey as a whole. Notice the patterns, connections, and themes that emerge. Reflect on the overall trajectory and the wisdom gained from traversing this path.*

9. *Reflect on the perspective that you are not a human being having a spiritual experience but a spiritual being having a human experience. How does this inform what you are now facing in life? Record your insights. What actions can you take to embody the insights you've uncovered? Perhaps you'll choose to share your experiences with a trusted friend or engage in practices that deepen your connection to the divine. Embrace the process of surrendering to the unfolding of your journey. Allow the insights you've gained to guide you as you continue on your path, and remember that every moment of reflection is a step towards greater awareness, acceptance, and ultimately, a more fulfilling experience of life.*

Remember, this exercise is a personal exploration of your spiritual journey. There are no right or wrong answers, and it's an opportunity for self-reflection and deeper understanding. Embrace the process and allow yourself to be open to the insights that arise as you map your spiritual highlights along your life's timeline.

CHAPTER 9

KNOW THYSELF

Today is non-refundable.

– CRAIG LOUNSBROUGH

THE CANCER'S BACK, DAVID. AND IT'S ON YOUR FEMORAL ARTERY." My doctor delivered the news heavily, but it wasn't anything I didn't already know. My symptoms had returned, initially minor but increasingly consistent and intense – rapid heartbeat, stomach churning, profuse sweating. I looked at him with a mixture of acceptance and determination. I understood the implications and the challenges that lay ahead.

"We'll need to admit you this week and start you on beta blockers to lower your blood pressure. It will take about a week to reach a level that allows us the most flexibility. Given that it's affecting a major blood vessel, we need as much leeway as possible. This will be more difficult than your first tumour."

Imagine having a bomb inside your body. It's called paraganglioma, a small yet potent cluster of cells filled with a volatile combination of dopamine, catecholamines and adrenaline. The trigger that causes the tumour to explode is emotions – anxiety, stress, anger, passion, anything that could activate my adrenal gland. Any intense experience of being alive could lead to my demise within thirty seconds. That's why keeping my blood pressure as low as possible is crucial; when the tumour is surgically removed, it tends to trigger a spike in my blood pressure. Without control, many patients die on the operating table.

I consider myself fortunate to have survived four of these tumours over the years and encountered countless close calls where smaller explosions dropped me to the ground in agony, rendering me unconscious. Little did I realize that this particular tumor would stop my heart for fifteen minutes, leading to the most impactful event of my life: a near-death experience.

For a brief moment, I glimpsed another realm and experienced a profound sense of wholeness, connection, integration and joy. The memory of that experience remains as vivid as if it occurred just yesterday. I delve into this extensively in my first book, *Beyond Surviving: Cancer and Your Spiritual Journey*, and will provide a summary of these phenomena in Chapter 26.

My cancer can only be treated through surgery. Paraganglioma grows slowly and is unaffected by chemotherapy and radiation – the primary treatments for lymphoma, leukemia, and the various other monsters found in a cancer ward. Therefore, a skilled surgical team must disarm this bomb and remove it from my abdomen.

Obviously, I had a good team; I'm still here! And cancer became a good teacher, one from which I'm still learning how to discern the seeds of self, how they are planted, and how to engage compassion to build the trust required to allow vulnerability and transparency. These two qualities open the windows of the soul, not so much for the therapist to peer through as for the patient. I've come to understand that this is the heart of spiritual care. We support authenticity and engage more sublime realities to assist in repairing archaic wounds, revealing the darkness we all constrain. These wounds ache to be revealed and, astonishingly, are hidden pathways to glory.

A health crisis amplifies all this. Suddenly, life feels fragile. Suddenly, the storm has come, and it stirs up the subconscious seabed of material suppressed over a lifetime: information and experiences we have not been able to integrate into the ego – how we have not loved well or been well loved. All lessons boil down to this: to discover that we are more than we imagined, more than the story we tell ourselves about ourselves. The truth that awaits is so fantastic it feels like fiction. So much easier to be comfortable with the mess instead. But the crisis has come, and those swells bring material from the depths of darkness and shove the unfinished homework of life in your face, challenging your sense of worth, identity, role, and significance. Here's the existential crisis. It's spiritual distress.

That's what I look for when I enter a patient's room, especially as spiritual issues rise to prominence as death approaches.[141] I'm always amazed at how rapidly they allow me into this inner world. Perhaps it's because I arrive with credentials in hand. More than the title of reverend, more than being a chaplain, it is the recommendation from a nurse or doctor that sells the encounter. They are my unwitting agents in the project of grace. I am grateful and humbled for their support – it's an honour to be part of the healthcare team. In the patient's eyes, though, my ordination comes not from the church or the hospital badge but from having survived cancer four times. I have street cred, which I hold with utmost respect and caution, for I also represent an unrealistic hope since my cancer is dramatically different from those I serve. Just because I survived does not mean they will.

Nonetheless, I share some common ground with my patients: I know what it's like to have cancer, to receive the diagnosis, to witness your family's worry, to wonder if you'll make it, and to reflect on your life in the dark of night. Worse, I know what it's like to have it happen repeatedly, each time raising the bar. I know what it's like to live daily with death. I know cancer from both sides of the hospital bed, and I have a sense of life from both sides of the veil.

What I do not know is the long road of pain and suffering that most cancers (and many treatments) cause. With my cancer, death comes in a moment. It does not scrape my body bare, does not devour my organs, does not leave me nauseous or gripped by prolonged pain. With this cancer, death snatches me in seconds and sends me to the great beyond with what feels like a single, swift punch in the gut. All the same, I represent

---

[141] Stanworth, Rachel. *Recognizing Spiritual Needs in People Who Are Dying*. Oxford Academic, 2011, https://doi.org/10.1093/acprof:oso/9780198525110.001.0001.

hope because I'm still standing. I see it in the patient's eyes, widened all the more by my sequels. "If he can do it, maybe I can too." At the very least, my words have traction. That's good because most of the time, the patient isn't quite sure why I'm there. Is it to check their religion, talk to God, or pray? No, I'm here to help you awaken to what you truly are.

A WINDOW TO THE SOUL

On a Greek mountainside stands an ancient ruin inscribed with eternal wisdom: "Know Thyself." Like a dying person, the temple of Apollo at Delphi looks frail and ruined against the lush trees around it, yet it shines with a mystery one must be patient in discovering. Opening this gift is a lifelong assignment accelerated by crisis and suffering. And it isn't easy. How can I know myself when I am blind to so much of who I am and how I function? Massive motivations dwell in my subconscious, influencing me in ways I cannot comprehend. My biases, desires, and wounds... all subtly influence behaviour and reality, for I see the world as I am, not as the world is. Even more ironic, I am the person most likely to deceive myself because of that subconscious material. Research in human behaviour shows I will tend to overestimate how well I'm doing (the Dunning-Kruger effect) or over-berate myself on what a mess I've become (negativity bias). Can I ever honestly know myself? This is the comedy and tragedy of the human journey.

As mentioned, the task of spirituality is not only to experience a healthy connection to life, wonder, and mystery but to be authentic – to know yourself as you truly are, without self-deception. It is to develop the ability to discern when the soul or the self leads, and when you follow the voice of love and awareness or the ego-identity. When one is aware of self (even more when one is aware of how one is aware, a quality called interoception), then one can work wisely and compassionately with whatever arises within. You arrive home within yourself – compassionate, integrated, whole. We will explore how to do that later.

Two other maxims are inscribed at the temple of Apollo, which follow "Know Thyself." They are "Nothing to Excess" and "Certainty Brings

Insanity." The first doesn't sound like much fun, but it is the path naturally taken when one recognizes and integrates their darker side. The second is a reminder that, in the words of French philosopher Emile Cartier, nothing is more dangerous than an idea when it is the only one you have. That's worth considering when discussing medically assisted death. I hope this book helps you see such an ultimate act from several angles.

Knowing yourself is no small task. It may be the greatest challenge we have in life, for we are talking about more than preferences, patterns of behaviour, or even the subconscious and how it influences your thoughts and feelings. Ultimately, the spiritual assignment is to know yourself as awareness itself.

To get started, I offer a simple tool to help you become more self-aware and integrated. It's called the Johari Window. (No, this is not some cryptic Greek term taken from a temple. It comes from the first names of the psychologists who devised it: Joseph Luft and Harry Ingham.) We'll explore this as it pertains to a person considering MAiD, which means opening challenging conversations about your experience with illness.

The Johari instrument looks like a window with four glass panes or quadrants (Figure 2). Quadrant 1 is the *Open* area or arena. This contains information about yourself that you and others know. For example, you now know I am an author, chaplain, cancer survivor, and someone who wants to discuss the spiritual dimensions of MAiD. You also know from my picture on the back of the book what I look like, my approximate age, and perhaps a bit about my style. All this is in the public arena, so it is part of my persona.

To explore the quadrant, consider what aspects of your identity and experience with illness are shared by you and those caring for you.

Quadrant 2 is what you know about me, but I do not know, so it's called the *Blind* area. We pick up this information through non-verbal cues, tone of voice, and observing behaviour. Here is where trust in our relationship can help me better understand myself, especially as aspects

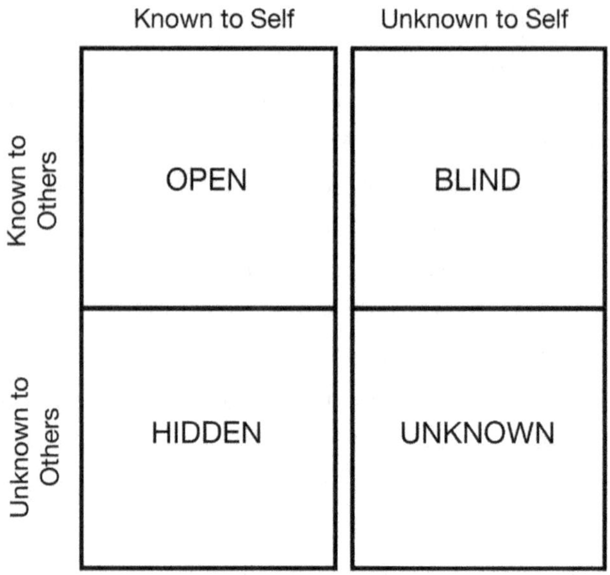

Figure 2: Johari Window

of my shadow – the hidden side of every human psyche – unintentionally come into play in my relationship with others and myself.

To explore this quadrant, ask someone caring for you what aspects of your experience with illness they have noticed you may be blind to, especially how these affect you considering MAiD.

Quadrant 3 is the *Hidden* area or façade. Here lies information about myself I keep hidden from others. This includes feelings, past experiences, fears, secrets, etc., that we appropriately keep confidential but reveal as the relationship grows. Healthy boundaries and ego-integrity require that the content in quadrant 3 is always kept private, and this becomes the main content we work with as we contemplate our life.

To explore this quadrant, consider what you keep hidden from those who care for you as you face mortality. How does this protect them? How does this protect you? How do you feel as you share this with others?

Quadrant 4 is the *Unknown* area. Here is all the information that no one is aware of – not you or others. Note that this area can contain traumatic past experiences or events that have been suppressed for decades. However, hidden qualities, capabilities, and unknown strengths and wisdom lie here. While many worry that this area contains only darkness, the great spiritual surprise is that it includes our light – more than we can imagine. I like to think of this window pane as having no outer boundary; it is infinite, for here lies the mystery of your connection to all of life. Since the information in this quadrant is not accessible through rational thinking processes (as the ego's integrity – who you think you are – will require keeping this material suppressed), we access this through listening to the body (somatic awareness), dreams, music, art... all the side-doors and hidden entrances to the subconscious.

To explore this quadrant, reflect on what physical, mental, and emotional sensations arise when you become still and watch your experience. What are your dreams like? This is best explored with someone you trust.

I offer this tool and approach to spiritual care through the lens of authenticity because of my near-death experience. I was temporarily transformed into a state of identity marked by absolute congruity, integration, transparency, and connectedness. No aspect of myself was suppressed, and there was no part of me I was blind to. I knew myself as I was fully known by that Presence, which I can only call love. I was more real than I have ever been in this physical form, and this led me to assert that love is not an emotion but the highest state of consciousness in which we are completely connected. If so, your spiritual health is not determined by what you believe but by how you love. Dying presses upon us this final assignment: to be serious about love, graceful in its practice, and courageous in its wisdom.

EXERCISE 9: JOHARI WINDOW

Time for another conversation. Ask someone you trust to help you know yourself more completely by doing the Johari Window exercise together. Afterwards, reflect on the central questions of the heart: Do I love well? Am I well-loved?

CHAPTER 10

THE SLIPPERY SLOPE

Heed the spark, or you may dread the fire.

– MILES FRANKLIN

MAID WAS MEANT FOR THE DYING. IT WAS MEANT FOR THOSE near the end of life who described their suffering as intolerable. But Amir Farsoud wasn't dying. And he wasn't sick. He was poor. And he was scared. The fifty-five-year-old suffered from chronic back pain and was soon to be on the streets as the rooming house where he lives was for sale. His income of $1,169 a month makes for meagre dining after paying the rent. Physiotherapy that supports some quality of life is an impossible luxury now. Fearing homelessness, he applied for MAiD and was reluctantly approved by his first physician assessor. Farsoud's argument was clear. "I would die, one way or another. It was just a question of, 'Do I have to take a bus to Toronto and jump in front of the subway, or will you be kind enough to do it?' "[142]

Here is a man who considered death to be better than poverty and struggle. And when his logic swayed a doctor, it almost brought him the tragic relief his despair demanded. Yet, just as all hope seemed lost, sharing his story manifested the miracle he needed: $61,000 raised through

---

[142] CityNews Staff. "Ontario man not considering medically assisted death anymore after outpouring of support." CityNews. Nov. 17, 2022, ottawa.citynews.ca/2022/11/17/ontario-man-not-considering-medically-assisted-death-anymore-after-outpouring-of-support-6114759. Accessed Feb. 21, 2023.

a community GoFundMe campaign. It seems there are options, after all, like compassion. Like community. Like common sense.

Mr. Farsoud stands among many as an example of the slippery slope, a perspective that takes a lot of heat when applied to MAiD, and for good reason. If employed as a logical argument that warns of inevitable outcomes, it is inherently flawed. But when there is evidence that dire consequences of the initial action are highly likely to occur, then the slippery slope argument has integrity. Therefore, stating that allowing MAiD for the dying will result in the government culling the elderly and frail to save money is nothing more than a rhetorical device driven by fear. But stating that allowing MAiD will likely lead to its use in non-terminal cases is not only a reasonable concern, it is an actual one. A growing number of MAiD cases demonstrate exactly that; originally meant for those facing a difficult death, MAiD is now being used for those facing a difficult life.

I review the slippery slope here not because I agree with it but because it is so often employed in discussions (more often arguments) on this contentious issue. And while relaxing eligibility for MAiD means we are sliding down the slope, I assert that MAiD should not be permitted for a very different reason: it is an inappropriate intervention, a medical procedure used to treat a spiritual condition. As much as it is dismissed in public debate, we need to consider the slippery slope nonetheless when it is informed by more than logic, such as experience, wisdom, and prudence, for logical reasoning alone does not capture the complexity and nuances of real-life situations.

The slippery slope stems from a concern not only for the vulnerable and frail in society but for the health of our country and our world. It proposes that MAiD undermines the ethical principles that strengthen the foundations of culture and preserve the integrity and health of humanity. Remove these principles, and society slides to chaos and harm at best, malevolence and evil at worst. Of course, the slippery slope only has traction if MAiD is understood as ethically wrong or at least questionable in the first place. Otherwise, expanding the practice merely adapts to a culture's needs. As I'm trying to deepen the conversation here, we first need to acknowledge that opposing camps may never agree due to how they read the map. Let's briefly identify why.

While, academically, there are several moral theories, in reality, few people operate on a single or cohesive one.[143] This can lead to heated debates over issues like MAiD and even a fundamental breakdown in our most intimate relationships. Such was the case with Jack Sorenson, a Nova Scotia man who suffered from severe chronic obstructive pulmonary disease (COPD). Every breath was a struggle, and he was tired of struggling.

His wife, Katherine, empathized with his suffering but felt his request for MAiD was rooted in anxiety and mental delusions. She also had a moral opposition to MAiD as she was a devout Christian, while Jack was an atheist. So extreme were these tensions that she took the issue to the courts, which delayed the procedure for two months, but did not prevent it. In a measured response of grace and acknowledgment, Katherine said, "I've had a wonderful life with Jack. There have been, as with any marriage, lots of varying opinions between the spouses and I thought we did a pretty good job of reconciling two pretty opposite views... until this issue came up of end of life."[144]

---

[143] For example, a Utilitarianism approach would assert that the moral acceptability of euthanasia should be determined by the overall happiness, well-being, or reduction of suffering it brings. This perspective claims that euthanasia can be justified if it minimizes the suffering of the patient and their loved ones.

From a deontological perspective, euthanasia is evaluated based on moral principles and duties. Opponents of euthanasia within this framework may assert that the inherent value and sanctity of life make intentional killing morally impermissible, regardless of the potential positive outcomes or the individual's suffering.

Virtue ethics considers euthanasia in the context of character traits and virtues. While it may not provide a definitive stance on euthanasia, it prompts reflection on the qualities and motivations of the individuals involved and how they relate to concepts like compassion, empathy, and respect for autonomy.

Living by a moral theory demands a high level of rational reflection and consideration. Truth is, most people base their perspective on their gut, which is heavily influenced by past experiences and future fears.

[144] Grant, Taryn. "Husband, 83, Dies With Medical Assistance After Wife's Court Bid to Stop Him Fails." CBC. Oct. 6, 2020, https://www.cbc.ca/news/canada/nova-scotia/nova-scotia-medical-assistance-in-dying-jack-sorenson-bridgewater-couple-court-1.5751454. Accessed May 1, 2023.

ETHICS

JACK AND KATHERINE SORENSEN HAD DIFFERENT LENSES THROUGH WHICH they read the map of life, resulting in opposing positions. Katherine's faith meant ethics rooted in her faith and the gift of life guided her, while Jack's decision was driven by his personal morals, pragmatic principles and fading resilience. Yet deeper dynamics were at play that could have resulted in greater understanding and intimacy. Getting there would require considerable time, guidance and discernment. How to find common ground?

Intricately woven into relationships and contextual dynamics, morality adapts its contours based on circumstances. In the crucible of a war zone, the absolute injunction "Do not steal" transforms into a nuanced consideration when faced with the spectre of starvation. Similarly, the stark commandment "Do not kill" takes on shades of relativity when hunting becomes a means of survival. The once unequivocal mandate of "Do not harm" now finds its relevance tethered to the poignant suffering of the dying, demanding a profound understanding of the nature of that distress. In this complexity, the letter of moral law must live into the spirit of its promise. This is going to get complicated!

Navigating this complexity is challenging, as morality has two edges: descriptive (what's right) and normative (why it's right). Descriptive morality guides how we should behave, while normative morality tries to explain why certain moral beliefs are justified. The catch is that normative morality often draws on big concepts like ethics, religion, or philosophy, while descriptive is based more on the lived experience of a person and a culture.

Can people with different views on morality, like descriptive or normative, talk and find common ground? Yes, but it's tough. We need respect and insight to get past our assumptions. These conversations aren't just about finding answers; they're about digging into what we assume and why we value what we value so we can ask even better questions. In this journey, we're not just figuring out what things are but also who we are – with all our biases, fears, hopes, and the mysteries that keep us curious.

No wonder ethics lies at the heart of medicine, guiding professionals through the challenging landscape of suffering and vulnerability, power and autonomy, all of which come to bear when a person becomes a patient. Seven core medical ethical principles guide this practice:

1. Autonomy: Respecting another's right to self-determine a course of action.
2. Beneficence: Taking positive action to help others, the core principle of patient advocacy.
3. Nonmaleficence: Avoidance of harm; a core consideration in medical decision-making.
4. Veracity: Telling the truth with complete, honest disclosure.
5. Confidentiality: Building trust through respected privacy.
6. Justice: Appropriately distributing limited resources, emphasizing non-discrimination and fairness.
7. Fidelity: Keeping one's word, doing as promised.

The practice of medical ethics is not the application of rules but the careful consideration of these seven principles in the complex world of making decisions about human action. Ethics are lived out through our relationships, so they will shift with the culture over time. Those shifts are accelerating with technological advancements which blur the line between life and death and extend life far longer than ever. And they do so in a culture that is mutating through technology at a pace few realize. These changes will drastically affect the story we tell ourselves about what it is to be human, and this will impact our sense of right and wrong, of what is healthy for humanity. In the process, will we come to understand what is perennial truth, what is fundamental to life and death?

Euthanasia sits at the centre of such storylines. It is among the core elements pervading all aspects of society, from the definition of a person to the nature of marriage, from the most personal principles to the purpose of civic institutions. At the very least, cultural storylines tell us who we are, where we come from, what we stand for, how things should be organized, and our connection to nature. But the storyline has changed so quickly that we've lost the narrative.

Is it any wonder? Stefan Timmermans, the medical sociology editor of *Social Science & Medicine*, points out, "While questioning the inevitability of death, modernity has added anguish to it. Security of small victories over some acute, devastating disease enhanced insecurity in light of the ultimate demise."[145] Our medical success has painted us into an existential corner from which the dying demand an early exit, the secret door by which they can escape their suffering. No surprise, then, that MAiD appears, at this time, in this setting.

MAiD arises from humanism, a non-theistic philosophy that affirms the worth, dignity and autonomy of the individual and the right of every human being to the greatest possible freedom compatible with the rights of others. It is guided by reason and scientific inquiry and motivated by ethics, compassion, and fairness.[146] Humanism's primary arguments in favour of MAiD are autonomy, liberty, minimizing pain and suffering, and the idea that there is no morally relevant difference between taking steps to hasten death vs. natural death when suffering is deemed intolerable by the one dying. When there is more struggle than blessing ahead, why endure?

To this, the slippery slope argument asks, have the principles of medically assisted death shifted faster than anticipated and moved beyond the intention of the original law? Does even embarking, in any way, down the road of assisted dying result in a sinkhole in the foundation of our humanity? To find out, let's look at the trajectory of MAiD as it has developed in Canada and the Netherlands, where euthanasia has been practised the longest.

New changes to the Canadian legislation came into effect on 17 March 2022.[147] In Canadian legislation, the waiting period between when a dying patient is approved for MAiD and receiving the lethal cocktail that ends their life has been removed. And now a broader group of people are eligible

---

[145] Timmermans, Stefan. "Death brokering: constructing culturally appropriate deaths." *Sociology of Health & Illness* 27.7 (2005): pp. 993–1013. https://onlinelibrary.wiley.com/doi/pdf/10.1111/j.1467-9566.2005.00467.x Accessed April 17, 2022.

[146] Humanist Canada. "What is Humanism?" 5 April 2023, https://www.humanistcanada.ca/about/humanism/. Accessed April 7, 2023.

[147] "Canada's Medical Assistance in Dying (MAiD) Law." Government of Canada, Department of Justice, Electronic Communications. May 26, 2023, www.justice.gc.ca/eng/cj-jp/ad-am/bk-di.html. Accessed April. 7, 2023.

to request and receive MAiD, people who were not permitted when the law was introduced. This includes those with an illness that is not terminal; it can be any medical condition the person deems intolerable.

Bill C-14, when passed in June 2016, included a provision that the MAiD law undergo a five-year review beginning in June 2020, but expansions of the law proceeded faster than the reviews could be done. A key provision, that natural death is reasonably foreseeable (a phrase that lacks effective meaning, as no predetermined time is required), has been split into two tracks for MAiD. The first track is based on someone whose natural death is deemed to be reasonably foreseeable. For these cases, Bill C-7 removes the ten-day reflection period and reduces the requirement from two independent witnesses to one witness, and it permits a person who was previously approved for MAiD to die by MAiD even if that person loses their ability to consent at the time of death.

The second track is based on someone whose natural death is not reasonably foreseeable. The main difference is that these people will be subject to a ninety-day reflection period. Determining whether a person qualifies for MAiD based on the first or second track will be difficult to determine and will be inconsistently applied based on the lack of definition for the phrase "natural death is reasonably foreseeable."

The Canadian government has considered calls to relax the safeguards yet again to allow MAiD for those with mental illness and mature minors. That's concerning, especially with the incredibly high rates of clinical depression and anxiety disorders in our culture. For so many, their end is infused with hidden trauma; a staggering percentage of us are scarred by abuse and seared with anxiety. That makes MAiD a radically inappropriate response; just as we don't treat mental illness like a lung infection or broken arm, we don't treat existential distress by killing the patient. That is, if you see MAiD as treatment. That was the position of Dr. Mauril Gaudreault, president of the Quebec College of Physicians, as he presented to a parliamentary committee in November 2022. He described MAiD as "a form of care. It's a medical procedure that may be appropriate in certain circumstances… It's not a matter of politics, morality or religion."

Well, euthanasia is a moral matter, and MAiD is not just another medical procedure. It is unlike any medical procedure that has ever been practised. It was originally intended to be only for those suffering unbearably near the end of life (and as the legislative bodies envisioned that, it was predominantly physical suffering. They had little framework for the existential dimensions and how they could be treated). But MAiD has now moved to a very dark place in Canada. Some advocates would like it extended to include children as young as twelve. The Netherlands already allows assisted dying for twelve-year-olds, while Belgium has no lower age limit. Deliberately taking a small child's life is unlawful everywhere else in the world, even when the child is terminally ill and asks a doctor to end their suffering.

For someone too young to vote, drive, or legally consent to sex to nonetheless be granted the power to insist on their own death is one of several troubling aspects of Belgium's policy.[148] The Dying with Dignity Canada website states, "In the Netherlands, assisted dying for children has been legal since the original legislation was implemented in 2002; data from between 2002 and 2015 has indicated that seven children had an assisted death in the Netherlands. In Belgium, assisted dying for children has been legal since 2014, and data from 2016 and 2017 showed that three children received medical assistance in dying."[149] Small numbers, yes, but shocking nonetheless. Just because something is legal doesn't mean it is ethically acceptable or, in medicine, clinically appropriate.

The legislation also insisted that a person be able to give final consent just before the procedure, but now a person need not be conscious or competent to receive the injection as long as their desire for it is documented. However, for those who work with the dying, it is treacherous territory to venture into, as we see the desire to die fluctuates considerably as one

---

[148] Lane, Charles. "Opinion: Children are being euthanized in Belgium." *Washington Post* https://www.washingtonpost.com/opinions/children-are-being-euthanized-in-belgium/2018/08/06/9473bac2-9988-11e8-b60b-1c897f17e185_story.html Accessed Feb. 20, 2022.

[149] Dobec, S. "Mature minors and MAiD: A deep dive into the issues of the Parliamentary Review." Dying With Dignity Canada. https://www.dyingwithdignity.ca/pr_mature_minors. Accessed Feb. 20, 2022.

approaches the end of life. Even those swimming in the abyss of cognitive impairment respond affirmatively to the kindness they receive. Yes, some are trapped in suffering. Yes, there are nightmares one would not wish on their enemies. Yes, some conditions seem worse than death. I know this landscape well, having cared for elderly patients who called out endlessly through the day and night, unaware of where they are, who they are, or that they matter. My own grandmother was transformed by Alzheimer's into a violent, tormented soul who my mother cared for until death. And, as you read, my mother endured a state of limbo for years.

I've also seen people, most people, in fact, who do not choose MAiD but live into the wilderness waiting, the expanse of desolation which they manage day to day. I asked one frail veteran how he imagined his days ahead when told he had dementia, and he replied, "I don't. Tomorrow is tomorrow. I am here, today. This is where my life is. And I have good care. I'm all right." His heroism clearly did not stop on the battlefield.

This is not a simple matter. And it is not about rules and regulations but our relationship with each other, ourselves, with life and death. The ground is shifting ever faster, and with the procedure being granted to impoverished people with psychological illnesses and multiple social challenges, the state now offers a ramp for people to run off the cliff rather than addressing life disabilities and economic inequalities.

Les Landry, age sixty-five, is an example of how this is embraced when society fails to care for those in need. He lives simply in rural Alberta, facing PTSD from child abuse, epilepsy, three strokes, and depression. "There's a tipping point where you can't afford to live," he says. "MAiD is the new society safety net." Landry has already received a signature from one doctor and is waiting to get a signature from the second. He has said that if he is denied the second signature, he will shop around until he gets it.[150]

[150] Subramanya, Rupa. "Scheduled to Die: The Rise of Canada's Assisted Suicide Program." *The Free Press* (Oct. 11, 2022). www.thefp.com/p/scheduled-to-die-the-rise-of-canadas. Accessed Dec. 30, 2022.

Naheed Dosani, a palliative physician who provides street-based care for this population in Toronto, has seen cases like this rising, and it causes him significant moral distress.

> I think of the people I have cared for over the years, like "Bob," a man in his fifties with multiple sclerosis and complex wounds. He was referred to our palliative care team to manage complex pain. Despite optimizing his pain and providing expert wound care, he pursued MAiD. Why? Because his progressive disease and its complications on his mental health led to an alcohol use disorder, which led to him losing his housing, which led to him losing his family and, ultimately, being alone.
>
> Conversely, I have witnessed how treating the social determinants of health for the people I care for can make a tremendous difference in whether someone pursues MAiD. "Mary," a woman in her thirties, is an example. She was on the streets living with untreated HIV, dealing with a substance use disorder and no health-care team to meet her needs. Mary wanted to die through MAiD. However, after addressing her emotional and physical pain, supporting her with housing, income, harm reduction services and providing the psychosocial support that all Canadians deserve, she changed her mind because she now has a better quality of life.[151]

The government is not so inspired. Justice Minister David Lametti has considered expanding MAiD to teenagers and said he "was not worried about the floodgates opening with respect to mental disorders."[152]

---

[151] Dosani, Naheed. "If medically assisted death becomes more accessible for Canadians, we have a moral obligation to make living well – through housing, mental health supports – accessible too." *Toronto Star*, (Feb. 11, 2021). https://www.thestar.com/opinion/contributors/2021/02/11/if-medically-assisted-death-becomes-more-accessible-for-canadians-we-have-a-moral-obligation-to-make-living-well-through-housing-mental-health-supports-accessible-too.html Accessed Nov. 2, 2022.

[152] Raj, Althia. "Canada is now No. 1 in world in terms of MAiD. We should think twice before expanding it." *Toronto Star* (Nov. 21, 2022).

Lametti is not the only one casual about the matter. A Veterans Affairs Canada (VAC) case manager offered it to retired corporal Christine Gauthier, a former Paralympian engaged in a years-long fight for a home wheelchair lift. She described the VAC agent she spoke with as saying, "Madam if you are really so desperate, we can give you medical assistance in dying now."

Her response was sharp and accurate. "I can't believe that you will… give me an injection to help me die, but you will not give me the tools I need to help me live."[153]

That is only one of several cases to which Prime Minister Trudeau has appropriately responded, "It is not the place of Veterans Affairs Canada, who are there to support those people who stepped up to serve their country, to offer them medical assistance in dying."[154]

We will undoubtedly hear more of such cases, as several studies have identified issues with MAiD practice. As well, there is a growing accumulation of narrative accounts detailing people getting MAiD due to suffering associated with a lack of access to medical, disability, and social support. The Canadian MAiD regime is lacking the safeguards, data collection, and oversight necessary to protect Canadians against premature death.[155]

Canada, known worldwide for its kindness, is now the world leader in euthanasia. Even more disturbing, we are the global epicentre of harvesting organs from patients who have undergone MAiD.[156] The assessment protocol for organ donation is done separately from the MAiD assessment and only once the person has been found eligible for MAiD. On one level, that makes sense and may give those who choose assisted death an even greater sense of purpose in their passing. But, on another, it feels subliminally dystopian, as it may significantly influence the decision to proceed

---

[153] Boynton, Sean. "Trudeau says assisted dying offers to veterans 'unacceptable' as cases mount." Global News. Dec. 2, 2022 https://globalnews.ca/news/9321582/veterans-affairs-maid-cases-trudeau/

[154] Ibid

[155] Coelho, Ramona, et al. "The realities of medical assistance in dying in Canada." *Palliative & supportive care* 21.5 (2023): 871-878.

[156] Mulder, Johannes, et al. "Practice and challenges for organ donation after medical assistance in dying: A scoping review including the results of the first international roundtable in 2021." *American Journal of Transplantation* 22.12 (2022): pp. 2759–2780.

with MAiD.[157] That dark shadow is jarringly exposed by Ross Douthat of the *New York Times*.

> The rules of civilization necessarily include grey areas. It is not barbaric for the law to acknowledge hard choices in end-of-life care about when to withdraw life support or how aggressively to manage agonizing pain. It is barbaric, however, to establish a bureaucratic system that offers death as a reliable treatment for suffering and enlists the healing profession in delivering this "cure." And while there may be worse evils ahead, this isn't a slippery slope argument: When 10,000 people avail themselves of your euthanasia system every year, you have already entered the dystopia.[158]

It seems that this is the case with the Dutch guidelines for euthanasia which have, without exception, been broken time and time again.[159] Their rates have climbed to such an extent as to indicate that dying by lethal injection may become the norm in the decades ahead. Currently, one in twenty-five deaths in the Netherlands is by euthanasia, rising to one in seven in cities. Dr. Theo Boer, a Dutch ethicist who was in favour of assisted death but has now shifted his position out of concern for what he sees happening in his country, comments that this act has gone from a "last resort to prevent a terrible death to a last resort to prevent a terrible life."[160] Reading that, I realized my moral distress is similar to Dr. Boer's, for an eruption has occurred deep beneath the waters of life and death that we navigate. The resulting tsunami is not only building; it has crested. Forget the slippery slope. The whole damn landscape has exploded.

---

[157] Middleton, Claire. "Organ donation after MAiD: it's not that simple." *CMAJ* 191.38 (2019): pp. E1062–E1062.

[158] Douthat, Ross. "What Euthanasia Has Done to Canada." *The New York Times* (Dec. 3, 2022).

[159] Cohen-Almagor, Raphael. "Critical Remarks on the Dutch Policy and Practice of Euthanasia and Proposed Guidelines for Physician-Assisted Suicide." *New Medical Ethics to Integrative Bioethics*, Ante Covic, Nada Gosic, Luka Tomasevic, eds. (2009): pp. 197–216.

[160] "Death on Demand: In the West, assisted dying is rapidly becoming legal and accepted." *The Economist* (Nov. 13, 2021) https://www.economist.com/international/2021/11/13/in-the-west-assisted-dying-is-rapidly-becoming-legal-and-accepted Accessed March 4, 2022.

EXERCISE 10: PERSONAL EXPLORATIONS

TAKE A FEW MOMENTS TO SIT IN A QUIET AND COMFORTABLE SPACE. CLOSE your eyes and bring your attention to your breath. Allow yourself to become present and grounded in the moment. When you feel ready, engage with the following reflection questions:

1. ***Personal Values:** How do your values and beliefs intersect with the concerns raised by the slippery slope argument?*
2. ***Quality of Life:** How do you define and assess your quality of life? What factors are most important to you in determining the level of suffering or loss of dignity that would make you consider MAiD an option?*
3. ***Support Systems:** Have you explored all available palliative care options and support systems to manage your symptoms, pain, and emotional well-being? How confident are you in the adequacy of these options to meet your needs and alleviate your suffering?*
4. ***Future Uncertainties:** How do you navigate the uncertainties surrounding the progression of your condition and potential changes in legislation or societal attitudes?*
5. ***Discussion with Loved Ones:** Have you had open and honest conversations with your loved ones about your considerations regarding MAiD? How do their perspectives align or differ from your own? How might their opinions influence your decision-making process?*
6. ***Seeking Professional Advice**: Have you consulted with healthcare professionals, including palliative care specialists, spiritual care practitioners and ethics experts, to gain a broader understanding of the potential implications of MAiD and the concerns raised by the slippery slope argument? How has this input informed your perspective?*

Remember, these questions are meant to guide personal reflection. They should be considered with professional guidance from healthcare providers, therapists, and ethical advisors who can provide individualized support in exploring the complex decision-making process surrounding end-of-life choices.

Chapter 11

THE COMPASSION CONUNDRUM

If you can, help others; if you cannot do that,
at least do not harm them.

– Dalai Lama

Next to the hospital where I work is a park full of opportunities. It's a great place to stroll during lunch, especially on cold winter days, though instead of trees, the park is filled with tents–tents belonging to people experiencing homelessness. Often, among those tents, I see people with clipboards, engaging in conversation over cups of coffee. These government workers check on everyone twice a day, ensuring they are fed, warm, and safe. The park feels like a place of awakened humanity, where those with stability sit with those without. They make a difference not by fixing lives–the issues are too complex for easy solutions–but by sharing lives. It is the connection, not the response, that makes us better. Only then, from the foundation of empowering compassion, can any lasting action be initiated. But what if you've been trained to fix lives too frail to continue?

It can be argued that the primary task of the medical profession is not to prolong life or to promote health but to relieve suffering. Throughout medical history, the height of this was the pledge not to cause death, even if the act was deemed merciful. Enshrined in the Hippocratic oath, dating from the fourth century BC, this central medical creed is often cited as a primary reason for not providing assisted death. It appears to state it plainly: "I will use treatment to help the sick according to my ability and judgement, but never with a view to injury and wrong-doing. Neither will I administer a poison to anybody when asked to do so, nor will I suggest such a course." [161] All seems laid out in black and white.

Would there not be an exception for euthanasia? After all, its Greek etymology sounds desirable: *Eu* "good" + *Thanatos* "death." And assisted death was not uncommon in ancient times. We must remember the historical context in which the Hippocratic oath developed: political backstabbing was rampant, and those knowledgeable about poisons and potions were the preferred collaborators. Hippocrates was no fool, but a man of principle who had pride in his profession, so he wrote this oath with a promise that protected physicians from becoming infamous political assassins.[162] Though the oath forbids euthanasia, like all ancient documents from wisdom traditions, it is dangerous and inaccurate to make universal absolutes out of what are, essentially, high ideals for a culture, a community, and a craft. Many accounts of physicians providing assisted dying in ancient times remind us that this oath was sworn by those belonging to a particular school of thought within the medical arts. One could even say it is an oath of a specific sect or secret society. And the revisions continue: contemporary versions do not include the prohibition against abortion and euthanasia. And, while nearly every medical school worldwide has it as part of their graduation ceremony, few now swear it by the name of ancient Greek gods – continued cultural adjustment.

Hippocrates was one of many prominent teachers in the medical arts, each with their following and philosophy. So, the principles of his oath were not universal, nor were they written in stone. As his approach to care

---

[161] "Perhaps the Earliest Surviving Text of the Hippocratic Oath." Jeremy Norman's HistoryofInformation.com. Accessed Feb, 10, 2019. https://www.historyofinformation.com/detail.php?entryid=2239.

[162] Markel, Howard. "'I Swear by Apollo' – On Taking the Hippocratic Oath." New England Journal of Medicine (2004), 350:2026-2029. Accessed Feb. 10, 2019. https://www.nejm.org/doi/full/10.1056/NEJMp048092

rose to prominence and endured throughout the centuries, the Hippocratic oath was revised to reflect the culture and ethical development in the evolving art of medicine. Modern medical schools did not adopt the oath until after the Second World War – a response to the atrocities of Nazi Germany.

We are not Nazis, but neither is our culture immune from the perennial challenge of discerning the balance between suffering and purpose or how compassion is compromised when our response to suffering is misguided. The medical and political professionals advocating for MAiD reveal not some malevolent intent but a spiritual poverty and social failure to address suffering wisely. This is not about technology and what can be done, but about humanity and whether it should be done.

No wonder. Dying is difficult in Western society. Where other cultures provide deep spiritual guidance on the final road, ours is navigated by medical and clinical experts. Instead of prayers, silence, and contemplation by the bedside, we have a blaring television or phone apps to distract us. The hospital is not conducive to cultivating clarity of insight into the profound dynamics at play in the centre of one's being. Even more, our culture's spiritual poverty leaves most struggling with the chaos of psychic deconstruction and physical deterioration.

A personal note: it isn't easy to describe what it feels like to witness a MAiD procedure. I share here my experience, which may not be yours, and which sits in contrast to the many who share that MAiD feels like peaceful acceptance of a harsh reality, an attempt to add more meaning and significance to the dying process by having more control than natural death allows. To these people, MAiD is not a bad or scary thing, but a peaceful and humane practice that made the process of losing a loved one easier to get through. However, as one who has been with hundreds of natural deaths, dozens of deaths through withdrawal of life support, and several MAiD procedures, I am left with a disturbing and visceral sense of how we can become confused about what compassion calls us to be.

MAiD is not an execution, and yet a doctor injects a lethal dose of drugs into a person's arm with the intent to kill them. And it's not a remedy to suffering, as much as the words are often said afterwards, "Her suffering is over." It feels, from my vantage point, more like a way out, an escape. The long road of descending, of disintegrating, is finally, suddenly over. But something is amiss. You sense it, but few put it into words. You can be in the trenches for a long time and not realize what you're staring at. To watch good people do what has always been considered the darkest deed in the name of goodness feels like a corruption in our humanity. There is an existential disruption of identity in what it is to be a healthcare provider and what it is to be a human being. I found my unease difficult to directly identify, to accurately put into words, until I landed upon one that shocked me, yet resonated with massive recognition in my gut. MAiD feels… malevolent. It feels like a confrontation between the forces of humanization and dehumanization. It feels like something very dark masquerading as something noble.

I want to emphasize that this is my experience. Yours may be not only different but opposite, depending on your life journey and existential framework. But I walk away from every MAiD procedure increasingly sensing that this is the ultimate act of our cultural impotence to respond to suffering, especially as Canada stands among the top ten wealthiest nations.[163] The forces of dehumanization–politics, technology, and capitalism–seem to be rising, while the forces of humanization–literature, the arts, community service, and faith–are declining. MAiD sits within the muck of spiritual poverty, relational trauma, social dysfunction, death anxiety, and depression that marks an astonishing number of Canadian lives. It is an efficient but short-sighted and inappropriate response to suffering on a societal level that could not be felt more viscerally on a personal level. Perhaps that's why, as a spiritual care practitioner, I find this even more jarring, disorientating, and existentially confusing.

At some level, I knew that these injections were killing more than just the patient. They were killing our culture and draining the social capital of values and principles. The nature of medicine and the role of physicians have undergone a profound transformation as MAiD ends the

[163] Shorrocks, Anthony, James Davies and Rodrigo Lluberas. *Global Wealth Databook 2022* (PDF). Credit Suisse Research Institute, 2022.

mandate for doctors not to cause death. It also enacts a principle that states a person is valued not just for being human, but for their participation and contribution to society. Now, vulnerable, fragile, and weak individuals (such as those who are dependent, old, or sick) believe that they can maintain their dignity by ending their life rather than discovering it through the most challenging parts of life. I acknowledge that this may sound simplistic, and I am fully aware of the brutal and devastating situations that many feel trapped in. For these tortured souls, death feels better than life. However, their suffering calls upon all of us to provide intense love, fearless presence, and our full support. I understand that this may seem idealistic, but my heart is shattered in more ways than one.

Each time I have been involved in a case, I have noticed something even more troubling. Part of me was dying. I was becoming accustomed to it. It was becoming routine, just another task among many. During palliative care rounds, MAiD would be mentioned, noting that a patient had received their assessment and the procedure would take place at noon. The brief silence that followed felt like pressure on my ears, as if I had gone too deep underwater and run out of air. I think about the Netherlands and the frequency of MAiD there. Many of my patients ask about it or casually say, "At least I have that option if things get bad." Euthanasia has become an existential anesthetic; its effect is felt long before the needle enters their body. But is it truly a compassionate choice?

The problem may lie in our understanding of compassion itself. *Webster's Dictionary* defines compassion as a "sympathetic consciousness of others' distress together with a desire to alleviate it." The *New Oxford American Dictionary* defines it as "a sympathetic pity and concern for the sufferings or misfortunes of others." Surprisingly, neither of these definitions is accurate; in fact, they are distortions of the lived experience of compassion.

In the research paper, *Sympathy, empathy, and compassion: A grounded theory study of palliative care patients' understandings, experiences, and preferences,* researchers sought to identify the difference between sympathy, empathy, and compassion from the perspective of patients. In discussions with fifty-three people facing advanced cancer, the researchers discovered essential nuances that have significant implications for MAiD.

> Sympathy was described as an unwanted, pity-based response to a distressing situation, characterized by a lack of understanding and self-preservation of the observer. Empathy was experienced as an affective response that acknowledges and attempts to understand an individual's suffering through emotional resonance. Compassion enhanced the key facets of empathy while adding distinct features of being motivated by love, the altruistic role of the responder, action, and small, supererogatory [above and beyond] acts of kindness. Patients reported that empathy and compassion were beneficial, unlike sympathy, with compassion being the most preferred and impactful.[164]

So, contrary to the dictionary's definition, no sympathy is present in genuine compassion. Instead, sorrow and connection resonate in the heart, which initiates action only after these heavy emotions are allowed to live and breathe in one's being. After all, the word means *to suffer with*.

Compassion requires engaging in a kind, loving awareness to be present with things as they are. That's hard when you're swallowed in apprehension, fear, frustration, even terror. The challenge not to get caught up in these emotions, but to allow and observe them, seems ridiculous as we imagine it. It is, however, transformative when we participate in it. With that in mind, I would offer an alternative compassionate intervention not considered by advocates or opponents of MAiD. It is a spiritual secret, a surprising way to engage compassion–not by what we do for the dying, but by what the dying can do for others.

---

[164] Sinclair, Shane, et al. "Sympathy, empathy, and compassion: A grounded theory study of palliative care patients' understandings, experiences, and preferences." *Palliative Medicine* 31.5 (2017): pp. 437–447.

MAiD is an act done in the name of compassion but is more aligned with the efforts of sympathy and empathy. The famous Buddhist nun and teacher Pema Chödrön clarifies this: "Compassion is not a relationship between the healer and the wounded. It's a relationship between equals. Only when we know our darkness well can we be present with the darkness of others. Compassion becomes real when we recognize our shared humanity."[165] At no point is our humanity so intensely shared than through death. Here is the great equalizer. Here you stand on common ground with kings and paupers, the foolish and the wise, every human being that ever was, and those that will be. Chödrön emphasizes that at this point, the key is not to run from the dying process or fix it but to *sit with what is* through a meditation called *tonglen*. Our instinct is to avoid suffering and struggle; tonglen is deep engagement with these trials, with what scares you, even with what destroys you. This is accomplished through a compassionate connection with others who suffer as you do.

Tonglen is how the dying can practice existential *Aikido*, the martial art in which practitioners defend themselves while protecting their attackers from injury. At its heart, though, the goal of Aikido is to overcome yourself. How can you do this while dying? Identify your struggle, breathe in more from others, and send your blessing and compassion to them. Send out what you need for the restoration of spirit. Send out spaciousness, understanding, and solidarity. *"I am with you. I understand."* Doing this quietly, constantly, with every breath, becomes your anchor, your stability. It is an astonishingly powerful way to process existential and physical distress while dying.

Notice that the *patient* does this with their suffering; it is not something we do to alleviate suffering. (And it does not mean we go light on the drugs! The pain must be managed; you cannot care for the soul unless you first care for the body.) I've practised this with many at the end of life, and the effect is remarkable. By using their fear as fuel for connection and kindness, the dying person's experience of suffering can suddenly shift.

---

[165] Chödrön, Pema. *The Places that Scare You: A Guide to Fearlessness in Difficult Times*. Shambhala Publications, 2007.

They are building purpose into it, and that is empowering. It restores dignity; it activates agency; it manifests meaning. Here's the conundrum: the ultimate compassionate response to the dying patient is not to end their suffering but to use it to engage their compassion for others and shift their relationship to their own experience. In doing so, they heal and bless the world. Now, the dying person is not alone. They are taking the lead, meeting the same need for control that drives MAiD requests, but in a way that deepens their humanity instead of ending it. They are shining, and the world needs their light.

You may be thinking this is the move of a master, not of the average person. And you are right. Few of us have such existential agility. Few of us have been trained to engage our suffering and struggle in such a way. How could we possibly do it at death? And yet I have seen that lack of experience render such effective results precisely because the person does not know what to expect. They have no preconceived notion of the power of compassion, thinking of it more as a soft and tender expression, something nice, not something fierce. Yet, by its nature, compassion empowers a person to maintain balance in the storm of pain and suffering, life and death, and remain a stabilizing force not capsized by the tempest. Their keel remains deep in the water, and they can adjust their sails to use the gale of grief and sorrow to move forward to a more profound humanity. It's certainly noble to be such a force as a healthcare provider or family member, but it's transformative to be that as the one dying. There is a warrior of compassion within us all, what Buddhists call a bodhisattva. Perhaps death provides us with one more chance to be a hero.

EXERCISE 11: TONGLEN

Time to practise. Let's first acknowledge that it's easier to be compassionate to someone else than to be compassionate to yourself. Yes, if you're dying, you are an expert in suffering and dying. You know what it feels like, which makes you uniquely qualified to resonate with others in a similar situation. If you have cancer, if you are depressed, if you are spinning into despair, then you are perfect for this assignment. We're going to tap into your struggle as fuel not only for connection to theirs but to help shift your relationship to your own experience.

Tonglen means "sending and taking." It's a meditation from the Buddhist tradition in which you focus on what troubles you most and breathe in more of it from others. What you breathe back to them is your compassion, a mental and spiritual energy that says, "I get it. I understand. I'm with you." Tonglen has parallels in other spiritual traditions. The Roman Catholic practice is called redemptive suffering, in which you offer your suffering to God on behalf of those who suffer. You're using your woundedness to become a conduit of divine compassion. Tikkun olam *is a mystical ritual in the Jewish faith to restore the world's health and return the sparks of Divine light to their source. Islam emphasizes that Allah is the compassionate one – a descriptor used more than any other adjective when speaking of the nature of the One God.*

Tonglen is the practice of the warrior of compassion – the one who can transform suffering by the quality of their presence within it. Instead of avoiding suffering, we're tapping into it as the most potent energy of connection. It's an incredibly effective way to get out of your own way! We move naturally into ambiguity, into emptiness, a state without action or judgment. You can practise tonglen in the moment, for brief intervals, or as part of a formal meditation practice. I will be exploring tonglen specifically for the person considering MAiD.

Take a few moments to sit in a quiet and comfortable space. Close your eyes and bring your attention to your breath. Allow yourself to become present and grounded in the moment.

We begin by opening to and allowing whatever arises in the external environment, such as noise, and the internal environment, such as physical sensations, thoughts, and feelings. Don't spend much time on this; a few moments are sufficient. Allow what is to be present without resistance, even if thoughts and feelings are intense, even if the noise in your room is irritating.

Second, identify what troubles you most, what you struggle with. For the purpose of MAiD, identify the fear and distress driving the request. What do you want to avoid through assisted dying? What are you most scared of? How does your imagination present the loss of control as you descend into death? Where is this held in the body? Notice how considering these struggles affects breathing, gut, and heart... notice if your head swims, and if you feel warm and anxious. Good... we're tapping in.

Third, breathe in more of it. Think of anyone else in the world who is in the same situation, considering MAiD. Breath in their distress, their anxiety, visualizing it as darkness, heaviness, even a sense of claustrophobia. Then breathe out feelings of radiant light, calm, and expansiveness. Breathe in the negative energy, the material you know all too well, and breathe back compassionate energy, kindness, and understanding. No need to fix it, only to connect. Remain in this compassionate alignment until the visualization synchronizes with your breathing.

Finally, expand your compassion. Extend your intention to two people, then ten, then a hundred. Expand it from those dying in your local area to the entire country. You know what it is like. There is no one better qualified than you to do this. Remain in this amplified alignment for as long as the visualization remains synchronized with your breathing. The goal in this is not to help you feel better or change your experience but to help you be real and change your relationship to your experience.

You may be wondering if this makes a difference. Yes! Research demonstrates that compassionate meditations affect those you are aligning with. One examined the effect of distant intention on the autonomic nervous systems of cancer patients and their partners. Each was connected to galvanic skin response monitors, and despite the distance between sender and receiver, their metabolisms synchronized and settled into a more optimal state. "Directing intention toward a distant person is correlated with activation of that person's autonomic nervous system. Strong motivation to heal and be healed, and training on cultivating and directing compassionate intention may further enhance this effect."[166,167]

The implication of this is exciting and unnerving. It means you do not stop at your skin. It also means there's no such thing as a private thought. Your intentions, especially as energized by compassion, create an energy field that ripples out to affect the local environment, specifically those to who you are connected through love. Remember, love, or its more objectively detached correlate, compassion, is not an emotion but a state of consciousness. Love connects consciousness. Perhaps, more accurately, it dissolves the illusion that we are disconnected since everyone and everything arises from the Ground of Being.

Sit now in quiet wonder. Sit and contemplate your connection to all that is. Accept and dwell in your mystery, your majesty, your remembering of what you are. Be still with this. Finally, end with gratitude, not so much through words like "thank you" as with shining light from your heart. Let it put a smile on your face. Let it lift you and expand... even explode you with joy. This is your birthright. We are all destined to become enlightened. We are all, beneath the muck and mess of the mind and perceived self, absolutely glorious.

For a guided experience of tonglen, go to https://soundcloud.com/davidmaginley/tonglen

[166] Radin, Dean, et al. "Compassionate intention as a therapeutic intervention by partners of cancer patients: Effects of distant intention on the patients' autonomic nervous system." *Explore* 4.4 (2008): pp. 235–243.

[167] Radin, Dean I., and Roger D. Nelson. "Evidence for consciousness-related anomalies in random physical systems." *Foundations of Physics* 19.12 (1989): pp. 1499–1514.

CHAPTER 12

TERMINOLOGY

Words are events.

– URSULA LE GUIN

PACIFICATION. IT'S A TERM USED TO DESCRIBE MILITARY ACTIONS AS a process of bringing peace, stability, and development to the local population. It was coined by the United States government to describe its efforts in the Vietnam War. The reality, of course, was far different. Defenceless villages were bombed from the air, the inhabitants driven out into the countryside, the cattle machine-gunned, the huts set on fire with incendiary bullets, and napalm scorched the land. The euphemistic language attempted to downplay the severity and violence of the United States' actions, creating a false perception that they were working toward the betterment of the Vietnamese people.

As the war escalated and casualties mounted, journalists and anti-war activists began to question and challenge the euphemisms used by the government. They sought to expose the true nature of the conflict, shedding light on the devastating consequences of "pacification" for innocent civilians.

These efforts to unveil the reality behind the rhetoric played a significant role in shifting public opinion and galvanizing opposition to the war. The power of truth and accurate language helped to mobilize a movement that ultimately contributed to the end of the conflict.

Medical Assistance in Dying. Should we not just say euthanasia? But that upsets people. Euthanasia has baggage, and we are Canadians, after all. Is there not a more tactful term? We certainly found one less emotionally charged. Yet, when dealing with the ultimate act – ending a person's life – do we not need emotional energy? Is this not the time for the poet and the storyteller as much as for the ethicist and the technician? What term not only accurately describes the act but adequately imparts its significance?

The United States has chosen *Physician-Assisted Death* (PAD). That's adequate as it identifies who provides the drugs and the result. Similarly, *physician-assisted suicide* describes the nuance when patients administer their own lethal dose. Europe does not recoil at the term euthanasia, and it seems accurate in its description and intention: to provide a good death (comfortable and on the person's terms).

In Canada, we have chosen MAiD. It had to be a term that reflected the decision to allow nurse practitioners, not only doctors, to perform the procedure. Ironic that it's called MAiD. That's a person who comes in to clean up the mess we've made. And that mess is considerable: lack of distributed palliative care; lack of skills in having honest, difficult conversations about the end of life or stopping treatment; and, of course, our culture's inability to face death with wisdom and deep insight. After all, death is not a medical issue but a spiritual one.

MAiD is also a euphemism, a term stripped of emotionally charged language. A euphemism can be helpful in the right circumstances: "I'm sorry for your loss" is appropriate in conveying empathy compared to "It's so terrible that your husband killed himself." But euphemisms often have a dark side in marketing and political debate: they can be crafted to desensitize us to moral impact and obscure factual clarity.

A euphemism clouds reality. We can all say that we want medical assistance in dying – clean sheets, excellent pain management, and compassionate nursing. That's called palliative care, which maximizes comfort without accelerating death. MAiD is doctors and nurse practitioners intentionally ending a person's life, whether hours, days, weeks, or months before one would naturally die. Is it killing? That's a term I squirm at using, for I know doctors who perform this, and I do not want to call them killers. I do not see them as killers. But I am left in moral distress because at the heart of moral responsibility is the ability to name one's actions accurately. Do we then need a different term to describe this procedure accurately? Is it killing, or is it assisted suicide? Well, in this situation, we have a person who is willing to end another person's life and a person who wants their life ended. The *Merriam-Webster* definition of "kill" is "to cause death." That may be done legally or illegally, morally or immorally, as reflected in the nuances between first-degree murder (pre-meditated), second-degree murder (an intentional murder not pre-meditated or planned), voluntary homicide (a form of manslaughter), and involuntary homicide (a less culpable state of manslaughter, such as if a driver accidentally hit a pedestrian). Note that "killing" itself need not have a moral context – a soldier kills in battle, an intended murder victim kills in self-defence, a drug dealer kills his competition, and a doctor kills a patient. Whether "killing" carries criminal culpability (the drug dealer), civil culpability (the doctor), or is righteous (the intended murder victim) depends on the context and circumstances.

A further nuance is realized when we discuss the removal of life support or letting a person die by stopping treatment. In both cases, suffering is reduced by stopping what is termed "futile care" - medical interventions that, if continued, would actually increase and prolong a person's suffering. This is in accordance with the ethical mandate to do no harm by letting nature take its course. It is the discernment of where the role of medical treatment ends, and the role of compassionate care becomes the singular focus wherein we sit as witnesses and fellow travellers into mystery.

Upon this continuum, proponents of euthanasia have successfully asserted their place on the moral spectrum. Unlike the other nuances of killing, this one is grounded in championing personal dignity, a term distorted by a desire for extreme autonomy. Yet, what is being asked here is not the right to die (there is no such thing, and claiming it is akin to claiming your right to be biological or three-dimensional), but the right to be killed. Dr. Donald Boudreau of McGill University, and Prof. Margaret Somerville, founder of the Centre for Ethics and Law at McGill, explore this in their article "Euthanasia and assisted suicide: a physician's and ethicist's perspectives." As I agree with their assessment that this is the most critical ethical conversation of the twenty-first century, it is wise for me to let them make the point in their own words:

> The "right to die" terminology is used in the euthanasia debate to propose that there is a right to have death inflicted. Death is inherent to the human body, vulnerable, and inexorably aging; death can be accelerated or temporarily delayed but never thwarted. The inevitability of death is an explicit, necessary, noncontingent, and universalizable phenomenon true for all living beings. There is no "right to die." In contradistinction, there are fundamental human rights to "life, liberty and security of the person."
>
> It's odd to hear advocates speak of MAiD as a right. You do not have a right to any medical intervention; instead, the healthcare system establishes best practices to treat your condition. Additionally, where there is a right, there is an obligation; therefore, were a "right to die" to exist, a logical consequence would be that some other person or agent would have a duty to inflict death (especially if the requisitioner were physically incapable of accomplishing the act themselves). Pro-euthanasia advocates rely heavily on this logic and have used it to impose responsibility for carrying out euthanasia onto the medical profession.
>
> The claim to a right to die must be distinguished from a "right to be allowed to die"; for instance, by refusing life-support treatment. The right to permit the dying process to unfold unimpeded flows from and is a consequence of persons exercising their right to inviolability, the right not to be touched without their informed consent. It does not establish any right to die in the sense of a "right to be killed."[168]

[168] Boudreau, J. Donald, and Margaret Somerville. "Euthanasia and assisted suicide." *Medicolegal and Bioethics* 4.1 (2014): pp. 1–11.

These nuances are not trivial – they are fundamental to our orientation towards life, suffering, death, decency, and destiny. Despite this, MAiD has allowed death to be considered a viable "treatment option" for those who find certain types of dying unacceptable. It has shifted death from an ineffable human destiny to a legislated human right. This is emphasized in arguments supporting individual autonomy in deciding when one's suffering becomes intolerable and when they choose to die. However, in places where assisted death has been made legal, the process works differently. Due to the necessary safeguards, the authority to decide who is eligible for this procedure rests with the assessors. If someone wishes to seek medical assistance to end their life, they must apply and appeal to a bureaucracy to determine their eligibility. The notion of absolute self-determination and individualism must acknowledge the necessary dependency on others at the end of life.[169] That's not you claiming independence and asserting your right. That's you appealing to an authority that is set above you. It is the relinquishing of your right to life to other people.

Furthermore, what is being sought is not only the right to end one's life, but also involving others in the process. MAiD results in unique forms of sociality and dependency that require terminally ill individuals and their caregivers to collaborate in orchestrating death. It is not the individual, but the MAiD assessors, who decide who will live and who will die, despite their deep compassion and good intentions. The purpose of the assessment is solely to determine eligibility and competency, not to address the existential distress that often underlies MAiD requests. While the assessment may identify this distress, it remains an unaddressed opportunity for deep preparation for the most significant event in a person's life: its end.

For several reasons, any of these assessments will be deeply flawed from their inception. First and most apparent, the assessors are not experts in existential distress. They have to take the patient's word at face value.

[169] Filene, P. *In the Arms of Others: A Cultural History of the Right-to-Die in America.* Chicago: Ivan R. Dee, 1998, p. 212.

Yet, the expressions, "I don't want to burden my family," "I don't want to become dependent," and "I don't see any purpose in suffering longer," are invitations to profound conversations on how to engage the *functional* process of ego-deconstruction, which facilitates opening to deeper dimensions of being (we will explore this in-depth later). What appears on the surface to be a request to end life is, underneath, a request to find meaning in suffering. Resistance to this deconstruction only increases existential distress. But most people are not aware of that dynamic. And the dying individual may not be interested in those conversations, especially when they are still problem-focused, especially when an injection seems to provide the solution. (And, let's be honest – few have ever wanted to do the work of engaging suffering as a process of transformation! Some seem to be natural at it, navigating the road with grace, but most have a very rough time.)

Second, medicine is, first and foremost, a technical discipline. The MAiD assessors and providers come from any medical specialty, so while they may be experts in neuroscience, family medicine, or gastric surgery, they are not trained in treating existential distress and have limited training in ethics. They likely have little experience being with the dying throughout the dying process. Research reveals that when healthcare professionals are called to respond to suffering, there are high levels of avoidance, denial, intellectualization, emotional disconnection, and intensified attempts to control processes that are not controllable.[170] It follows that doctors are under-qualified to make the normative judgment in assessing the appropriateness of euthanasia for a patient.[171]

Due to the primacy of patient autonomy and competency in declaring their pain intolerable, we have nothing else to go on. But can a person suffering such total pain of mind, body, and soul, indeed, be an expert in their condition? Anyone so compelled by existential distress that they

[170] Chen, Chuqian, Amy YM Chow, and Suqin Tang. "Professional caregivers' bereavement after patients' deaths: A scoping review of quantitative studies." *Death Studies* 43.8 (2019): pp. 500–508.

[171] Symons, Xavier. "Suffering, Euthanasia and Professional Expertise." *Solidarity: The Journal of Catholic Social Thought and Secular Ethics* 6.1 (2016): p. 5.

want someone to end their life is experiencing an overwhelmingly (and understandably) negative stance on fundamental questions about their existence: if it has meaning, value, and dignity. As such, they cannot engage their suffering as a process of further transformation through the graceful and grateful release of self. We see this inability through its psychosomatic effects – typically feelings such as weariness, numbness, futility, anxiety, hopelessness, helplessness, and a loss of control. As the provenance of these feelings is existential, not psychological, the appropriate referral would be to spiritual care professionals, who use a vocabulary distinct from psychology or medicine (and the patient would have to accept such a referral).

An additional ethical conundrum arises: physiological and psychological suffering is an *empirical* phenomenon. It can be measured using diagnostic tools. But existential suffering is an *axiological* state (pertaining to why something has value). This is not measurable by anyone except the one dying. It is not verifiable. How can it be assessed to justify ending a life? The appropriate response is to process this distress, not end it by ending everything. As the fear of future suffering, rather than the suffering itself, often drives requests, do we kill the person because they are afraid? Doctors need to practise epistemic humility not only as deference to a patient's wishes but as recognition that they are not qualified to treat existential distress. MAiD becomes a grossly inappropriate action in addressing suffering.

There is yet another paradox at play here. Suicide, although legal, is a form of ending a life that is culturally taboo and highly pathologized. On the other hand, MAiD is a form of ending a life that, while illegal throughout most of the world, is constructed as an act that can be publicly supported and understood. One might conclude, then, that suicide is destroying your life for distorted reasons, while MAiD is ending your life for reasonable ones. Yet, as requests for assisted death are driven by the existential distress boiling beneath the thin veneer of civilized composure, we know reason has very little to do with it. There is no emotion more primal than fear. There is no trigger more potent than death. Compound that with grief, physical deterioration, and likely hidden trauma, and what you have is a psychologically vulnerable population unable to accurately articulate their existential pain. It does not matter how educated and informed we are in this situation: even the most brilliant mind cannot speak through a crying heart. But they can appear calm, controlled, and quite reasonable during a MAiD assessment. They conceal the anguish, presenting as competent, because they want to be approved. They want to escape. Beneath that lies the brokenness few assessors would explore. In the end, suicide and MAiD are driven by similar distress: loss of meaning, spiritual suffering, and hopelessness. Yet this can be effectively treated, as we will explore in Chapter 18. The tragedy is that we have not yet stepped up to the challenge.

This clarification of language and terms is critical to our conversation, so it's helpful to listen to the voice that may be playing out in your mind right now. Here's how it might run: Does not a person have the right to choose how they respond to their suffering? Do we not have autonomy in this most important event in life? Well, yes, but only in relation to the public good, which changes over time. For example, smoking in public places was once acceptable, but no longer; the harm to others is now understood to be too great. OK, then, how could my choice for MAiD harm others? In several ways:

> MAiD normalizes a new relationship to suffering and death by normalizing assisted suicide, all the more appealing because it leaves the act to another, one in authority, one who is an expert: the doctor. Such trust is evident in the fact that 95 percent of euthanasia applicants ask the doctor to perform the act, even though they have the option to do it themselves.[172] While suicide was decriminalized in Canada in 1972, it remains a criminal offence to assist a suicide or counsel anyone to commit suicide – an interesting conundrum, to

[172] de Bellaigue, Christopher. "Death on demand: has euthanasia gone too far?" *The Guardian* (Jan. 18, 2019). https://www.theguardian.com/news/2019/jan/18/death-on-demand-has-euthanasia-gone-too-far-netherlands-assisted-dying Accessed Jan. 2, 2022.

> say the least, when talking about MAiD. Because suicide is an individual, self-administered act, its impact is limited to the person and their immediate social circle. (Suicide as an act of political protest is radically different, done for the benefit of societal reform, not to escape living.) In contrast, MAiD is a societal construct, with effects that are both insidious and far-reaching, impacting everyone, whether they realize it or not, especially as MAiD poses to society that a difficult life is not worth living and a difficult death is devoid of meaning, instead of the message that both call on us as a community to support the least among us through the best within us. One is a way out, the other a way through. But, now with MAiD legalized, that way is not on the radar for an increasing number of the dying. They remain unaware of the potential of counselling and compassion to restore their Ground of Being. All they feel is that it is crumbling. Life is disintegrating before their eyes. What power would something as "fluffy" as compassion, counselling, and community possibly hold in the face of such overwhelming despair? (Interestingly, it was thought suicide rates would decrease after its adoption. The opposite has proven to be true.[173])

More terminology problems: dying with dignity is a term that speaks to the desire to restore and maintain self-worth at the end of life. However, this term once again belongs to the realm of the ego. It is dignity defined by who you think you are, who you want to be, your appearance, your agency, your autonomy, self-determination, and personal will. Your body, your life, your choice. This is a natural and completely understandable assertion in today's culture, but from a spiritual perspective, it's all part of the ego's narrative.

---

[173] Jones, David Albert. "In Europe, suicides rise after 'right-to-die' is legalised, says bioethicist." BioEdge: Bioethics News from Around the World. Feb. 19, 2022. https://bioedge.org/end-of-life-issues/euthanasia/in-europe-suicides-rise-after-right-to-die-is-legalised-says-bioethicist/ Accessed Feb. 27, 2022.

In contrast is the deeper dimension of being, found through vulnerability, compassion, silence, contemplation, and surrender to what is by allowing it. This is a spiritual practice; admittedly, few of us do well. Stephen Levine sums it up concisely: "Detachment means letting go… non-attachment means… letting be."[174] In this expansive state of non-attachment, your self-worth is no longer determined by what you do, who you are, or even who you believe yourself to be. Your worth–and thus your dignity–is inherent in your existence. As your life nears its end, this becomes the dominant truth, while all else falls away.

The experience of dying with dignity depends on the dying person knowing that their loved ones, carers, and strangers perceive them to be fully human, regardless of their frailty. However, the more one asserts one's will to preserve the ego's identity of self, the more this will feel like an abstract proposition. This should come as no surprise, given our spiritual poverty and unfamiliarity with the language and process of ego deconstruction at the end of life. These dynamics are well captured by the often-irritating aphorism: a bad day for your ego is a good day for your soul.

This truth is actualized only through the last thing you may want to do: allow it all. Turn toward what is, without control, but with acceptance of the whole mess within: all the fear, all the anxiety, all the grief, all the apprehension of suffering ahead, and all the power of how that mess *increases* your suffering in the present moment. You can't get away from it, so you may as well turn toward it with kindness, curiosity, and compassion. This is what Pema Chödrön means by *the wisdom of no escape.* For beneath it all lies unfiltered awareness as a singular expression of life in this vast cosmos. Beneath all the turmoil lies your true dignity.

"Hmmm," you may be thinking. "Then somebody give me a shovel because I don't know where to dig, how to dig, or how long it will take to uncover that dignity you speak of." Well, you're holding the shovel right now. Let's dig.

---

[174] Levine, Stephen. *A Year To Live: How To Live this Year as If It Were Your Last.* Harmony, 2009, p. 95.

EXERCISE 12: THE POWER OF WORDS

Take a few moments to sit in a quiet and comfortable space. Close your eyes and bring your attention to your breath. Allow yourself to become present and grounded in the moment. When you feel ready, engage with the following reflection questions:

> *What emotional effect do each of the following terms have on your perception of and considerations around the end of your life?*
>
> - *Medically assisted death*
> - *Withdrawal of treatment*
> - *End-of-life options*
> - *Dying with dignity*
> - *Comfort measures*
> - *Assisted suicide*
> - *Natural death*
> - *Euthanasia*
> - *Kill*ing
>
> *How would you describe MAiD in direct terms?*

CHAPTER 13

PALLIATIVE CARE

We cannot change the outcome. But we can affect the journey.

– ANN RICHARDSON

HARRIET SCOTT BELIEVED THAT STAYING PHYSICALLY ACTIVE AND maintaining her weight would keep her healthy. Then she was diagnosed with terminal liver cancer, with only two months to live. Harriet was determined to prove her cancer doctor wrong – she would not allow someone else, even fate, to determine her time of death. She had been in control all her life and wanted to die that way, too. A natural death without any pain would be preferable, but if she suffered in the future, she planned to take things into her own hands. This is because thirty-eight years ago, she watched her mother suffer terribly from bone cancer and become addicted to morphine. Harriet was forever imprinted with that memory, and combined with her independent determination, her desire for assisted death was quite understandable.

She planned her funeral, wrote her obituary, and discussed these openly with friends and family. Harriet planned to die before the pain became intolerable, as she was already well past her "best before date," the date her oncologist said she would die. Harriet had no spiritual wrestling on the matter, for she was an atheist. "There's nothing. Nothing. I think it's just over. I don't think I'll have to pay for the sins I've committed, all the bad things I've done. It's just over." Her main concern was Ron, her husband, who had Parkinson's. Overall, though, life became peaceful. Their grieving had been processed smoothly. Sitting on the deck, they enjoyed their coffee, the cream of extended days, and the clarity that comes with a plan.

"I don't want to die when I'm having a good day," she said. "But I want to die when I can still do it." And she did not want to put her husband in the position of making that decision. "If I have uncontrollable pain, I'll do it."

Weeks later, she woke with intolerable pain in her belly. She ended up in the hospital, where pain relief was readily available and much better managed. All the same, it was difficult for her to rely on others, her nurses, and the medical system. Death anxiety was eroding her composure. "It's more scary now. I wanted more time. It's happening too quickly, and I'm a bit annoyed. It's not happening according to my plan."

What was the most important part of that plan? Seeing her son, Adam, who wanted to travel home from Europe immediately to be at her side. Ever practical, she insisted he complete university. "There's no point in him coming if I'm unconscious. I just want to hold him, have physical contact, maybe talk about the past, but he doesn't want to do that. I tend to keep wanting to apologize for bad parenting and my mistakes. I just want to hug him and hold him and have him be my child a little bit longer."

And she did. A blood transfusion extended her days to the one she had marked on the calendar, the day her son arrived. She looked strikingly different, a withered form with sunken cheeks and hollow eyes. She held his hand and said, "I saw the calendar and felt such a peace. So at peace. My journey is complete. So happy," she whispered. In the end, finding the peaceful death she wanted meant not going it alone. The next day she died by MAiD, surrounded by love.

Harriet's story echoes the experiences of many facing terminal illness. Dreading the suffering ahead, she did not realize how physical pain could be controlled under palliative care, nor that much had changed in the thirty-plus years since her mother's death. Above all, she could not comprehend how love could alleviate her existential pain until she experienced the unexpected peace and happiness that enveloped her through her son's presence. The central element of death could not be less medical:

it's all about love. Everything – our identity, accomplishments, dreams fulfilled and those left untried… all boils down to love. One can certainly argue that it's about the experience, too, but the experience is hollow without company.

Harriet's death is marked by all the themes common to the modern mind as the final day approaches. She wanted to be in control. She wanted her dignity intact. She wanted to protect her husband and son from the final disintegration of her being. She wanted death on her terms. She had no knowledge of the natural process by which her ego-identity, so dominant throughout life and even more at the end, would be whittled away through dying. She only knew she did not like it. She did not want the wilderness, the transformative fields of chaos. And, in her maternal instinct to care for her son, to protect him from the final breaths, she did not know that in her dying, she would teach the ultimate lessons of life: to say the final words, to feel the weight of grief, and to engage it as a healthy expression of love. And, with good palliative care, how to trust the body's processes in dying. She only knew that she hated the dependency, loved her son, and that MAiD appeared to be so sensible.

These are the lessons end-of-life medical professionals know well, which makes it all the more ironic that the field is so misunderstood. The public tends to see it as the last stand, so moving to palliative care gets labelled as giving up. This arises out of the confrontational language around cancer – the fight, the battle, the brave soul, the feeling that one must do everything possible, instead of everything reasonable, to extend life for the sake of those you love. You can't let them down, so you can't give up. How unfortunate, as palliative care can make such a difference, transforming the dread of dying into the depth of living to the very last moment.

Palliative care emerged from the way death became medicalized in postindustrial societies. *Palliate* means "serving to mitigate or alleviate" suffering. Technology and specialization in Western cultures removed death from the home to "treat" it in hospitals and other institutions. In the 1950s, physicians in Britain and the United States started approaching the care of terminal patients with a resolve to provide active care to the end of life – a significant improvement over the standard line, "there's nothing we can do." As the decades progressed, respect for patient autonomy improved as well. Previously, the doctor wouldn't even say the word cancer out of concern that the stress would cause more suffering. Now informed consent lies at the heart of medical care. (BTW, that's also why I'm writing this book. If you're considering MAiD, the ultimate act, you should be fully informed of its nature.)

Dame Cicily Saunders started formal palliative care as a wartime nurse, ironically because of her first-hand experience with assisted death. That experience was visceral, as recounted by David Clark in his book, *Cicely Saunders: A Life and Legacy.* She had been caring for a young boy, about five years old, suffering from a brain tumour. His constant crying was met with an imperious command from the professor of pediatrics: "I do not expect to see that child when I come back next week." Cicely Saunders writes,

> That night, the houseman came in and wrote up a large dose of an opiate and, between the two of us, we gave it. I mean, the Night Sister knew about it… I don't remember which of us gave the injection. But I knew it was wrong. I felt helpless and I really had to back up the houseman. We were just stuck, but, of course, thinking about it now, there were no alternatives. There was no palliative medicine. It didn't exist. The child didn't, in fact, die that night. We had to repeat it and he died the second night. It's extremely vivid to me now. I can place that cot exactly where it was in the ward. I think it may have been one of the roots of why I wanted to do something about palliative care.[175]

Despite Dame Cicely Saunders's strong opposition to euthanasia, many patients now request it as part of palliative care. I often encounter this in our unit, where the boundaries between palliative care and MAiD can blur. Some palliative care physicians perform assessments,

[175] Clark, David. *Cicely Saunders: A Life and Legacy.* Oxford University Press, 2018.

and the procedure can be carried out on palliative floors. Is it not, then, part of our service?[176] Not according to the World Health Organization, the Canadian Hospice Palliative Care Association, or most palliative care associations worldwide.[177,178] This position stemmed not only from the view that medicine must not hasten death but from the experience of Dame Cicely Saunders and the other founders of hospice and palliative care.

Physicians who carry out the procedure often do not even specialize in palliative care – they may be neurologists, orthopedic surgeons, or family doctors. All medical doctors of all specialties can provide MAiD. This means not all (and I would not be surprised to find that very few) are familiar with what it's like to be with the dying, let alone know how to handle the existential distress that fuels the request. That's a problem not only for the patients and their families but the docs as well. Will this be the primary lens through which they experience dying?

How ironic that palliative care has its roots in preventing euthanasia. Even more ironic is that both address a person's primal need to feel safe in the face of death, one through excellent end-of-life care and the second through ending life. To add to that irony, polls show that about while 85% of Canadians want to die at home, over 60% die in a hospital.[179] Fewer than 30% of Canadians have access to high-quality hospice palliative care, despite 90% of all deaths in Canada potentially benefiting from it.[180] And,

---

[176] Excellent guidelines for healthcare professionals are available to help guide that discussion. See "Canadian Hospice Palliative Care Association. *Hospice Palliative Care and Medical Assistance in Dying (MAiD) in Canada: How Will They Co-Exist?* June 2017. https://www.chpca.ca/wp-content/uploads/2019/12/ chpca-maid-booklet-eng-12page-final-web.pdf. Accessed Jan. 10, 2021.

[177] International Association for Hospice and Palliative Care. "Statements on Euthanasia and Physician Assisted Suicide." https://hospicecare.com/policy-and-ethics/ethical-issues/statements-on-euthanasia-and-physician-assisted-suicide/ Accessed Jan. 10, 2021.

[178] Radbruch, Lukas, et al. "Euthanasia and physician-assisted suicide: A white paper from the European Association for Palliative Care." *Palliative Medicine* 30.2 (2016): pp. 104–116.

[179] Statistics Canada. Table 102-0509. Deaths in hospital and elsewhere, Canada, provinces and territories, annual, CANSIM Accessed Dec. 20, 2020.

[180] Quality End-of-Life Care Coalition of Canada and Canadian Hospice Palliative Care Association. "The Way Forward National Framework; a Roadmap for an Integrated Palliative Approach to Care." Mar. 2015.

while the majority of people who receive MAiD do so while under palliative service,[181] the extent of that palliative care is poorly described in the research.[182] The issue is that Canadians' access to palliative care is not considered a fundamental health care right. In contrast, MAiD has been deemed a right through the Canada Health Act, even though deaths from MAiD account for about 3 percent of all deaths in Canada.[183]

The system is clearly in need of reform since palliative care delivered at home is far less expensive than a hospital stay and far better for the family. All can participate in providing care; all can be a part of the most significant event of life and the most profound expression of love. Generations have done this from time immemorial, with children, elders, and everyone in between playing their part in providing a dignified death.

How far that is from today's reality, for multiple reasons: depersonalized care, mismanaged medical technologies, institutionalized dying, and diminished patient and familial control of the dying process. Courtney Campbell, Professor in Religion and Culture at Oregon State University, concludes from this that it is "ethically premature to conclude that the primary way to remedy the medicalized culture of bad dying is allowing physicians to be directly involved in ending the life of the patient."[184]

It is, therefore, important that we identify identify the systemic aspects where solutions lie. First, ensure clear conversations with families so that their loved ones transition to palliative care instead of an intensive care

---

[181] During 2021, the majority of MAiD recipients (80.7%) received palliative care. This compares similarly to 2019 and 2020 (82.1% and 82.8% respectively). Of the MAiD recipients who did not receive palliative care, 88.0 percent had access to these services if they required them. "Fourth Interim Report on Medical Assistance in Dying in Canada." Health Canada. https://www.canada.ca/en/health-canada/services/publications/health-system-services/medical-assistance-dying-interim-report-april-2019.html. Accessed Dec. 29, 2022.

[182] Chochinov, Harvey Max. "Medical Assistance in Dying, Data and Casting Assertions Aside." *Journal of Palliative Medicine* (2022).

[183] "Fourth Interim Report on Medical Assistance in Dying in Canada." Health Canada. https://www.canada.ca/en/health-canada/services/publications/health-system-services/medical-assistance-dying-interim-report-april-2019.html. Accessed Dec. 29, 2022.

[184] Campbell, Courtney S. "Focus: Death: Mortal Responsibilities: Bioethics and Medical-Assisted Dying." *The Yale Journal of Biology and Medicine* 92.4 (2019): 733.

unit, where patients and families will often insist on doing everything possible, resulting in more suffering and prolonged death. Treating pain, reducing suffering in all dimensions, and maximizing quality of life is the wisest path, especially as we can foresee most deaths coming. Every year one in one hundred Canadians dies from one of the top four causes: heart disease, cancer, diabetes, or COPD. Eighty percent of those are people over the age of sixty-five. We know these diseases well, so how people decline and die is fairly predictable. Why, then, do so many people – three in five – die in hospitals, where they often end up in intensive care units receiving unnecessarily aggressive treatment? Better to train our doctors and staff in having difficult conversations about the end of life and clarifying goals of care. Better to promote advanced care directives and engage creative ways for families to use them early in the disease trajectory.

Second, since the goal is to decrease hospital admissions, increase resources for home palliative care teams, specifically for the psychosocial and spiritual care practitioners who specialize in addressing and treating existential distress. This is a far more economical way to provide care, as some indices show that over 60 percent of health care costs are incurred in the last six months of a person's life. In the last 180 days of life for patients with cancer, Canada had the highest per capita hospital expenditures at USD 21,840, compared to the United States, Norway, Germany, Belgium, and the Netherlands.[185] Counselling at the end of life decreases the existential distress driving the demand for these extreme and expensive interventions.

Third, increase the number of hospice beds. Hospices are centres that specialize in providing the absolute best care at life's end. Though it may sound bold, hospice care truly offers the highest standard of comfort. When you're dying, you deserve to be pampered! Most hospices in Canada are built through philanthropic giving and fundraising. While the government partially funds their clinical operation, it is estimated that more

[185] Isenberg, Sarina R., et al. "The association between varying levels of palliative care involvement on costs during terminal hospitalizations in Canada from 2012 to 2015." *BMC Health Services Research* 21.1 (2021): pp. 1–12.

than 50 percent of the overall operating expenses must be raised year after year to make up for shortfalls, and many of them rely on volunteers.[186]

Fourth, increase home care services. This nursing support goes above and beyond, taking on the basics of cleaning, food preparation, and daily tasks, as well as providing companionship and medical care for the dying individual. This team plays a significant role in palliative care, but it is grossly underfunded and operates as a hybrid model, charging for most of its services. Without adequate coverage, practical support like this is unrealistic for many.

Fifth, allow palliative care and active treatment to overlap. In most provinces, a referral to palliative care is not done until treatment to manage the disease has stopped. This leaves a person in limbo for a brief period (that does not feel brief!), wondering who is caring for them after the news that treatments are no longer effective.

Sixth, increase funding for psychosocial care to help patients and their families engage the non-medical aspects of dying. This must include psychospiritual therapists, trained to address the existential aspects of dying. Those therapists must be well-versed in ego-deconstruction, the transformative fields of chaos, and the transpersonal dimensions of consciousness that follow. We must be able to provide a coherent roadmap of your transformation.

Finally, there's the elephant in the room, the most significant player at the end of life: long-term care facilities. Here the costs quickly run into thousands per month, where the estate is spent on quality of life in the final years. Yet only 6 percent of residents receive palliative care.[187] Canada ended up with the worst record for COVID-19 deaths in long-term care homes compared with other wealthy countries.[188]

---

[186] "Fact Sheet: Hospice Palliative Care in Canada." Canadian Hospice Palliative Care Association. https://www.chpca.ca/wp-content/uploads/2019/12/new_fact_sheet_hpc_in_canada-summer2017-final-en.pdf Accessed Dec. 20, 2020.

[187] "Access to Palliative Care in Canada." Canadian Institute of Health Information. https://www.cihi.ca/sites/default/files/document/access-palliative-care-2018-en-web.pdf. Accessed Dec. 20, 2021.

[188] "Long-term Care and COVID-19: The First 6 Months." Canadian Institute of Health Information. https://www.cihi.ca/en/long-term-care-and-covid-19-the-first-6-months. Accessed Dec. 20, 2021.

The way forward rests on the willpower to make fundamental changes to our health care system. Ultimately, reforming end-of-life care requires a deeper understanding of both the physical and existential dimensions of dying. Only by addressing these comprehensively can we ensure that every person's final journey is one of dignity and love. While there now is a National Palliative Care Strategy, whether it will receive adequate funding is yet to be seen. Creative delivery of these services is more possible than ever, with remote or virtual medical appointments now common and cost-efficient. However, actual human contact and support are what's needed. It is essential to the human condition when leaving this world. At life's end, it needs to be imparted in person, hearts ready, all hands on deck.

EXERCISE 13: MAKING A PLAN

Making a plan for the ultimate trip is best done early. Explore how at advancecareplanning.ca. You can also print and do the exercise in the document "What's Important to Me," found at bit.ly/3MoRgAT.

PART 3

MAiD AND MEANING

CHAPTER 14

A DISTANT SHORE

Sunset and evening star,
And one clear call for me!
And may there be no moaning of the bar,
When I put out to sea.

– ALFRED, LORD TENNYSON

PANCREATIC CANCER WASTES NO TIME. ONLY A FEW WEEKS LAY BEtween diagnosis and death. The swelling came first; a duct was occluded by the tumour. Scans showed the dark mass extending from the head of the pancreas, and given his ninety-one years, the path forward for this patient seemed clear. But the man I was sitting with was no ordinary patient, and this would be a death unlike any I had ever known. This man was my father. A retired naval officer and perpetual pragmatist, he looked at the doctor and asked the key questions plainly: how long do I have, what suffering should I expect, and what can be done to mitigate it?

"I would expect a couple of months, maybe three," came the reply. The doc knew my father could handle it straight, no chaser. "The pain should be manageable, as it hasn't spread to the intestine or stomach. If there's no nerve involvement, then we'd manage your discomfort with injected morphine. I would imagine the bile duct could become blocked, resulting in jaundice and fatigue. You likely will also have more fluid building up in your belly, and while this can be drained through a needle, eventually, we leave it at the end. You'll become tired, more dependent on others, and then pass." He paused, letting emotional weight register in his expression and allowing the words to sink in.

"Right," said Dad. "Right." His eyes became distant, as if seeking a far-off shore. He shifted in his seat. "Well, that sounds like I'm heading out. We should set things up to make sure it all goes smoothly." He looked at me, nodded. I could see the goodbyes already beginning, the realization of leaving this world. "I presume, then, that I won't be seeing you anymore, doctor. Thank you for your service; I appreciate all you've done." Then the pause, the sigh.

The doctor waited a bit longer before responding. "I'm sorry I couldn't do more. I'm sorry it turns out this way. It's been an honour caring for you."

Dad smiled. "Well, ninety-one years. Not bad! It's been a good run. A good run. Thank you." He rose. They shook hands, and the doctor gave me his card in case we had any questions later on. We moved quietly to the fresh morning air. The sunlight played upon Dad's face as we sat in the car, oddly accepting of this final chapter. I was grateful to be there, to hold the moment with as few words as possible. This also allowed me to embrace my own grief, to quietly contemplate the gift of this man.

The ride home was marked by a mixture of life stories and strategies for what to do next. I knew the palliative care team in his area, and he knew he wanted to die at home, surrounded by family and friends. This was just as the pandemic was unfolding, and he joked that it would be better if he left early in case he got infected, making his condition worse. I assisted him from the car to the door, to his favourite chair. And then, I did something I rarely did with my father. I sat close, held his hand, gazed and waited. And with that, he raised it. A slight hesitation, then a soft tremor in his voice... "If it gets too difficult, I could use MAiD. I know you're involved in that at the hospital... I'm just thinking of how rough it could get for everyone. What are your thoughts?"

Gulp. Already? Well, who could blame him? He knew time was short, and he understood that suffering could escalate suddenly. "Can you tell me more about what you feel?" I asked. "What specifically are you most concerned about?" I wanted him to go deeper, to help him process his fears, his grief, to speak his imagination into being, so we could explore it together and discern the deeper themes within it. Easy enough to do with a patient, but here, again, was my parent considering an early exit. And, here again, I felt the lump in my heart, my throat, churned up by the prospect of bypassing the hard work of dying.

"I'm concerned about the pain. It's hard enough. . . ." He paused. "It's hard enough going through this weakness, this swelling. But what if it becomes more than I can bear? And, more importantly, puts you all through utter misery?"

My response came as fast as it had with my mother. "We would welcome the role of supporting you through the misery, Dad. We would be honoured to be at your side every step of the way and to do every awkward thing there is to do. Besides, we can ensure you're too drugged to be embarrassed." Ah, humour. If comedy is tragedy in hindsight, I was getting ahead of myself.

He smiled at that. "But what would it mean? What does it look like? You've seen it. Tell me."

Again, straight, no chaser. "That's a great question for the palliative care team. They are the experts in pain, suffering, and how to make sure you're comfortable. They will also guide us in how to care for you."

"But what have you seen?" he pressed.

"Well, with pancreatic cancer, I have seen considerable pain when it gets into the nerves, as your doctor mentioned. Pain meds do well but leave you sleepy and drifting. It will be on you to tell us accurately how much pain you're in and not to be shy about taking meds like morphine regularly, every four hours, even if you're comfortable. The purpose of those meds is to stay ahead of the pain. You don't want to chase it. If it doesn't go into the nerves, as is the case with you, the swelling from fluid buildup in your abdomen is the main issue. That fluid is coming from the cancer cells, which are growing rapidly. Draining is straightforward but is done in the hospital. I hope that means day trips, but you might have some overnight stays."

Too many words. I paused. "This is an excellent conversation to have with your palliative home-care team. They can address it far better than I can. But I'd like to understand what you imagine it would be like to lose all autonomy and depend on us."

"I trust you can do it. I'm grateful you can do it. I want you to do it. But I've never done it before... as far as I know... what is this thing you talk about... deconstruction?"

"Ah, that's the stuff you're going through now. Dying gradually diminishes your role in the world. In the end, your identity is reduced to the essentials: thoughts and feelings, as you lie in bed, eventually unable to lift even your head. People naturally resist this, even resent it. They understandably get frustrated, sometimes more demanding. They wrestle with their grief, get angry at times. It all depends on your personality, your life story, your acceptance of the process. Yet, even with full acceptance, it feels like sinking to rock bottom. Your body is also disintegrating, slowly shutting down. You stop eating, drinking, and moving except for breath, which is laboured. We turn you to prevent sores and skin abrasions, to shift the weight of bones on the bed."

I was being graphic because he deserved to know. Dad had read my first book, which had plenty of examples of what dying was like and the mystical shift with nearing-death awareness. We discussed my near-death experience, the nature of my work and the accounts I hear monthly from my patients. He was familiar with such hope, but this was walking the road, this was the entrance to the wilderness. You do not rush this stage.

"It's hard, Dad. It's really hard. And it's why many request MAiD – to avoid the suffering they imagine to come. But, the drugs will keep you as comfortable as possible. And I hope the love and care will help you feel safe. You sleep a lot. Eventually, you undergo a shift in consciousness, often a profound sense of peace, expansion, and then transformation into wonder. But this usually takes far longer than you want it to. Even with the best of care, it is a challenging experience." Time to pause again.

"Well... sounds quite unpleasant. But I guess if it's going to happen, I have the best around me to do it." My father's assessment: ever practical, always balancing the worst of what could happen with how we can respond to it. "What I worry about most is the pain. And if you say it can be controlled, then that's what I'll go on. I'll discuss it with the doctor."

"OK. I hope you can always feel that you're the captain of the ship. The medical team and we are your crew. Just tell us what you need, and we'll jump to it."

I offered this encouragement because my father has always been tied to the sea. Born on a small Caribbean island, he joined the Merchant Marine in his teens and served in the British and Canadian navies, then the coast guard. The sea was his life. A captain, a nautical historian, and a man who preferred things to be upfront, this final voyage stirred within him profound sentiments of gratitude for family and friends. Getting things shipshape meant he made sure to say all the important last words through letters and phone calls, emails, and in-person visits. Expressions of gratitude and love, forgiveness and goodbyes were the order of the day. And, for us, his children and grandchildren, extended family and friends, caring for him became the order of our day. My two sisters focused on physical care. They had the experience of supporting our mother for so many years at home, lifting, turning, and washing her aging form. My older brother, an accountant, took care of the estate as executor. The younger was a gopher for everyone and had been an excellent support for our father, living with him for the past two years. I did what chaplains do – I counselled and witnessed the love pouring into the apartment.

It only took a few weeks, as the doctor had assessed. Dad's strength evaporated as the fluid built up in his abdomen, and we knew the time was short. Children took turns staying the night and dividing the day into shifts of care. Movement from bed to bathroom was always with assistance, and he was gracious with our taking over every aspect of personal life, actually enjoying the constant company. That company included one who was a profound gift in the last two years of Dad's life. He had met Susan at a community dance, something our father enjoyed immensely. Interest in this "much younger woman" grew into a deep friendship, an unexpected companionship that made a ninety-one-year-old feel like he was fifty again. For us, his children, it was one more way our father showed us that life is to be embraced and that gratitude and a bit of mischief can make one feel young again.

"What a wonderful way to end," he said at my side one Sunday afternoon. "I'm very content, you know. It's been a great life... not without setbacks, but you can't let those define your days. And you're all doing so well with this; you all seem to know exactly what I need. Hopefully, the rest will go smoothly, and I'll leave in my sleep. That would be good." His voice was soft, the accumulating fluid making breath shallow, and words all the more precious.

"How have you been sleeping, Dad? Any dreams?" Here was the chaplain, assessing for shifts in consciousness as death approached. The early indications often manifest in dreams, a side-door entrance to the soul that bypasses the ego, which guards the front door of the self against anything that threatens its existence. My father paused, then his eyes softened and suddenly teared up. He looked at me and shifted in the chair.

"Actually, about two weeks ago... I had the most wonderful dream. All the dogs I have ever known came to me. All of them. And I felt such love, such gratitude from them, such joy." The tears began to fall. "It was an open white space; it was... wonderful. And it felt so real, so intense. Do you think it was real?"

I smiled. Pets often appear in dreams during the process of dying, and communication with them is reported as astonishingly clear and joyful. This was a sign that the process of shifting to a transpersonal state of being had begun – the wisdom wired into my father to leave this world was emerging. "Yes, yes, I encourage you to trust it was real. And they will be among the company of all who have died, waiting to receive you with great love, joy, and open arms. It's going to be quite the reunion."

Dad wept softly, an expression of astonishment upon his face, and breathed a heavy sigh of relief. "Amazing. Amazing. This is what you've been talking about, but I didn't know I'd see my dogs."

"Well, you know what Will Rogers said: "I don't want to go to heaven if there aren't any dogs."[189] He smiled, and I appeared intelligent and witty. Win-win.

Dad gave himself to death with little resistance but with much gratitude. He made sure to share how proud he was of all of us. He unpacked his life through stories of his career and his adventures, which my sister wisely recorded. And he gave away his repository of knowledge in naval history through his vast collection of books, carefully considering the best individuals and organizations that would appreciate them. He had written three on the Canadian Coast Guard and was an expert on nautical esoterica, especially vexillology – the study of flags. Passing on this legacy enabled Dad to give himself entirely to the final release: that of his body.

Days later, he lay prone in his bed. We turned him on request every hour or two as the fluid pressed uncomfortably upon his organs. A nurse also stayed the night and drew up the medications, but we administered them at the scheduled time. Sleep had, indeed, become the order of the day, with intermittent periods of consciousness. We made sure someone was always at his side, able to affirm the love and attend to his needs. Some of us slept in the living room on the couch, on the floor, in the recliner.

I recall one time sitting at his side. My father opened his eyes to see my appreciative gaze. "Hi," I said softly.

"Oh…" he said. "Every time I open my eyes, I see someone smiling."

"Yes," I replied. "Which means you're still here. But you're doing it, Dad. You're moving toward transformation. We love you. We're all together, gathered in the living room."

He closed his eyes. "Good… good… good… ." It was the last thing I heard him say. Rising from his side, I returned to the family and the hot pizza that had just arrived while a sister spelled me off. Stories and photo albums, memories and quiet music, card games and confessions of

---

[189] The actual quote from Will Rogers is "If there are no dogs in Heaven, then when I die I want to go where they went." https://www.goodreads.com/quotes/18943-if-there-are-no-dogs-in-heaven-then-when-i Accessed June 27, 2021.

teenage foolishness marked the hours until sleep called us away. As it was so crowded, I decided to take a room at a hotel. Stars shone in the clear sky, but the road seemed darker, the velvet blackness swallowing my headlights. Afterwards, I wished I had stayed at the house to share what would happen. But, it seems, it was not something for me or anyone else to witness except the newest companion in his final years.

Four a.m. Susan was at his side; his best friend, love's unexpected gift to a man who had ridden the waves of life for almost a century. Dad lay in deep unconsciousness. He had not stirred for hours; his breath was soft and shallow. The air seemed still. And then, it happened. His eyes popped open. He raised his head and shoulders. His face lit up, ecstatic. "Yes, yes. I understand. I'm going now." And then, sinking back, his eyes closed, body heavy once again. Susan sat in shock, skin tingling. Should she wake the others? Should she gather the grieving to witness the final breath? For some wise and hidden reason, she did not. She gazed at her friend, opened to the mystery, held his hand, sent in the love, and waited. All her attention was on him, and she gave herself calmly to the moments ahead.

Stillness. Breathing. An hour passed. Then, again, he opened his eyes. This time, he pulled his hand away with force as if the physical sensation was too crude and incongruous with what he was now witnessing. This time, he sat up... well, more like he bolted up... astonishing, given his deterioration and the fluid swelling his belly. Then, throwing his arms up and out, he grasped for an unseen embrace at the ceiling, trying to reach someone. Looking to a hidden land, his face ecstatic with awe, he called to them. "Yes, come, come to me, come to me!" Susan, witnessing the joy, was struck by this sudden vitality. She knew she was not alone. She knew his welcoming party was just beyond her vision. And then, his body shut down again. He slumped back to the bed, back to the deep sleep before death, and never awoke again.

It was 6 a.m. when my phone rang. Everyone was up. Dad's breathing had changed yet again, and there was obvious distress this time. He moaned. He winced in pain. We arrived within minutes; medications were administered but to little effect. We had breakthrough doses and a massive amount of morphine drawn and ready. But neither the nurse nor we were comfortable giving them without the doctor's go-ahead. Fortunately, she responded to our text immediately and said, in no uncertain terms, "Don't be shy with the meds!" We administered the breakthrough dose, and he sank into sweet narcotic slumber.

We were so grateful he was unaware, for the abdominal fluid was pressing upon his stomach, pushing digestive juices up. It gurgled in his throat and began to flow from his mouth. We cleared the thick, dark brown gunk with sponges, filling the small garbage can. There was no disgust, no hesitation, no comment at all. This was an act of love. This was the least we could do.

Our father wanted to avoid this in his consideration of MAiD – the utter dependency, the pain, and the descent into darkness while his body slowly dissolved. He could not imagine this stage of dying. And, with MAiD, we do not even allow it. We have the power to prevent the process, which, as we have explored, brings great comfort to the ego and the perceived and experienced self. Yet, in our effort to control this chaos, I would assert that we limit ourselves. We fail to imagine or realize the deepest dimension of our being; we sabotage the wisdom wired into us from birth to emerge through the final stage of life into something more ineffable, something more sublime. This is marked by the most remarkable quality, for the dying have an even more astonishing power within this frailty, subtle and supernatural in its perfection. When pain is controlled (perhaps even when it is not), they can wait until everyone is where they should be. More than that, they seem to discern where everyone will be. It's as if they orchestrate us into place. Sometimes, this means getting family members away from the bedside. Whether this is to protect them or shun them, I don't know. Often, it means getting them close. I've seen countless patients exercise this, an arrangement we only realized in hindsight. It makes one wonder what abilities lie latent within us through the decades, only to be awakened when the ego has been sufficiently dissolved. I trust this ability enabled my father to remain with us a bit longer, for one brother had returned to his home, an hour away, to get a good night's rest. The decision seemed reasonable at the time but infuriating when we realized the last breath was imminent. One sister, ever wise, assured us that if Dad wanted all his kids to be present, he'd hang on. And he did just that. It was 9:30 a.m. before we heard our brother's car pull in. And these ninety minutes enabled us to move to ever deeper levels of liminal time. Grandchildren practised the art of holding space, a central skill of the vigil. All of us were gifted with the infuriating homework of navigating anxiety, working with worry, breathing into the edge of the abyss, surrendering to suspension. Only in this state could we experience how we were held by grace – God's infinite wisdom, kindness, and mercy. It is difficult to describe… but it's much like a loving parent enfolding his anxious children and the soft words of comfort ensuring you are safe and that all will be well. "I've got this," came the whisper, felt in the heart. "I've got you."

Dad seemed to sense the change as we gathered around his bed, for within moments, his breathing became even softer.

"It's happening," I said. My sister squeezed my hand as another said the essential words the dying must hear.

"Thank you, Dad. Off you go. Off you go. Love you." I think we all echoed that, but I was also aware that the air seemed thicker, as if there was pressure on my ears. I sensed how very different this felt from all my patients and realized this was the first time I had experienced the death of someone I loved. Here was grief from the inside. And, here was my father, about to enter the realm I had only touched upon in my near-death experience thirty years earlier. Suddenly, secretly, I was envious of the joy, of the astonishing authenticity and integration he was to know. I remembered it all as if it had happened yesterday. One aspect of this temporary transformation is that it never fades but leaves you homesick, heartsick, for what you saw, what you were, what you fundamentally know and yet cannot explain. Let me try, nonetheless.

Here, in this incarnate form, we are fractured, fumbling creatures. Our awareness, the perceived self, is like the tip of an iceberg. The ego is blind to the enormous material of the subconscious, the suppressed material that lies beneath the surface. I cannot truly know myself from within my own experience or even know my world as it truly is. The apparatus of my senses filter that external reality – eyes only receive a tiny fraction of the light spectrum, and ears hear a paucity of the frequencies around me. The brain's wetware is a reducing valve, processing only what is required for biological survival. But in death, we undergo a transformation, an expansion of awareness to realize all that is, all that we are. No aspect of ourselves is hidden… we are integrated, authentic, whole, and awake. This is why many who have a near-death experience call that state "home." Finally, we are home – no longer a stranger to ourselves or others, no longer separate entities. We are one, yet we remain aware that we are unique expressions of that One. I tasted this at twenty-seven years of age. Now, at ninety-one, my father would become that, any moment now… any moment…

His breath paused. The seconds slowed to a snail's pace. I felt my heart beating and imagined his slowing, stopping. Another breath, even softer. It was like listening for a sonar wave to return, indicating a Presence somewhere out there in deep time. Another gentle exhalation. Then… nothing. It was as if his soul, the life within, was so amorphous and sublime that it could only be carried away on a whisper, on the trailing edge of a feather's current, on that final, gentle breath. One moment he was there; the next, he was gone.

We hovered around him as if lifted slightly from the earth by his exit. Silence. I then placed my hand upon his forehead and said the prayer I say too often through the weeks at work. While all those are said sincerely from the heart, this time was intensely personal. This time felt so different.

"Gracious God, receive our father. Transport him on the wings of angels to the wonder that awaits. Receive him in the arms of love, the company of saints, and the embrace of all who have passed on. And may you be with your dogs, Dad. May they run to you, lick you, and love you. May you know you are home." I breathed into the words and sank into the sorrow that swelled within me. "Thank you, Lord, for giving him to us to know and love. Thank you for his guidance, his joy, and his spirit; thank you for everything. Thank you, Dad. Thank you." The tears were close. Pause,

pause… I swallowed… it felt hard and sharp in my throat. "Loving God, we pray Dad has released his body with gratitude and his life without regrets. May he let everything go but the love. Let everything go, knowing love will always connect us, Dad. Go off on new adventures. But watch over us if you can. Guide us in our days until we see you on the other side. Thank you. Love you. Love you."

My family is eclectic and varied in their beliefs. Some are atheists; some are agnostic; some are out there "on the fringe." Most feel there's more to life than meets the eye. All allowed my prayer and invested themselves in the words as they could, sensing this was the right thing to do; some formal ritual that marked the transition and assisted Dad in letting go… that helped us in letting go. Closure. For me, the professionally religious one, the prayer could not be complete without the benediction, ancient words from the book of Numbers which the Lord instructed Moses to have Aaron and his sons use to bless the children of Israel, a special pronouncement of security, grace, and peace. I felt my father would want this, as he was raised and remained Anglican, and it marked the end of every worship service he attended and every worship service I have presided at. Making the sign of the cross upon his forehead, I echoed the energy of generations past.

"May God bless you and keep you. May God's face shine upon you and be gracious to you. May God look upon you with favour. . . ." I could not finish. The tears erupted as my body went limp. Steadying myself against the bed, I felt the hands of those beside me on my back, words of comfort and encouragement at my side. I sank and sat at his side, giving myself to the grief. It was enough. Those tears completed the prayer better than my words could, as did the embraces which followed. We consoled each other, knowing we had loved him well, and walked by his side to the valley of the shadow of death, and then, once there, discovered the light needed to navigate that wilderness shone from within.

The space we inhabit after a person dies feels distinctly different. Infused with relief and realization, we immediately feel the void of the one around whom we have orbited for days, to whom we were drawn since diagnosis. Gradually, our energies shift from attending to him to attending to each other. We sat together in the company of a corpse. This shell both draws and repels us, so I could not help but admire every member of my family as we took turns sitting silently at its side. Now, even in this lifeless form, our father was teaching us about our mortality. He was teaching us how to engage with this experience with even greater compassion. He was teaching us about the gift of ordinary moments, to say "I love you" often, to release that which is not of love, and to travel lightly through this world. Our father imparted these ultimate lessons of life through his departure. We found the courage not to shrink away but to contemplate. One of life's greatest lessons is to learn how to abide with death and become familiar with its shape, gravity, and dense silence. And we had plenty of time to practice; the funeral home had been called, but they had two other bodies to pick up, one of which was over an hour away. This would give us all day, into the evening hours, to witness the transformation to come.

The biological process of death does not stop when life leaves. We are bone and flesh, but more than that, we are mostly liquid, and that liquid shifts over the hours ahead. Immediately, we noticed the skin change as blood ceased to circulate. It becomes pale, somewhat translucent. Warmth evaporates quickly, veins and arteries collapse as blood and lymphatic fluid yield to gravity. The body sinks into the bed. Muscle tension is released. The cheeks and eyes become hollow, and the shape of the face changes. And, of course, the body becomes stiff. This spurred us to do what has been done through the ages when a family member dies, which is rarely experienced in our modern Western culture. We prepared the body.

Washing our father was a final act of reverence, of respect. Brushing his hair, removing his rings, and selecting his best suit, which he had chosen to be cremated in. I was happy to help with that part – more hands were needed to lift this wooden puppet, animate his arms into his shirt and jacket, and select the naval pin for his lapel. We stepped back and nodded – quite presentable. And then, we sat to process our grief through breakfast and binders of photographs, which brought memories to life. Kindness, calmness, and laughter indicated we were in good shape, deeply connected, and reflective on life. I felt exhausted, so I stepped out for some air, to stretch and make some calls. And, in that simple choice, I missed the final mystical moment of the day.

In the apartment, as the family sat in a circle sharing stories, an unexpected visitor entered through an open door, a sacred gift wrapped in a cliché – a massive brown dragonfly as big as an adult's hand. It flew in confidently, then slowly circled the audience, pausing in front of each astonished human. One circuit, weirdly intentional, and then the creature headed for the exit. However, it was too high, bumping against the ceiling. As with Dad, everyone encouraged it along with words of guidance.

"Lower, lower, to the left. That's it. Almost there! Yes!" As it left to the vast blue sky, they cheered. A final goodbye? A salute to indicate he was well? A way to say thanks? Dragonflies have long been a symbol of transformation and rebirth. When they told me about it on my return, one part of me was astonished, another quietly skeptical. Which is weird… the pastor, the chaplain, the "expert" in death and the near-death experiencer still had a bit of a doubting Thomas in him – just another example of how incredulous we are until we experience these things first-hand. We cannot help but remain among the incarnates, embedded in this world and limited by it, even as we graze the edge of the other.

As if to make up for my loss, there was yet one more thing that happened almost a week later. As I relate this final account, I am struck by how subtle these indicators of the afterlife are. It's as if anything more substantial would violate the laws of free will or compromise our ability to do our homework in love and trust.

I was restless, so I went for a walk with my wife in Point Pleasant Park. This woodland by the sea has always symbolized my father, for it was here that he trained cadets in the diffusing and disposing of bombs… clearly without any incidents. And here, near the entrance, is an anchor from the HMCS *Bonaventure*, a Canadian aircraft carrier on which Dad served as flight direction officer, talking the planes in. And I was baptized on board in one of the ship's bells, as is naval custom.

Then… as I leaned against the anchor for a photo, a Canadian frigate entered the harbour behind me. These ships specialize in anti-submarine and near-shore surveillance, something Dad also experienced as the commander of a fleet of minesweepers. I thought the vessel would head to the naval base ahead, but instead, just as it passed the anchor, it turned and headed back out to sea. We got the shot with the ship and a grateful, grieving son leaning against the remnant of the vessel on which the ceremony of life, death, and resurrection took place. Through the ritual of baptism, we affirm we are one in Christ and that even death cannot separate us from God. We are anchored to that foundational love by grace. All of it – life, death, and new life... joy, sorrow, and resurrection... even suffering itself into death – merges us with the mystery from which we flow. It was as if Dad was saying, "Missed you at the house, so here's one final wave as I head out. See you on the distant shore, my boy."

EXERCISE 14: YOGA FOR GRIEF

As challenging as it is to deal with suffering, grief can bring us self-knowledge, opening us up to more love and a more profound presence. This understanding invites us to allow our grief and realize it is there to heal the pain. It is not something understood by the mind, for it resides in the body, so that is where it is best processed.

Many yoga poses may help you cope with sadness and loss because of the focus on breath work and restorative postures. This practice emphasizes the liberation of emotions rather than physical flexibility and helps us cultivate awareness of areas of struggle or pain held within the body and mind. Within this compassionate space, emotional energy is released through intentional movements, breathwork, and vocalization. The intention is to create heartfelt openness and a connection to what emotion is being suppressed and held in the body.

If you are ill and in bed, an alternative is to stretch your body, tightening every muscle you can, holding that for a few seconds, releasing, then repeating. As you do so, and if you are comfortable, add your voice to the practice by moaning or making an 'ahhhhh' sound with gradually increasing intensity.

Consider consulting with a healthcare professional or yoga instructor before doing these exercises; do not continue them if they are painful or cause discomfort.

Child's Pose

Practicing Child's Pose (Balasana) is an excellent stretch for your back and hips, where we unconsciously carry stress, and can feel deeply comforting as if you're releasing a tight knot in the core of your being. Kneel on your yoga mat or a thick towel with feet together and knees shoulder-width apart.

1. *Lower your upper body toward the floor so your forehead rests on your surface.*
2. *Keep arms reaching in front of you.*

3. *Hold the pose, focusing on inhaling and exhaling deeply and completely, to release tension.*

Reclining Bound Angle Pose

Practicing Reclining Bound Angle Pose (Supta Baddha Konasana) can be grounding and is also a good hip-opener.

1. *Lie on your back with your chin tucked slightly.*
2. *Draw soles of feet to meet, allowing knees to splay left and right toward the ground or upon yoga blocks.*
3. *For added emotional support rest a hand over your heart and another on your belly as you breathe deeply.*

Supported Bridge Pose

Practicing Bridge Pose (Setu Bandha Sarvangasana) is a restorative move that also strengthens the legs and back.

1. *Lie on a mat or towel with your legs bent and feet on the floor.*
2. *Gently push off your feet, lifting your pelvis off the ground while keeping your shoulders glued to the floor.*
3. *You can slide a yoga block underneath your hips for support.*

Remember, these poses are to be done gently. If there is any discomfort or pain, ease back or stop altogether. Consider consulting with a physiotherapist or yoga teacher to learn more and deepen your practice of processing emotions through the body

Chapter 15
EXISTENTIAL SUFFERING

Suffering = Pain x Resistance

– Dr. Kristen Neff

Robert was pounding the mattress with his fists. The whole bed shook under his massive frame, heavy with frustration. "I've travelled the world, run major corporations. I've made millions, had thousands of employees… I've done great things all my life… but now I lay here in this decrepit hospital while my daughters worry and sit and ask me what they can do for me. What's the point? I'm going to shrivel up and die. Die! What the hell is wrong with putting me down?" This was in 2010, before MAiD. Robert was one among countless who have cried out from their deathbed, "You wouldn't do this to a dog; why do it to me?" He stared through me, paused as tears welled up. Was this the first time he had cried? That he would do so with me was an honour. I let the silence sink in, so the vulnerability could leak out. He closed his eyes, his voice becoming a whisper. "I can do nothing."

He had a point. Why not make the trip smooth? Why endure such turbulence when taking flight? Before answering, let's recall that physical pain is rarely why people request MAiD.[190] They want it because of

[190] "Data Reveal More About Patients Who Request Medical Assistance in Dying." Relias Media. https://www.reliasmedia.com/articles/146584-data-reveal-more-about-patients-who-request-medical-assistance-in-dying. Accessed March 10, 2022.

the subjective experience of dying, the emotional and cognitive impact of the experience as opposed to the objective reality of it. The Grim Reaper awaits, and you cannot escape. No wonder facing finality can erode self-worth, increase suicidal ideation, and amplify physical symptoms such as pain or nausea.[191,192]

This is existential suffering – the hopelessness, futility, meaninglessness, disappointment, remorse, and complete disruption of personal identity. It is death anxiety, and it is inevitable. Existential issues are endemic to the human condition, and at no point are they more overt than when a person insists on controlling their death. Their road of existence has come to the borderland, this line in the sand where life passes through the sieve of time. How strange to find the story we have been so casually living now comes to an end. Where did the years go? Is this truly the final chapter? We only realize how we have unconsciously inhabited our days as we approach permanent unconsciousness.

Perhaps there is an afterlife, perhaps we continue, but even that is conceived only within the limits of our mortal mind, built on concepts from our culture. What's "out there" beyond tomorrow is either oblivion or mystery. It's nothing or everything. The bounded finite has run up against the unbounded infinite. What can we do but grasp for what we know – this life, this love, this self about to end? Suffering exists as a consequence of that tension, where we discover our mortality is complex beyond our understanding. We cannot encapsulate it, though we sure think we can, as evident in the affirmations, "It's my life!" "It's my choice!" Subjectively, yes, that is how it seems. And we defend this even more when the integrity of our identity is threatened by the ultimate situation wherein our diminutive stance in the scale of the infinite is amplified: at death.

Existential suffering is strewn along the road in many forms under the guise of worry, mental distress, and feeling disorientated or powerless.

---

[191] Kissane, David W. "Demoralization: a life-preserving diagnosis to make for the severely medically ill." *Journal of Palliative Care* 30.4 (2014): pp. 255–258.

[192] LeMay, K, and Keith Wilson. "Treatment of existential distress in life threatening illness: A review of manualized interventions." *Clinical Psychology Review* 28 (2008): pp. 472–493.

So many times, I've seen people wrap their distress in frustration, anger, or bitterness and hurl at the nurses who compassionately care for them. Commenting on the toll this must take, a nurse nodded and said, "Yes, but he's grieving, and this is the only way he knows how to express it. I can absorb his pain because I get to go home at the end of the day." (I work with amazing people.)

When your life is falling apart due to terminal illness, these existential potholes damage your alignment and compromise your ability to absorb the bumps. The early ones, like losing a favourite toy as a child or gaining a new sibling who threatens your primacy in the family, challenge identity integrity without much real risk. Major ones like betrayal, the death of a loved one, or severe illness threaten the whole structure of identity, of feeling safe on your road through the world. Then, when your end approaches, the car is headed to the cliff.

Think of Robert, saying he could do nothing. With MAiD now available, you can do something; you can have someone shut the car off before you experience the free fall and the impact of the end. Yes, the injection will cause you to die, but it does so by putting you to sleep first. So much gentler than the death one's imagination provides. And it seems to meet the desire of the dying to remain in control as they face the end. It gives them what they want. But does it give what they need? Does it give society what it needs? The request for MAiD is the statement, "I do not want to die in that way!" Here's the challenge: can you engage such vulnerability in dying to make it not only acceptable but desirable? Can you employ it as the greatest lesson of growth, love, and humility? Can you allow the not knowing and not controlling to be the central path to your true self, the conscious awareness beneath the body, and mind, and story you have lived? This is the question central to suffering and our existence. If we get that wrong, we lose meaning; we lose our bearings, and we lose ourselves.

Can you do this as you die? Can you do this at the ultimate moment of your life? Can I? I'm not sure. Even having faced cancer four times, I'm not sure I can answer that with integrity unless you ask it of me while I suffer. And, eventually, I will, for we all will. What I do know is that as deep and dark as the pit of despair may be, we can endure it far longer than we can imagine from here and be transformed in ways we cannot imagine as we fall. My patients have taught me that. Before we explore this ability, let's stay with suffering to become familiar with its difference from pain.

Physical suffering is relatively easy to identify and somewhat straightforward to treat compared to the deeper dimensions of distress. I say "relatively" and "somewhat" because physical pain is not isolated to the body. It is intimately entwined with psychological and spiritual suffering. As they increase, the pain of the flesh increases.[193] It's as if these non-physical aspects of suffering act as an amplifier, distorting the perception of pain in such a way that narcotics cannot touch. And there is no one way that people deal with this. The essence of suffering is the intrapersonal self-perception rather than the characteristics of the threat itself. Thus, two persons with a terminal disease having equivalent medical and symptom profiles may have very different experiences of suffering.

In addition, we're conditioned to hate our pain, to treat it as unwanted and fix it. When it comes to physical pain, that's understandable, but when it comes to existential pain, that's damaging. Physical pain is the body sending an alert to you to pay attention and remove yourself from danger. It says something is wrong and in need of repair. Existential pain says the same thing about the soul. It is asking for mercy, kindness, embrace, and softness. It is asking for the restoration of meaning and belonging through compassionate presence and purposeful engagement. But we are unfamiliar with this spiritual medicine. We are unfamiliar with the language of our soul's pain, so we suppress it, distract from it, and do anything to avoid being swallowed by it. Worse, we conceive of it as a threat to be fixed instead of an invitation to deeper connection and compassion. In the past, the goal of medicine was to "cure sometimes, relieve often, and comfort always"[194] by accepting the limitations imposed by disease but taking pride in its potential to relieve and comfort. Now,

---

[193] Robinson, Kathryn L., CD Connelly, and JM Georges. "Pain and Spiritual Distress at End of Life: A Correlational Study." *Journal of Palliative Care* 37.4 (2022): pp. 526–534.

[194] Li, Weimin. "Precision medicine: to cure and relieve more." Precision Clinical Medicine 1, no. 1 (2018): 3.

medicine embraces the responsibility to eradicate suffering, even at the expense of eradicating the one who suffers. This means providing death as a medicalized treatment. Existential suffering demands deeper investment than that.

What does this suffering feel like? That's difficult to describe unless you've been there, but psychological symptoms include panic, anxiety, depression, sadness, and paranoia. Existential aspects include demoralization, despondency, dependency, difficulties being on the decline, loss of will to live, hopelessness, loss of purpose or meaning, loss of dignity, mental exhaustion, feeling battle-weary, and death anxiety. At least, that's the consensus. As spiritual distress can be defined as "the impaired ability to experience and integrate meaning and purpose in life through connectedness with self, others, nature, and/or a power greater than oneself,"[195] and existential distress is the inability to find sources of meaning, purpose, hope, agency, comfort, strength, and connection,[196] we can treat them as the same. Academics will split hairs here, as there is no widely agreed-upon definition of existential suffering. So complex is its form and so cultural its expression that its specific nature can only be summed up in the terms "total pain," "existential distress," or the more familiar phrase, "misery."

In his excellent article "The Nature of Suffering and the Goals of Medicine," Dr. Eric Cassel writes that suffering is a

> … specific distress that occurs when impending destruction of the person is perceived and continues until the threat is done or the integrity of the person can be restored. A person is an embodied, purposeful, thinking, feeling, emotional, reflective, relational human individual existing through time in a narrative sense. Generally, all of these parts are consistent and harmoniously accordant. Suffering, in which all of

[195] "Spiritual Distress." ScienceDirect. https://www.sciencedirect.com/topics/nursing-and-health-professions/spiritual-distress. Accessed Feb. 15, 2023.

[196] Bruce, Anne, et al. "Longing for ground in a ground (less) world: a qualitative inquiry of existential suffering." *BMC Nursing* 10.1 (2011): pp. 1–9. https://bmcnurs.biomedcentral.com/articles/10.1186/1472-6955-10-2. Accessed Feb. 15, 2023.

> these parts are affected, destroys the coherence, cohesiveness, and consistency of the whole. It is in this sense that the integrity of the person is threatened or destroyed.[197]

"Perceived destruction of the person." That accurately describes what's beneath the surface when desiring an early exit. Their very identity in this world is eroding – who and what they *think* they are will end. That's a key point – the dying person is identifying completely with their personality, with the experience of self they have been used to for decades. Spirituality states that the perceived self is not fundamental but more like clothing the soul wears. In fact, spiritual teaching asserts that ego is a *mistake* that consciousness makes when it attaches its identity to experience. Spiritual practice is, then, for nothing less than knowing yourself as you truly are – a particular expression of universal consciousness (or source, God, *Brahma*, life, etc.). Awakening to this nature allows you to have experience without confusing it with your identity. But few in our culture relate to the self from such an observational orientation. We state, "*I am* a mother, artist, or successful businessperson." Even more, we say, "*I am* angry, frightened, grieving. *I am* dying." The spiritual surprise is that the only truth to those statements is the words *I am*. That is what is fundamental; that is what is eternal. The rest is impermanent.

We'll explore this in depth later in the book, but for now, let's admit that this is universal. It's the human condition. So, when the integrity of the person's identity is so threatened, controlling how one's destruction comes about with MAiD ironically restores integrity, activates agency, and empowers one to reclaim the shattered pieces of self and say, in the words of Paul Anka, "I did it my way."

I sat with a woman for who this process was unfolding with patterns I recognized as classic, but she could only experience as tragic. Life was abruptly ending, just as she was hoping for five more years. Five years… it seems long enough to be enough, especially compared to two months.

---

[197] Cassell, Eric J. "The nature of suffering and the goals of medicine." *Loss, Grief & Care* 8.1-2 (1998): pp. 129–142.

That's the prognosis the doctor had just given her moments before. Gina's body seemed deflated in the chair.

"It doesn't seem real. I thought I could live a bit longer. I don't know what to feel."

I sat and sighed, extending my heart to encounter if only a fraction of her experience. I, too, sunk back in my chair, shaking my head. "Oh… oh…" then silence. "Everything is different now. The texture of life is different."

"Yes… yes…" Her eyes could read mine; her heart could feel mine connecting. That was critical. When you've been told you'll die, you don't want the person across from you turning away. You want them turning toward your fate. You want them holding the space because yours is collapsing – your future is imploding, your yesterdays compressing. And then she said something that gave her present moment purpose. "But I know what I want."

"What's that?"

"I want to die at home. I want to go home. Surrounded by my friends. I want a party. We're all artists, and we know how to party. I want colour and laughter and stories and wine… and fireworks. I want fireworks!"

Brilliant. Utterly brilliant, I thought. In all my years, no one had said that. It made me want to be there. "And I want MAiD. Just do it like I had to with my dog."

Here it was, with almost predictable timing. Now that it's "acceptable" (some would say even favourable to natural death), MAiD is becoming the fallback when considering one's demise. Engaging that directly, however, is pointless because it's not about one's choice. It's about what's beneath that desire which, for Gina, was a bedrock of grief and disappointment.

"Your dog? Do you have a picture?"

The image showed a true companion, a border collie whose smile shone from the screen. Having had dogs most of my life, I appreciate their unconditional love. "That's a wonderful friend. It will be good to see her again."

"Do you think?" Gina's eyes grew wide. People don't expect clergy to talk of dogs in heaven.

"Oh, yes. Doesn't it seem only right? After all, they love better than we do. And God is love, so they say."

"Well, that actually makes me feel a bit better. That would be wonderful." Gina teared up, indicating more than grief. There was a backstory here. There always is. She hadn't mentioned a family.

"Have you been alone long, Gina?"

She shook her head, held my gaze. Here I was, a stranger who had just entered the room, a man and representative of the church. But she had opened up… to me. I was honoured by the gift of her brokenness. Our discussion explored the fragile nature of the human heart, our longing for love, and our defences against it. Her journey through life demanded resilience and independence for emotional survival. From childhood to this day, it seemed she always had to scrap for a place in this world. Though a diminutive figure, at five feet even, I know her spirit was ten feet tall. It was no surprise she wanted MAiD.

"What are you most afraid of, Gina?"

"Losing control. I can't stand the idea of lying around, dependent on others. That's not how I've ever lived, and by God, it's not how I'm going to die!"

Her eyes were fierce, her voice strong as she sat forward in the chair. I wasn't going to mess with her! And there was no time. Gina would be discharged the next morning, so she could spend her days as she desired while she still had the strength to walk, to eat, to care for herself.

Here it was: the anesthetic of control. MAiD was so effective in relieving her worries and strengthening her resolve. It felt like an impenetrable wall before me. Vulnerability was not in her vocabulary. Gina sat defiant, a perfect example of how suffering arises from our relationship to the frailty of life. This is why a person can suffer tremendously without being in any physical danger or pain. We suffer when our dreams fall apart, when our children make reckless choices, and when we lose a loved one. Suffering is never one-dimensional; it is entwined with a web of factors through which our personhood is built: the past and our personal story, culture and societal norms, identity, and roles in family and work. Beyond this, there is our connection with our body, with the subconscious material that invisibly influences our behaviour. Finally, and fundamentally, there is our connection to nature and reality itself. The tangled web of suffering extends into one's political identity, the secrets we hold, the shame and the dreams, and the transcendent aspects unarticulated but felt at the core. There is a dimension of suffering when any of these are sufficiently compromised or shattered. And unless that suffering is adequately addressed, it will only increase.

When all these dimensions of personhood come to an end through death, the scale of that suffering can become unacceptable to the person. We become overwhelmed imagining that final breath. So we resist, refuse, explode, withdraw. We engage in the language of conflict against death, resilience, and resistance, of doing whatever it takes, even when the disease has taken everything. Such an orientation to dying can only invoke one lesson: that to fight a battle is to invite another. But death is not a failure, and it is not your adversary. In fact, gracefully moving toward our disintegration decreases suffering by reducing resistance to what is and opening to the ambiguity (and the surprise) of what will be... of what you will be. The more present we are to our experience, even the experience of dying, the less will be its hold on us.

What is being expressed by the shattered soul is not a desire to die; it is a lament. This weight of sorrow is central to the human condition, for it arises from a longing for wholeness, for connection, for safety, for love. In that, lament is a noble quality of the human spirit. It testifies to the inherent goodness of a person, for the capacity to grieve can only manifest through the part of us wired for connection and completion. But we don't feel it that way. We feel it as a crushing sorrow, a wail in the storm of life now disintegrating. Lament is a cry longing to be received by more than the void, more than the meaninglessness. It longs to be received in the embrace of compassion, the presence of others who see the broken and descend to embrace their frail form.

When imagining the suffering to come and lamenting the loss of dignity and self-determination as death approaches, suffering is, then, understandably alleviated by the option to choreograph one's exit. So great can this relief be that it is experienced as empowerment, which feeds the conviction that it is not only one's right to choose assisted death but also the best choice available. This is due, in part, to a misunderstanding of the feelings that motivate the desire for an early exit. These are as rich and varied as they are debilitating: grief, sorrow, anger, frustration, sadness, loneliness, despair, depression, rage, melancholy, impatience, anxiety, bitterness, fear, helplessness, incompetence, yearning, and withdrawal, to name a few.

These are outward expressions of the injury, not the injury itself. How often we need to remember this, defaulting to helping a person feel better rather than engaging those complicated feelings as doorways to a deeper understanding, a more nuanced articulation of what gives meaning, of what is an area of wisdom, growth, and new awareness. While running the danger of sounding triumphant and idealistic, nonetheless, throughout time, the best of our humanity has been found as we engage suffering in such a way that it fuels adaptation, resilience, and, in the face of death, compassion and solidarity with all who suffer. No wonder dying is the most significant opportunity for spiritual growth a person can ever experience. But that growth is private; it cannot be imparted. It can be supported, but it is sourced from within. One cannot force a flower to open.

Suffering is experienced only at the edge of our comfort zone, only at the limit of our ability, only when our options have crumbled and we seem to have nowhere to turn. At no point is this more intensely felt than at death, yet even there, a fundamental principle still holds: that on the other side of suffering is greatness. You will not feel it while you struggle. You will not know it as you endure. You are reaching for something you cannot understand; it must remain a vision, a hope, a trust, a faith that you are more than you seem. This significance will be found only as you fall apart. You cannot find peace within yourself until you overcome yourself. This is challenging, to say the least. I do not want to give the impression it is anything less than the hardest thing in the world. You may even feel that it's like being stuck in a kind of hell, and you can't process it. It's too much. Your mind keeps defaulting to the thoughts, "I hate this. I don't want this. I can't do this." The first is a judgment, the second a truth, and the third a lie.

People have been dying since the dawn of time. The mental and emotional struggles are so much greater than the physical. But the mind has a tactical advantage over you all the time. It knows your fears and insecurities. It knows where you don't want to go, so it will guide you away from that. It always controls you... until you notice it doing so. With that single manoeuvre, you now have your thoughts; they don't have you. You now have your feelings; they don't control you. You now have this experience, but it is not you. You are, however, soon to experience what *is* you. It requires the rest to fall away.

This will not make sense to many people. We are strangers to our spiritual nature, defaulting to God being "someone" in the cosmos instead of the Ground of Being from which the universe, and you, arise. Awaken to that and you awaken to yourself. Yet it also means that you must go to the shadow within to find real peace and enlightenment. You must speak that darkness into the world, out of hiding, and have it naked before you. Here is engagement with your grief and anger, and the fear that wears that anger as a mask.

There is no algorithm for transformation. There are no specific steps you must do, but there are guides that lay it all out, such as the 15th-century guide, Ars Moriendi ("The Art of Dying"). This Latin text offered advice on the protocols and procedures of a good death, explaining the stages we go through to "die well" according to Christian precepts of the late Middle Ages. For simplicity, I'll summarize that guide as it parallels Kathleen Singh's map of ego deconstruction.

The first stage, Belief, is marked by impatience and irritability as death unfolds in an undesired manner; it's taking too long, and the ego finds it intolerable, for it's not just that we don't want to die... we don't want to die in this way.

The second stage, Social Contract, involves worldly concerns and the burden of care, leading to attempts at self-preservation through controlling behaviour and expressions of despair. The dying person may swing between emotional outbursts and sinking into silence – both manifestations of misery.

The third stage, Ego Saint, revolves around preserving personal dignity as one fears the perception of frailty. Here is the loss of personal (not fundamental) dignity - the insult of mortality to the integrity of the perceived self, the ego. Our body is becoming unrecognizable as the dying process scrapes us to skin and bone.

The fourth stage, Philosopher Charlatan, witnesses the inadequacy of lifelong beliefs in the face of this disintegration, fostering a search for hope and defending faith amidst internal doubt. Faith statements become theodicies, defending God's goodness and the mysterious purpose of our suffering. We're trying to put handles on the chaos because the alternative is meaninglessness, despair, and the obliteration of hope.

The final level, Disillusionment, brings desperation and self-doubt. Here is a driving force behind requests for MAiD. Paradoxically, all these stages serve as invitations for self-examination and self-awareness, for tender engagement with one's woundedness and frailty. We practice through self-forgiveness and the release of self-narratives, culminating in final integration through surrender. Near-death awareness emerges, offering an opening to the spiritual realm just on the other side of the transformative fields of chaos.

The imagined unbearable waiting in the liminal realm is described as akin to a night passed without the sunrise. Ego remnants dissolve, and confusion alternates with stillness. Loved ones may go unrecognized, and the distinction between body and mind fades away. The ensuing stillness precedes apparent unconsciousness, increased apnea, and an opening to the Ground of Being, where the body ceases to serve as the instrument of consciousness.

Breath becomes a key indicator of the soul's calibration to transformation, with periods of rapid, shallow breath resembling the soul's unpacking for the final journey. Attachments dissolve, and the dying open to their original state of being, reaching the most profound stage of human consciousness.

I have felt this countless times as patients die. An energy flows from their head as I say a blessing, my hand close to their crown. There can be electrifying sensations that make my skin tingle and catch my breath. Family members have witnessed light leaving the body, a shift in the air, and a vibrant, dense silence enveloping the space.

What the dying experience can only be inferred from the accounts of near-death experiences, which we'll explore in chapter 26, and from the insights of the world's spiritual traditions. They describe a disconnection from the body, sometimes seeing it from above. Often there is a compassionate detachment, even disinterest, in what was once your form. Other times, as noted earlier, there may be disorientation and anxiety, but this is rapidly supplanted by the encounter with the Light; brighter than anything experienced on earth, yet comforting to gaze at, and infused with Love. Bliss saturates the soul, as everything that formed a self in this world, separate from others, disintegrates. We are released into the Ground of Being from which all emanates.

Becoming lost is a requirement of this process. Relinquishing control is necessary. Only the contemplative mind can navigate this rough sea with grace. Only the contemplative mind can bring forth the deeper dimensions of consciousness as a process of opening, of awakening, which is why a sense of meaning and transcendence, the feeling that you are part of something greater, is the most powerful way of restoring, even resetting the integrity and infinite dignity of the person. It shifts the Ground of Being from the self to the world, to the story of your life, to the generations to come, or, in the mystical traditions, to the universe and the spiritual dimensions. Pain and loss, even death and dying, can be transformed by this transpersonal dimension.

It's important to point out that this need not be religious or even spiritual; people for millennia have died for a cause, their country, and for ideals. Those secular aspects of transcendence powerfully place one's identity and significance in something more significant: one's community, convictions, and principles. They give meaning to dying as they provide one something to die for.

I recognize that some choose MAiD for precisely that reason, adopting MAiD not only to relieve their distress but to help others, to advocate on their behalf, to make a public statement that, when facing not only an imminent death but an unacceptable life, one should have the right to choose how and when they die. In the context of terminal illness, I hear staff, nurses, family members, and the public speak of this as an act of great courage. And no wonder – the patient is turning toward death, not away, and doing it on their terms, often with calm gratitude and complete acceptance of its reality, but not of its process of deconstructing the self for transformation. I certainly appreciate the depth of their distress and the passion of MAiD advocates in pressing the matter of how we respond to suffering. I'm even grateful their efforts have brought death out of hiding and pushed conversations on dying to new heights. However, those conversations have little depth. They have not considered the illuminating aspects of ego deconstruction and demonstrated no awareness of the gift of disappearing to the self as the final stage of human development. For the dying, their distress is too great for them to articulate such ephemeral notions. Introspection is unrealistic when grasping for a life raft in a raging storm. With MAiD on the table and its concomitant effect of calming existential distress by restoring power and agency to the ego, such insights are likely to become even rarer.

Here's a foundational example. Suffering is to the mind as pain is to the body. Pain indicates that something has gone wrong in the body. Suffering indicates that something is in danger in the mind. It arises from a threat to your identity, and it is here that spirituality asserts an astonishing principle: that you have allowed yourself as an expression of the Gound of Being to become personalized by experience and belief. Just as a toothache tells you to go to the dentist, this spiritual suffering tells you to address those attachments and beliefs, correct them, and wake up to what you truly are. This is its function. This is why we can engage suffering to accelerate our realization that we are not our body, thoughts, feelings, or even our experience. We are consciousness, we are awareness itself. I appreciate that this sounds abstract, and I promise to offer exercises to demonstrate it's nature. For now, I propose that the belief that we are all separate selves in a world of things is a universal delusion of humanity. There is no such thing as "separation" in a non-dual, fully integrated reality that arises from consciousness. I also acknowledge that few spiritual traditions overtly teach this fundamental lesson, that you are not a thing in the world, but a thought of the world. So, how could we expect the average person to realize this, especially as they are dying? As we will see, it is precisely because they are dying that they will realize it. In the end, we all will, for dying will either walk us or drag us to our awakening on our final day.

Existential Domain	Description	Clinical Manifestation
Mortality	Awareness of the inevitability of death and a wish for life to continue.	Anxiety about dying and the afterlife; concern about separating from loved ones.
Freedom	Reality that humans must always choose and all choices have consequences.	Regret about past choices; unresolved conflict with one's self or others.
Meaninglessness	Struggle to find meaning in life despite the universal reality of death.	Loss of purpose; questioning the meaning of illness, suffering, or faith.
Isolation	Sense of isolation from part of a larger community (family friends, work, church, etc.).	Feelings of abandonment by community or God; a sense of disconnectedness

Figure 3: Existential Suffering

Clearly, significant aspects of existential suffering are spiritual (Figure 3). However, that may go down poorly with some. While there is significant overlap, and existential suffering is a universal human experience, many patients in this modern age may not identify as spiritual. They may even resist the term due to moral injury or intellectual irrelevancy. The religions of old have little sway upon generations whose identity is shaped more by the cellphone than the church pew. To further complicate matters, the term spirituality carries different meanings for different individuals. Therefore, I would argue that existential suffering is a secular term for spiritual suffering because both describe the threat to a person's identity and their place in the world. As death approaches, these two terms become synonymous.[198,199] But what does "spiritual" truly mean? For some, it encompasses a connection with nature, while for others, it is a deeply personal relationship with the divine. An increasing number of people see spirituality as an abstract, unexamined notion, more an incidental mystery than a core principle of reality.

Nevertheless, at the end of life, we intimately understand their meaning. We feel it in the depths of our being, even though we struggle to find the precise words to describe the experience. Above all, we want to feel safe. As we approach the great unknown, we cannot imagine anything other than misery. That is why it is best to explore these feelings using simple, tender terms, like "Are you afraid?" "What is the most challenging part of this?" and "I am here for you." The words themselves may not matter as much as the quality of your presence. To effectively address spiritual distress, caregivers must be willing to enter that pain themselves and embody the compassion to embrace it. This can only be achieved by those who have experienced suffering themselves, as we must have traveled the difficult road to resonate at that depth with others still on the journey. Perhaps one cannot fully understand what it means to be human without having experienced suffering. When the dying can achieve this for themselves, their suffering shifts, and meaning arises from the darkness.

But how do we begin? Perhaps you are a healthcare provider, a support person, or a family member. You might be wondering how to determine the nature of existential distress when there isn't even a common definition. Maybe that's for the better – so complex, so human is this state that it's wiser to help the heart recognize it before words reduce it. Even more,

---

[198] Boston, Patricia H., and Balfour M. Mount. "The caregiver's perspective on existential and spiritual distress in palliative care." *Journal of Pain and Symptom Management* 32.1 (2006): pp. 13–26.

[199] Boston, Patricia, Anne Bruce, and Rita Schreiber. "Existential suffering in the palliative care setting: an integrated literature review." *Journal of Pain and Symptom Management* 41.3 (2011): pp. 604–618.

better to touch the soul through the question, "Are you at peace?" Here we begin to explore a state of openness, acceptance, congruity, and authenticity. We're talking about releasing resistance to what is. We're exploring the courageous step of forgiving the broken bits, the poor choices, and the ways in which we did not love well. We're even stepping up with curiosity about what is to come. These are spiritual conversations. This is how we come back to the better part of ourselves. This is where true hope is found: in connection, in belonging. This is the call to a deep encounter with self that terminal illness compels us to answer. It is an awakening to hope in its true form.

MAiD certainly brings hope that is satisfying to the ego, but in this guise, it is counterproductive, for it is hope that death will be smooth, and that suffering will be managed. All of that is in the future, even if that future is just the next moment. When hope in this form evaporates through the dying process, we are left with the here and now and no other. Hope as a posture of the mental ego is transformed into presence, a stance of the Spirit.

This is something I do not claim to consistently manifest in myself (check with me when my time comes!), but something I have experienced and witnessed time and time again from my patients: that we can give ourselves to suffering in such a way that love remains more potent than fear or the desire for an early exit. As Carl Jung stated, "What we fear most is where we develop next."[200] I'll plant that seed for now and return to the distress so we can more adequately appreciate the hard soil in which hope grows.

Existential suffering, by its nature, is subjectively determined. Only the patient can state its severity. And yet, again, by its nature, existential suffering is almost impossible for a patient to articulate accurately. Words will fail, for they rely on the frontal lobe. The suffering patient has long descended to the more primitive functional centres of the brain. They dwell beneath language. They swim in the darkest waters. It is the body now that speaks accurately, through sobs and sorrow, aches and visceral

---

[200] Jung, Carl Gustav. *Abstracts of The Collected Works of CG Jung: A Guide to the Collected Works of CG Jung*. Princeton University Press, 1976.

expressions of anguish. We sigh, we weep, we wail and curl into a fetal position (if there is strength to do even that). We sink to the bottom, where the detritus of our unfinished life temporarily swirls, then settles upon us. Yet there are others who state their suffering is intolerable and are approved for and receive MAiD while still reasonably independent, walking around, enjoying their meals and the beautiful connection of company, conversation, sunrise and sunsets.

There is an ironic twist at play here, a brutal surprise that can change our entire relationship to that which we are straining to avoid: suffering is exponentially amplified by the rejection of one's actual state. It is the resistance of the ego to an unwanted reality. By straining against what is, we feed what might be. Most of the time, when this happens, our imagination becomes more painful than what is happening in the present moment. That's a bold thing to say when talking about dying, but an accurate assessment when talking about MAiD. No wonder even having the option brings peace of mind – with the injection comes the power to make death what we want it to be: simple, predictable, controlled.

As if the heat of distress wasn't hot enough already, we also have to factor in that over a third of palliative patients wrestle with unresolved trauma. MAiD is intoxicating in its power to anesthetize the massive material of fear, distress, and unresolved darkness beneath conscious awareness. "[PTSD] is more common in the dying, their families and the bereaved than you might think," says Dr. Louis Heyse-Moore, a retired consultant in palliative medicine, counsellor, and writer. He found that a third of clients with bereavement issues referred by a hospice for counselling had PTSD.[201] We're dealing with more than a terminal illness here. One's entire life story is compressed and processed at its end. With that, trauma is reactivated: that sense of helplessness, that fear of the nightmare, the abyss of oblivion. But now, in the face of death, you have a way

---

[201] Heyse-Moore, LH. "Is Psychological Trauma in Palliative Care Underdiagnosed and Undertreated?" Abstract. 1[st.] European Conference on Somatic Experiencing, Denmark, 2015.

out; you have the final word as to when and how. You have control now when you didn't then. No wonder MAiD is so attractive.

EXERCISE 15: AN EXISTENTIAL EXPERIMENT

Take a few moments to sit in a quiet and comfortable space. Close your eyes and bring your attention to your breath. Allow yourself to become present and grounded in the moment. When you feel ready, engage with the following exercise: (You can also listen to a guided session at https://soundcloud.com/david-maginley/Exercise15)

> *Notice your body, and what it feels like supported by your chair or bed. Observe any sensations it may have: the feeling of feet resting, the weight around your hips, any sensations in your back and neck. Lightly be aware of your body.*
>
> *Now do the same with your feelings. Notice any emotions. If you are calm and relaxed, that is an emotional state, so notice the energy of it, the sensation of it. Mentally, step back from your emotions and notice how they are held and expressed through your body more than your brain. Your body sends the emotional signal to the brain, but that's where the emotion is named or identified. Feel the calmness, or any other emotion, in your body.*
>
> *Now observe your thoughts. You can do this even while reading this book. Mentally step back from your thoughts and observe them flow. This is a very slippery experience; you may get caught up in your thoughts every few seconds during this exercise. Notice when that happens; even observe it happening.*
>
> *Even further, step back now and observe yourself having this experience. Do it lightly, without effort. It's like opening your hand and dropping a feather. Open yourself and drop the attachment to who you are. Observe the experience of being you. Observe yourself as one having this experience.*

So, who or what is having this experience? Sense the space of this, the ambiguous nature of it. Allow the openness of it. Can you describe what it is like? Take a few moments to sense this state. You are not your body, feelings, thoughts, or experience. You can be aware of these, so that is what you are: awareness. You are an individual awareness. I've heard people describe this as an awakening to an expansive reality, a spaciousness of being. And everyone gets uncomfortable with it! Save for a few exceptionally experienced meditators, we are only able to touch upon this briefly before the ego asserts itself and fills the space with its small, convincing voice. Ego cannot abide such disposal. It shoves its way into awareness and states, "I am! This is me!" What would it do if it discovered it was not the self? Can we treat the ego as a required part of the human journey and keep it healthy by keeping it in perspective? ***Ego is functional as a process through which consciousness has experience, but dysfunctional as a construct that identifies with experience.*** *So convincing and persistent is its form through attachments that this becomes the ultimate spiritual assignment. In the end, you can't take your ego with you, for what you're headed to is the Ground of Being.*

CHAPTER 16

EACH IN THEIR OWN WAY

Death should take me while I am in the mood.

– NATHANIEL HAWTHORNE

THREE PATIENTS LIE IN THEIR BEDS, SEPARATED BY WALLS BUT BONDed by a mutual trajectory: they are all about to die. One will pass peacefully surrounded by love. She has embraced mortality as an opportunity to go out shining and is fortunate to have excellent pain management from her medical team. One plans to check out early – it's been challenging to control her pain and nausea, and she sees no point in facing what only looks like misery ahead. And one has already left but is trapped between worlds, his family refusing to remove the life support that runs his body like a robot, an empty shell. But that's not how he appears to them, so they're betting on a miracle.

JANET

THE FIRST ONE WAS EASY. THE ENERGY OF JANET'S ROOM IMMEDIATELY struck me. Drawn curtains blocked the winter storm brewing outside. Small lamps discreetly placed low to the floor bathed the room in a golden light while soft music flowed from a speaker in the corner. Personal photos and items were thoughtfully placed about her, and a beautiful quilt transformed her hospital bed into a cocoon. It seemed to portray her impending transformation: a spring-like scene of flowers, butterflies… new life.

Her daughter was reclining comfortably on a cot while her son sat at the foot of the bed, eyes sleepy with a tender sorrow, a notebook on his lap. He had been chronicling the days, the special moments, and his mother's words. They came less frequently now with advanced disease and were made all the more precious because of it. Janet was now floating on fentanyl, a powerful pain medication that blocked the agony of her breast cancer. She smiled with ease and didn't bother with the effort required to open her eyes when I greeted her. Instead, she offered her hand, which slipped quickly into mine as I sat by her side.

"You're David. I've wanted to see you." Her words slid lazily from her lips.

"Nice to meet you, Janet." My voice was deep and warm, thanks more to the remnants of a cold than my compassion. Still, it opened her eyes and widened her smile. "You seem to be doing this very well. Good music, good light, good love."

"And good drugs," she added. Her kids laughed.

"Yeah, don't be shy about that. So, you know I'm with spiritual care, checking in to offer support and help people struggling with the ultimate moment of their lives. From what I can feel, you're not going to give me much work there."

Janet squeezed my hand. "It's all good. All good." I could see there would be little unpacking for her journey, just a few questions to assess her well-being.

"Any concerns? Any questions as to what it will be like when you die?"

"Well, I've heard you've done this before, so maybe you could give me a hint?"

Clearly, the nurses had been talking. Sharing my near-death experience with patients is always an honour, but I only do so if invited and appropriate. The spiritual care practitioner must be discerning in nurturing the expression of the patient's spiritual beliefs and not prematurely presenting their own.

"Hmmm. Well, each person's experience is unique, but most are marked by an expansion of consciousness as they move into a realm of indescribable love. Many are greeted by the spirits of loved ones, and there are other beings, too – angels, celestial entities. You may have a welcoming party waiting."

"Did you have one?" Janet asked.

"I was met by someone who felt like my best friend. Incredibly powerful, wise, and compassionate. It seemed I was finally home. Intense joy, profound love. I've missed it ever since. Say 'hi' from me when you get there."

She closed her eyes. "Shame one has to die to do that."

"But it's an honour to help as you do. As long as we have physical pain under control, you can trust that you're wired for this. You know how to go, so lie back and soak up the love. As long as we keep ahead of the pain, you can give yourself to this process." Then, looking at her children, "You all seem to be doing that quite naturally."

"That's good to hear," her daughter sighed. "We've never done this before. But Mom's pretty comfortable, so we've been able to talk about life, all the adventures we've had." Tears softly fell as she spoke.

It's rare to have such plain discussions at death, and wonderful when everyone in the room is on the same page. No one was hiding, no one was suppressing any aspect of their experience, no one was protecting anyone else from the truth. As difficult as it was losing their mom, her kids were able to be authentic. I admired how their courage embraced their vulnerability – no emotional masks were needed in this room. They had, after all, been practising her death for some time, long before the word "palliative" was mentioned. This was anticipatory grief, the repeated rehearsal of saying goodbye. And, since they loved her, to part with something of themselves as well. Janet had been doing similar homework from the moment of diagnosis, but hers was a different form of grief – contemplating what it's like to say goodbye to everything and everyone. So great is this departure that it can only be done in small and accidental increments. This is preparatory grief, and the most challenging part of it is leaving those we love.

There's such great wisdom at play here; it's no wonder we all struggle to access it. Grief is love with no place to go, so it leaks from the corners of our eyes and shuffles in the hollow of the heart. This sorrow, consuming at times in the quiet of the night, is the mark of a truly evolved being. A creature that grieves is a creature that connects and values others. We work best with such sorrow through solitude and social connection, through tears and exercise, through patience that time will bring us back to ourselves. What a wilderness… yet spiritual growth occurs in precisely such a landscape. Perhaps that is why we are, mysteriously and tenderly, all the more beautiful and noble for travelling it.

Janet died… radiant. Her skin seemed to glow, a sacred smile upon her face. Did she have a good death? That's a term often used to express a hoped-for ideal, but can it be used at all? If pain is controlled, if we are deeply loved and deeply loving, if we have forgiveness and reconciliation, if we release this body, and this life, with gratitude, if we are lucid to the end or die quickly in our sleep… our death may be described as good. Perhaps we need a better term. Janet's children still grieved, still sank into tears and a heartache that felt heavy on the chest and sharp in the throat. There was still some pain, much sadness, and plenty of diarrhea at the end. But there was also a beauty that surpassed anything Janet or her family could have imagined. David Giuliano, the former moderator of the United Church of Canada, spoke of this when reflecting on his own cancer.

"What happens when we are ill is sometimes so unbelievably beautiful. The tenderness that happens within families at that moment of suffering. That awareness of our humanity and our mortality that we keep at a distance most of the time. The kind of intimate, beautiful, sacred conversations that happen in those moments that we would never ever be open to at other times."[202]

Those who opt for medically assisted death seek those conversations too, but on their terms, not death's. They sometimes take beautiful and creative steps to experience a good death: suffering avoided, celebrations planned, love affirmed, calamity escaped. Too often, though, this

[202] Giuliano, David, as told to Andreas Laupacis, in Healthy Debate. http://healthydebate.ca/faces-health-care/cancer-religion-philosophy. Accessed March 13, 2019.

is carried out with no consideration of the conversations and connections Giuliano speaks of: that deep tenderness, solidarity with all who suffer, the breaking in of awareness that comes to us only as ego defences crumble. Instead, the MAiD procedure is carried out soon after the final evaluation of the patient's competency, with little psychological and less spiritual assessment, and no passage into the final breath that allows the not-knowing and permits grace to emerge (so slowly!) from the darkness. Ironically, those who qualify for MAiD are in the ideal situation to experience all of that and more: they have an environment for family and loved ones to be present, deliberate time to unpack one's life, repair the broken bits as best they can, and affirm the gift of love. Most importantly, they have optimal access to a multidisciplinary healthcare team and medication that can adequately, if not perfectly, manage pain.

And pain is paramount, both that which is experienced at the moment and imagined to come in the next. Here is a critical distinction: while pain is of the body and suffering is of the mind, the two are intimately entwined in a spiral dance of escalation and exhaustion. That was certainly the case with the woman three doors down.

OLIVIA

Advanced colon cancer can be excruciating; the stabbing gut pains and nausea were more than Olivia anticipated. And she had lost weight so quickly. It was easy to imagine withering away within weeks, dissolving to dust soon after.

She was hopeful surgery would be straightforward, though it was extreme. It's called a Sugarbaker – visible cancer is cut out, then your innards are excavated from your abdomen, into which heated chemotherapy is poured. The solution is sloshed around to clear all areas of microscopic cancer and then cleaned out with saline. While recovery can take months, this shake-and-bake approach is effective for many. It would not hold such promise for Olivia. As soon as the surgeon saw her organs, he knew the cancer was too extensive. He immediately closed her up, then sat with her in recovery with a heavy heart. His compassionate delivery of the bad news was a precious gift and helped Olivia feel genuinely cared for and truly seen as a person, not as broken parts. That approach was amplified in palliative care, where the focus on quality of life gave her time to go within and honour the short days ahead.

Except that she didn't know how to honour them. The days ahead looked dreadful because the day she had now was intolerable. We could not get the pain under control. This was due to several factors, not the least of which was the type of pain she endured. It emanated from nerves in her lower back, likely cancer consuming her kidneys and attacking the spine. The cocktail of hydromorphone and fentanyl worked only sporadically. Olivia was also underreporting the severity of her pain and postponing medication – a common issue. She did not like how they made her feel – sloshy, sleepy, sedated. If her days were numbered, she wanted to live them engaged, animated, doing something more significant than lying in bed, catheterized and comatose.

On top of that was how it felt like her body had betrayed her. Olivia had been a triathlete and a woman at the top of her career. Now a physiotherapist was recommending a walker. A nurse was washing and wiping her clean. No wonder she asked about medically assisted death. The initial assessment was done the day following her request, and the second ten days later. In between lay the only opportunity to engage suffering and discover if there was an optimal third way besides misery or the off switch.

"What's the point?" she asked. "What's the point of going through this when it's only going to get worse?"

I sat close to the bed, leaned in. "Yes, it's profoundly difficult to imagine anything of value or purpose coming from this. Not only do you continue to deteriorate, but you witness your family's grief and imagine them at your bedside in the last days."

"Exactly!" She sighed, suddenly on the edge of tears. "Exactly." Her voice became small. "My mother… my mother is…"

I let it hang for a moment, a witness to the sharp edge of grief cutting off her voice. "Your mom is heartbroken watching this. It's not right for a child to die before their parent."

Olivia nodded, her eyes wet with affirmation. "I feel so helpless."

"I want to introduce an idea that will be very difficult to live out, but I hope it will empower you to engage your suffering to build meaning: it is an honour to be with you as you die. It is your family's honour to love you into death, not to shrink back even though it's utterly heartbreaking. They long to hold you in love. Allowing them into your dying will require great vulnerability and trust. It means giving yourself to this process. The goal here is not to be calm or strong or protect them from this reality but to be real. You and they will become all the nobler for it. That's where true dignity is found, when we engage grief this way, as the greatest opportunity to love, not fix, the other person. This is how we bring the best of ourselves to the end of life."

Olivia was listening deeply, listening from the heart. There was truth here for her, in which the better part of her humanity was waiting. But a barrier had to be bridged first. "How can I do that when I'm in pain, when I'm lying here drugged up but still able to hear?"

"You're right. We cannot do this well when you're in agony. We have to get the pain under control first. That's the priority. For now, let's try something that doesn't involve a needle. What's your pain at now, out of ten?"

"Well, not bad; I had a shot just before you came in. About a four, I guess."

"Good. We want it fairly low at first so you get the hang of this technique. Close your eyes, gently breathe and quickly scan your torso. Check-in where the pain is concentrated."

It took her only a moment. "My back, my gut."

"Good. Now breathe into that area. Don't fix it, suppress it, or distract from it. Feel the pain deeply." I paused to allow her to move awareness into the sensation. "Try to sense the qualities of the pain: its shape, if it's moving, how the edges of it feel, how dense it is, what colour it is." I said this softly, slowly. The goal was to help her stay with that which she would rather avoid. "Stay with this for about thirty seconds." We sat together, soaking in the sensations. "Now shift your awareness to the sound of traffic outside, the voices in the hallway. Just observe these sounds for about twenty seconds." Olivia's face softened, and her breath moved easily from her belly. "How's your pain now?"

"Hmmm. Interesting." She opened her eyes. "Maybe one. I feel relaxed."

"Nice. We'll take relaxed!" That got a smile. "We often feel we have no control over our pain," I explained. "But we can shift our relationship to it, even reduce it, because while pain is of the body, suffering is of the mind. It all depends on the quality of presence you have with yourself. So, this little exercise is an experiment in mindfulness. The goal, again, is to be real, to be softly present with your experience without straining against it. When peace fills the mind, the body responds."

Olivia smiled again. "I like that! I can do that!"

"Yes, and do it often throughout the day. This is part of your training to stay with grief and pain."

"So, it's an assignment?"

"Oh, yeah. And there will be a test! I'll check on you throughout the week to help deepen your practice. Hopefully, this will help you get through until we find a more effective medical solution. To get that, I strongly encourage you to report your pain accurately and accept the medication, even if it leaves you floaty. It will be effective only as it stays ahead of the pain instead of chasing it."

I was so relieved to hear that did happen, but it took over a week of adjusting and experimenting to discover the best approach – a spinal block. Even that came with a hiccup that threatened to drain all hope: the procedure involves the injection of a solution that kills nerves in the pain area, but it takes a couple of days to do so. Olivia did have immediate relief, but that was from the local anesthetic used in the operation. When it wore off, she spiralled into agony for hours, too intense to mitigate through mindfulness. Her desire to die returned but then subsided as the block kicked in. We had bought her time and comfort to do the deeper work of dying well, but she did not like the new assignment.

"Death will deconstruct your ego," I said. "Your new task is to let it do so."

She raised an eyebrow. "What if I don't want to?"

"Perfect!" I replied. "Notice your resistance? The ego's defence mechanisms have automatically been triggered, which is good because it means we've begun."

We explored how dying gradually strips us of our role and identity. We can no longer work, support family, walk without exhaustion, or wipe without assistance. Dependency increases, and autonomy decreases. Vitality is eroded along with hope to finish the list – one more day at home, one more meal, one more word. Just one more. So, the ego fights back. Hers did so by seriously contemplating a trip to a clinic in Mexico, feeling disgusted at the indignity of her body, and resisting sharing her true condition with colleagues and friends. And, most of all, considering medically assisted death as a means to avert utter dependency. If she could not live on her terms, dying on them at least felt empowering and so much safer.

"Yes," I affirmed. "It would be wonderful to feel safe. Ironically, the spiritual path shows us that as we resist what is, we remain trapped, but as we offer ourselves in surrender, we experience freedom. This is not giving up, but giving your whole self to something greater."

As esoteric as it may sound, we are speaking here of the path of the mystics. Their spiritual practice – meditation, contemplation, service, and compassion – are means by which the ego is continually stripped away to cultivate union with God, union with Love (the two are synonymous). One hardly has to sit in a monastery to merge with Sacred Presence. Life inevitably will drag us down other pathways that render us raw before the Divine much more rapidly. So, while many speak of suffering as having a purpose (to awaken us to God), it's more accurate to see it as a process that challenges, then deconstructs ego-identity, which naturally uncovers a deeper identity, one paradoxically without "you," the self equated with your mind. That's what suffering does to us; any purpose will arise from what we do with it.

Being a sporadic meditator and an abysmal mystic, I can only turn to someone with proper authority to speak on this matter and do it justice. Mirabai Starr is an author, speaker, and seeker of God who experienced this infilling of the divine through the worst tragedy a parent can experience: the death of her fourteen-year-old daughter in a car crash.

> Grief strips us. According to the mystics, this is good news. Because it is only when we are naked that we can have union with the Beloved. We can cultivate spiritual disciplines designed to dismantle our identity so that we have hope of merging with the Divine. Or someone we love very much may die, and we may find ourselves catapulted into the emptiness we had been striving for. Even as we cry out in the anguish of loss, the boundless love of the Holy One comes pouring into the shattered container of our hearts. This replenishing of our emptiness is a mystery, it is grace, and it is built into the human condition.
>
> Few among us would ever opt for the narrow gate of grief, even if it were guaranteed to lead us to God. But if our most profound losses – the death of a loved one, the ending of a marriage or a career, catastrophic disease or alienation from community – bring us to our knees before that threshold, we might as well enter. The Beloved might be waiting in the next room.
>
> Suddenly, the sacred fire I have been chasing all my life engulfed me. I was plunged into the abyss, instantaneously dropped into the vast stillness and pulsing silence at which all my favourite mystics hint. So shattered I could not see my own hand in front of my face, I was suspended in the invisible arms of a Love I had only dreamed of. Immolated, I found myself resting in fire. Drowning, I surrendered, and discovered I could breathe under water.
>
> So this was the state of profound suchness I had been searching for during all those years of contemplative practice. This was the holy longing the saints had been talking about in

> poems that had broken my heart again and again. This was the sacred emptiness that put that small smile on the face of the great sages. And I hated it. I didn't want vastness of being. I wanted my baby back.
>
> But I discovered that there was nowhere to hide when radical sorrow unraveled the fabric of my life. I could rage against the terrible unknown – and I did, for I am human and have this vulnerable body, passionate heart, and complicated mind – or I could turn toward the cup, bow to the Cupbearer, and say, "Yes."
>
> I didn't do it right away, nor was I able to sustain it when I did manage a breath of surrender. But gradually I learned to soften into the pain and yield to my suffering. In the process, compassion for all suffering beings began unexpectedly to swell in my heart. I became acutely aware of my connectedness to mothers everywhere who had lost children, who were, at this very moment, hearing the impossible news that their child had died.[203]

We never think of surrender as an empowering act, yet by opening fully to what is as we die, we come into our most authentic selves. No longer suppressing any aspect of our experience or resisting any facet of our situation, we encounter what the spiritual traditions describe as grace. We've moved from the acceptance, *agreeing to,* which is passive, to surrender, *agreeing with,* which is active. It is acting in the moment instead of being acted upon by it. Now we are participating in the event of dying. It's not happening *to* us; it's happening *through* us. This existential orientation fosters stability and wisdom, it becomes a process of awakening. Surrender is infinitely more thorough and transforming than acceptance.

---

[203] Starr, Mirabai. *God of Love: A Guide to the Heart of Judaism, Christianity and Islam.* Monkfish Book Publishing: 2012, pp. 63–75.

I've seen this in my patients as they die. They describe an inexplicable connection with everything, an instinctive compassion that causes them to forget themselves. It is an astonishing and unexpected grace through which everything unessential to the self is burned away. This is the sobering course of terminal illness, a crucible through which we are transformed. This psycho-spiritual alchemy is the last process of human development. Perhaps such dynamics are accelerated for those who die suddenly in an accident. For the rest, slow dying defaults us to a passage of time in which the dying negotiate, accept, then surrender (sometimes on a moment-to-moment basis). No longer the centre of their universe, the ego dissolves, and they are finally free. How could this be cultivated in Olivia? Her walls needed to crumble. I knew just the tools to use: vulnerability and affirmation.

"Time for a new assignment. You mention you haven't invited friends or co-workers to see you. We've reflected on how this protected them and yourself from grief and sorrow. As they enter the room, they bring their awkwardness and anxiety, not knowing what to say, wanting to make you feel better. You then end up being the host and the patient, taking care of their feelings and your own."

Olivia nodded, then sighed again. "I dread that. I know they care, but what do you do with that?"

"Allow it, and take the lead. Here's the truth: they are coming to say goodbye because you're worth ending the relationship well. Instead of shrinking back, say it plainly. Say goodbye, and tell them what they mean to you, what you admire about them, and what you hope for them. Ask them for forgiveness for when you fell short of your best self. They will naturally reciprocate. You are exchanging a gift of affirmation, but it requires you to be vulnerable and transparent. Great courage is needed to do this, and you will find that by again listening to your body, where you're holding the anxiety and breathing into it. Let it be there. Trust it will relax, so you can truly connect. The quality of presence you have with yourself will determine your encounter with another."

To her credit, Olivia got right to work, inviting a co-worker in and discovering the gift of who she was to others and who they were to her. This built purpose into her suffering – she used the tragedy of her impending death to create meaning in the only place it would endure: her relationships. As she experienced this, with the pain now under control, she postponed medically assisted death… at least until the next crisis.

MARCO

JANET HAD EMBRACED DEATH CALMLY IN THE CARE OF HER FAMILY AND the medical team. No resistance to reality instilled clarity and comfort – she had a smooth trip. Olivia endured more turbulence as she struggled with suddenly shortened days and difficult pain management. She considered MAiD, as it promised to restore control over her athletic body once again, even if only to shut it off before it shut her off. But Marco would have no say in the matter. His family would decide if his life would end, and that notion was intolerable to them. How ironic that while some demand to wield the reaper's scythe, others hold it back mid-swing just as its grace would grant freedom.

It was a stroke that brought this giant down. A pillar of his community, a hero to his family, he suddenly seemed so small when his wife found him by the bed. 911 was called, CPR was given, and a pulse was detected, but there was no response in his eyes. Rushed to the hospital, Marco was plugged into our technology to sustain body functions. His family had insisted on this, as most would. And it worked. As the days rolled into weeks, his heart stayed strong, his blood pressure stable, his skin warm to the touch, and his chest rose and fell… but this was the work of the ventilator. And this would become a curse as the months stretched on, for a scan showed minimal brain activity. We did not think Marco was still there.

"But we can't give up on him," his wife, Emily, cried. "He never gave up on us!" Here was a story to be told. Marco had been a soldier, defending communities in Afghanistan from attack, witnessing the most brutal forms of violence, and then defending his daughters from assault when he returned to a disintegrating Detroit. They had to rebuild all aspects of life, and Canada seemed a safer place to do so. A relative in far-flung

Nova Scotia commented on how refreshing the ocean was, how plentiful the beaches. They made it here, they made here home, and they made a life driven by determination and principles. But now life was crumbling again. His daughters, safe and successful, supported their mom as she sat by his side, day after day, refusing to leave him alone for a moment. That was understandable for the first few weeks, but now it was five months!

As shocking as it may be, we often see this in the ICU: bodies artificially animated by the respirator, dancing the undulating line on the heart monitor for months on end. There is always an unfinished love story, always a theme of obligation to family, a deep sense of duty, an adherence to faith. The same was playing out here again. "Life is sacred, and God is good," Emily declared. Desperation was non-negotiable – they would not allow it. If God brought them through all that, God would provide a miracle now.

When our world is falling apart, we cast our prayers like pennies to heaven. But God is not a wishing well, and the heart can only bear so much hope before turning away to build walls around the wounds. What could I do but cast my own coin in? "It would be wonderful," I said, "if you got that miracle. But it's been almost six months on these machines. If Marco dies, I know there is another miracle – his transformation into love, his shining with eternal life. And, hopefully, his continuing to guide your life until you are reunited."

Emily gazed at him, stroking his arm. "I am nothing without him. He has to live."

Here it was again: the denial of death. Five floors up, one requested MAiD as a refusal to participate in the dying process fully, and here before me, death was denied for the same reason: neither could give themselves entirely to the finality. Neither would allow death on its own terms, clinging instead to their identity and role in this world. Same theme, separate courses. Would they have felt differently if death actually had meaning?

EXERCISE 16: THE BOOK OF MY LIFE

Materials needed:

1. *A cell phone*
2. *A collection of photographs that hold personal significance and evoke memories related to the grieving experience.*
3. *Pen and paper or a journal.*

Instructions:

1. *Set aside dedicated time and find a quiet, comfortable space to engage in this exercise without interruptions.*
2. *Gather the collection of photographs that are associated with the person, event, or aspect of your life that you are grieving. Choose images that hold emotional significance and represent different moments or aspects of your relationship or experience.*
3. *Take a few deep breaths to centre yourself and bring your attention to the present moment. Allow yourself to acknowledge and embrace any emotions that may arise during this process.*
4. *Take your phone and go to YouTube.com. Listen to the song, 'The Book of My Life,' by Sting. Selecting a video of this song with lyrics playing will help (bit.ly/428A08R). Pause and reflect upon your life, the memories behind you and the mystery ahead.*
5. *Begin by selecting one photograph from the collection that resonates with you in this moment. Take a few moments to observe the details, colours, and people captured in the image. Allow the emotions and memories connected to the photograph to emerge.*
6. *Write down your reflections and memories associated with the photograph. Share the story behind the image – what it represents, the emotions it evokes, and the significance it holds in your grieving process. Be as detailed and authentic as possible, capturing the essence of your experience.*

7. *Repeat this process with several other photographs, one at a time. Each time, select a new image and delve into the memories and emotions it brings forth. Write down your reflections and storytelling for each photograph, allowing yourself to express your thoughts and feelings fully.*

8. *After exploring multiple photographs, take a moment to reflect on the collective narratives that have emerged. Notice any common themes, emotions, or insights that have arisen through the storytelling process. Consider how these narratives contribute to your understanding of your grief journey.*

9. *If you feel comfortable, you can share your reflections and stories with a trusted friend, family member, or therapist. Sharing your experiences can provide a sense of connection, validation, and support as you navigate the complexities of grief.*

10. *Take a moment to honour and appreciate the stories and memories that have been shared. Acknowledge the significance of each photograph and the emotions they hold. Express gratitude for the opportunity to reflect, remember, and heal through this exercise.*

11. *Close the exercise by taking a few deep breaths, fully embracing the emerging emotions and insights. Remind yourself that this exploration of grief through photographs and storytelling is a valuable and ongoing process. Be gentle with yourself as you continue to navigate your grief journey.*

Remember, this exercise is a deeply personal experience, and there is no right or wrong way to engage with it. Allow yourself to express your emotions authentically and at your own pace. If you feel overwhelmed during the exercise, take a break, practice self-care, or seek support from a compassionate listener or grief counsellor.

Chapter 17
MEANING

It is a waste to be asking the question when you are the answer.
—Joseph Campbell

Carolyn confused me. She should have been wailing but was not. She should have been weeping yet was smiling. She should have been dead, or at least want to be. Carolyn had sickle cell anemia, a blood disorder that changes the shape of hemoglobin cells from smooth and round to sharp and curved. Each cell becomes a miniature scimitar that clogs blood vessels, cripples organ function, and causes excruciating pain. There is no cure.

We knew Carolyn well. She was, unfortunately, a familiar face on the unit. Pain crises were intermittent but intense enough to warrant admission for blood transfusions and plenty of narcotics. That she did not ask for these more frequently motivated my visit; the nurses were perplexed about how she managed such agony.

She lay limp in the bed, eyes closed. I paused to consider waking her when she softly said, "Come in. Come sit. How are you, David?"

"How did you know it was me?"

"Your shoes. You're wearing the brown shoes that click when you walk down the hall. I heard you coming."

Mental note: buy new shoes with soft soles. I sat at her side. "Got a question for you. I don't expect an easy answer, but I'm curious." Her eyebrow raised a bit. "How do you manage this pain when others would be crushed by it?" I didn't mean to make her heroic, and she didn't seem to be inflated by my words.

"My body is in pain. I'm not."

I picked my jaw up from the floor before she turned her head, eyes open this time. "Pain is funny, you know? It's like, sometimes, I can watch it. I can breathe and let it be what it is. I've been learning to allow it. Doesn't always go well, you know." Her smile was radiant.

I wanted her to teach me. I wanted to know the inner experience of such equanimity. I can do that well enough if I stub my toe, but this was a different league. What enabled her to change her relationship with her experience so dramatically?

Pain is perplexing. Research shows that dopamine, the brain chemical involved in pleasure, is equally involved in pain.[204] And, of course, anticipation and personal judgment can make both experiences more or less intense. Thankfully, when you're in pain, you're not powerless; you can reduce dopamine levels and thereby reduce pain through the quality of presence you have with it. Meditation seems to be the path by which you can regulate metabolic processes, even dopamine levels, thereby altering your perception of pain.[205] The challenge is fully showing up! That turned out to be the key for Carolyn. She would never call it meditation. For her, it was prayer, and through prayer, she found purpose in her suffering. "My Lord went through so much for others. Maybe I can go through this for others, too. I give my pain to God. I rest in God's grace."

This patient took the chaplain to church that day and taught him a thing or two about what it is to do more than believe in God. She taught me how to believe into God, how to use pain to open and merge with that

---

[204] "Pleasure and Pain: Study Shows Brain's 'Pleasure Chemical' is Involved in Response to Pain, Too." University of Michigan News. Oct. 25, 2006. https://news.umich.edu/pleasure-and-pain-study-shows-brains-q-pleasure-chemicalq-is-involved-in-response-to-pain-too/#:~:text=It's%20the%20first%20time%20that,intense%20stress%20in%20their%20lives. Accessed May 3, 2023.

[205] Mohammadi, Farzaneh, et al. "The effects of 'mindfulness meditation for pain management' on the severity of perceived pain and disability in patients with chronic pain." *Iranian Journal of Ageing* 6.1, (2011): 0-0.

ultimate underlying Presence. This shift offers us a staggering proposal: that while meaning and identity throughout life are found not through comfort, but in the lifting of a worthwhile burden, at the end of life it is found through surrender. This becomes the ultimate burden as we resist it, and the ultimate release as we engage it with gratitude. It is the letting go and the opening to the moment, God, mystery, source… life and death. (Ironically, I stubbed my toe the next day and cursed. I still have much to learn!)

Research verifies that unbearable suffering is equally present in those who request assisted death and those who do not. In a study on requests for euthanasia among cancer patients, "no differences were found in the prevalence of unbearable suffering for physical, psychological, social and existential symptoms, nor for overall unbearable suffering, between patients who did or did not explicitly request [euthanasia]."[206] What factor differentiated the two groups on such an intense and ultimate issue as ending one's life? Meaning. Those who found ongoing meaning within their suffering, which at times was more intense than those who requested MAiD, endured through to their natural death. For Carolyn, that meaning was found through her faith; for others, it's not so easy to identify. Sometimes the patient can't even put it into words. There is simply a knowing, a feeling, a trust, or a belief that this dark experience is marked by something more than nothing.

Meaningless suffering is an abyss. It strips us of our dignity and our humanity. It adds insult to injury and violates hope with the assertion that there is none. One feels this in the body and throughout the soul. Worse, it seems eternal, never-ending, and astonishingly powerful. "Finally, the illness that dominates everything will wipe out all life has to offer me," one patient said. "What I feared most is exactly what will happen to me. I won't belong anymore, the emptiness of existence, the lack of independence, being unable to do things myself, being at the

---

[206] Ruijs, Cees DM, et al. "Unbearable suffering and requests for euthanasia prospectively studied in end-of-life cancer patients in primary care." *BMC Palliative Care* 13.1 (2014): pp. 1–11.

mercy of others who I will have to beg to do the things I need in a way that's suitable for me."[207]

This blackness swallows you with an annihilation that threatens to continue long after you do not, for one imagines the immortality of sorrow and grief continuing in your loved ones, only to fade as the memory of you evaporates from this earth. Despair infuses your mind, your body, and your days. Even more, you know that your loved ones, too, will face this; they will deteriorate, they will die. Suffering reduces all of us to raw meat and bone and dust. Here is the embodiment of the existential wail heard in the book of Ecclesiastes:

> "Meaningless! Meaningless!"
> says the Teacher.
> "Utterly meaningless!
> Everything is meaningless."
> 3 What do people gain from all their labours
> at which they toil under the sun?
> 4 Generations come and generations go,
> but the earth remains forever.[208]

Here is the ultimate existential pain. This is why the spiritual, emotional, and psychological struggle with a life-threatening disease consumes one's energy far more than the physical aspects of dying. Imagination becomes the vehicle of sorrow as you envision the rocky road ahead and that of your loved ones without you. Your angst is, at least, contained. But theirs… theirs you have no power over. Theirs is their own. Worse, while their pain is not your homework, it still feels like your responsibility.

Here's how the inner voice runs: "I'm the cause of this. My illness, my dying, and worse, all the choices I made in life that contributed to this mess… it's all on me. If only I hadn't smoked, drank, ate junk, become

---

[207] Dees, Marianne K., et al." 'Unbearable suffering': a qualitative study on the perspectives of patients who request assistance in dying." *Journal of Medical Ethics* 37.12 (2011): pp. 727–734.

[208] Ecclesiastes 1:1-4

emotionally toxic… if only I had exercised, gone vegan, loved better or lived larger… if only I hadn't been so afraid, so selfish, so… something." It's too big. You'll never know. But you wear it for them because you care for them. You wear it because you feel helpless, and this at least puts handles on the chaos to give it some reason, some structure. You see it in their eyes and awkward words. You feel it as the ache in your heart, the tears on your cheeks in the quiet of the night, in the bathroom or the bed, where it's safe to shed the shell and sob into darkness.

No wonder many find it impossible to imagine anything good coming out of suffering. No wonder existential distress is the main reason medically assisted death is requested. We are choosing what is expedient over what is meaningful because we are terrified. This is a way out, an escape, a statement of the one power we now have over suffering and death: if we are to be destroyed or transformed by our end, at least it will be on our terms. No need to struggle any more than we're comfortable with. No need to enter the ambiguity, the wilderness and the wasteland. Now we have death on demand. Let's skip the misery and save everyone the sorrow.

That sorrow is difficult, if not impossible, to accurately describe, though fatigue, decline, negative feelings, loss of self, fear of future suffering, dependency, loss of autonomy, being worn out, being a burden, loneliness, loss of all that makes life worth living, hopelessness, pointlessness, and being tired of living are constituent elements of what the MAiD assessment form sums up as "unbearable suffering."[209]

Existential distress at the end of life often results in significant behavioural changes. Composure struggles to constrain such primal dimensions of our humanity. Obsessive-compulsive reflection, an inability to escape the deep grooves of negative thinking, hyper-vigilance to all of the body's sensations… these dominate the world within, all while retreating from the external world.

Research has found that people become far more judgmental and hostile as they die.[210] The animal within snarls and snaps when sufficiently

---

[209] Ibid

[210] Solomon, Sheldon, Jeff Greenberg, and Tom Pyszczynski. *The Worm at the Core: On the Role of Death in Life.* Random House, 2015.

threatened. I find that most people (particularly men) do not have the vocabulary to express their deepest feelings when approaching the end. This compounds the challenge of exploring such distress with loved ones (especially as they instinctively protect them from such matters). While I admire the tender compassion of the doctors I work with, the reality is that many healthcare providers may not even go there, as so many are unfamiliar with the spiritual dimensions of suffering. Compassionately embedding themselves at suffering's side has not been part of their medical training. Their own death anxiety, or discomfort with others' distress, can even result in superficial joking and encouragement to prematurely place a salve on the stress. It's sad. The patient is looking upon their doctor or nurse as an expert in dying, waiting for guidance or at least acknowledgment of their existential pain. The incongruent words, the silence or awkwardness received result in a secret loneliness. Suffering increases when it remains hidden – what we suppress, we give power to. No wonder an increasing number want MAiD.

And they will not appreciate you challenging their choice. The decision for MAiD, and the accompanying decrease in anxiety, is not to be questioned (though there is often anxiety about how the family will take it, resulting in some secretly exiting this world). It's a decision that sits at the core of our identity when facing death. MAiD feels empowering and calming. It is a relief, and not arrived at casually in any of the cases I have supported (though it often is brought up casually in the initial conversations, now that it's officially on the table. "I could always do MAiD if it gets too difficult.") One's resolve is additionally reinforced by the very same death anxiety that drove the decision. Studies show that when facing death, people like others all the more who share their beliefs and become more hostile in thought, if not in deed, to those who are different, who threaten their existential integrity.[211]

Ironically, one of the best ways to decrease existential fear of death is to be reminded that you will die… five times a day. Sounds depressing, yet with a wonderful book and accompanying app called *We Croak: A*

[211] Ibid

Handbook for Being Temporary, the reminders help one to lean into mortality in a way that amplifies life, deepening appreciation and connection. Its creator, Hans Bergwall, observes, "There's a difference between reacting to death around you and doing a death contemplation. There's something different about taking a deep breath, sitting with it, and leaning into it as a contemplative tool."[212] If only those requesting MAiD were given such a tool and spiritual guidance to work with their fear.

In a modern culture that celebrates the individual's autonomy and freedom of choice, the request for MAiD is not to be criticized or questioned. Who are we to instruct others on how they should face suffering and how they should meet their demise? Well, who we are is brothers and sisters in that enterprise. As much as one faces it alone, mortality is the universal ultimate that all humanity shares. Between birth and death, the storylines may be as varied as the stars of heaven, but they all begin and end the same: we enter, and we exit. At no other moment is there the opportunity or the challenge to discover who and what we truly are. This requires, above all else, vulnerability. Our vulnerability is not only fundamental to what it is to be human; it is desirable because what makes us limited also makes us lovable. The least within us is intrinsically tied to the best among us as we rise to meet it. This is how our limitations make us a community. Our frailty, especially as we suffer, evokes the response in others to come alongside, and not fix or rescue, but descend into the pit and embrace with the healing message, "I'm here." The apex of this is found at death. Suffering becomes our fuel. Suffering becomes the proving ground of our character and our culture.

[212] "WeCroak: The App that Reminds You of Death, an Interview with Hansa Bergwell." Ernest Becker Foundation. https://www.ernestbecker.org/wecroak-the-app-that-reminds-you-of-death

EXERCISE 17: FORGING MEANING

This exercise is designed to support individuals facing mortality and experiencing seemingly meaningless suffering. It aims to provide a framework for reflection and exploration, encouraging the discovery of personal meaning and fostering a sense of peace, acceptance, and connection.

Note: Each individual's journey is unique, and adapting this exercise to your needs and preferences is important. Feel free to modify or skip any questions that don't resonate with you or add additional reflections that feel meaningful to your experience.

Instructions:

1. *Find a quiet and comfortable space where you can reflect without distractions. Have a journal or a piece of paper and a pen ready.*
2. *Begin by acknowledging and accepting the reality of your mortality. Recognize that your physical and emotional suffering is part of this unique journey you are on.*
3. *Reflect on your current experience of suffering. Write down the specific aspects or situations that feel particularly challenging, painful, or meaningless to you. Allow yourself to express any frustrations, fears, or uncertainties.*
4. *Challenge your perspective. Consider that even in the face of seemingly meaningless suffering, there may be opportunities for personal growth, learning, and discovering hidden meaning. Ask yourself the following questions:*
5. *How can I find strength, peace, or acceptance within my suffering?*
6. *What lessons or insights can my suffering offer me at this stage of my life?*
7. *How can my experience of suffering deepen my empathy and understanding of others who face similar challenges?*
8. *Are there ways in which I can use my unique journey to inspire, support, or bring comfort to others?*

9. *Reflect on your values, beliefs, and spirituality. Consider the principles, values, or spiritual beliefs that have guided your life. How might these beliefs provide a foundation for finding meaning and purpose even while suffering? Write down any values or beliefs that resonate with you.*

10. *Seek connections and support. Reach out to loved ones, friends, or spiritual advisors who can offer companionship, comfort, and understanding during this time. Engage in conversations or support groups where you can share your thoughts, fears, and hopes and learn from the experiences and wisdom of others.*

11. *Cultivate gratitude and appreciation. Reflect on your life, relationships, or the world for which you are grateful. Find moments of beauty, joy, or connection and express gratitude for them. Embrace the present moment and cherish the experiences and relationships that bring comfort and peace.*

12. *Engage in acts of kindness and compassion. Consider how you can extend kindness, compassion, and love to yourself and others, even amid your own suffering. These acts can bring meaning, connection, and a sense of purpose to your life and to those around you.*

13. *Reflect on your journey. Regularly revisit your reflections and see if new insights or meanings emerge as you continue your journey. Consider keeping a journal to capture your thoughts, feelings, and moments of growth or connection.*

Remember, this exercise is meant to support and guide you in finding meaning and peace within your unique experience of suffering and mortality. Be gentle and compassionate with yourself as you explore these reflections. If you find yourself overwhelmed or need additional support, reach out to a therapist, counsellor, or healthcare provider who can offer guidance and assistance.

CHAPTER 18

TREATING EXISTENTIAL SUFFERING

And the day came when the risk it took to remain tight in a bud was more painful than the risk it took to blossom.

– ANAÏS NIN

KEVIN WAS IN AGONY. HIS LYMPHOMA HAD BEEN RESISTANT TO EVerything we threw at it. Now it was turning his blood to sludge and manifesting as tumors, multiplying exponent – mitosis gone mad. His liver, his lungs, even his brain were swarmed. Kevin's skin turned grey, his eyes glassy. He moaned and pulled himself upright. Sitting on the edge of the bed, he poured his panic into the nurse.

"Give me something now! Give it to me!"

The nurse could not, as Kevin had requested MAiD. So severe was his condition that the customary ten-day waiting period between the initial request for assisted death and the actual procedure had been waived to ensure he could still consent. He would lose that if she gave him any more medication. With the grace of accelerated approval, Kevin knew that he could request the procedure any day. The ball was in his court; we were all on standby for the moment he said, "Ready." It left his partner, Michael, in a state of suspended anxiety as he watched Kevin linger on the edge of the abyss, lapping up every eternal moment he could.

This man, who came into Michael's life only two short years ago and turned every day into an adventure, was always stubborn and a risk-taker. It seemed ironically appropriate that the type of cancer he would get was equally dangerous, especially as Kevin downplayed the symptoms and delayed investigations. That meant our treatments had been rushed and far more severe than a sixty-five-year-old should be able to tolerate. Each day, Michael would ask the unthinkable question: "Is today the day you will die?" Every day, Kevin would answer, "Not yet. Not yet."

Oh, how we wanted Kevin to listen, to comprehend the danger in that strategy. We explained how important it was to take the meds to stay ahead of the pain. We saw it building in his moaning, shuffling, and abrasive words. This man suffered but would not give in, even as his liver shut down and oxygen counts fell. But it was the bone pain that was the worst. The marrow was overrun with lymphocytes, the pressure within them excruciating. The issue was that cancer cells grow exponentially. That's a minor concern at the beginning but rapidly accelerates to catastrophe at the end. He did not appreciate the speed of this; exponential growth means cells are doubling. It takes only twenty doublings for his white blood cells to leap from the healthy average of 7,000 to an artery-clogging sludge of roughly a million. One exponential step beyond that would take them over a trillion. Today could be fair, tomorrow fatal.

That next day had arrived – suddenly tortuous, the pain escalated to an anguish we rarely witness. The doctor to administer MAiD had been called. He said he would be there as soon as possible. But the clock ticked slower and slower with every wail from Kevin's room. And the expressions of staff accustomed to death became marked by anguish as we gazed at the hallway, waiting for the man with the bag. What could keep him from the most crucial task imaginable? Travel – he was arriving from a community clinic. There weren't many to do the procedure in the first years of MAiD, and this man was the only one on rotation. He wasn't a palliative care physician or even in cancer care. He was a general practitioner – a family doctor. He didn't usually work in the hospital.

The nurses paced – all of them. The entire floor was filled with a silent tension, pierced by his anguish and torment. I stood by Kevin's room, submerged in the cries and the cursing.

His nurse came out into the hall, tears testifying to her compassion. She had been present for ten MAiD procedures, which all went smoothly. All of them were marked by peace, gratitude, and comfort. Not this one. This was a nightmare. Our eyes met with shared helplessness. "This goes against everything that I am," she whispered. "I'm here to provide comfort, but if I give him the drugs that would do that. . . ."

"He'll lose capacity," I finished for her. "Which leaves you stuck in moral distress."

"Exactly!" she exclaimed.

"What can we give?" I asked. "What can we do to take the edge off?"

"Nothing more than we have. Ativan, fentanyl… I'm scared to give him more. But his adrenalin is so high; it has little effect." She paused, breathed, and held her gut as another wave of tears washed through. Then the man with a bag appeared.

I like this doctor. He's got wit and a calming demeanour even in the greatest emotional storm. He is efficient and professional, considerate and kind. I've been with him for MAiD procedures. I've witnessed his sincere desire to alleviate suffering. And this he did in short order upon entering the room. I stood by the door, supporting Kevin's nurse, who needed a few deep breaths before entering to witness the final consent. The doctor's manner was polite yet efficient. He introduced himself, acknowledged the distress, and apologized for the wait. Kneeling by the bed (an insightful and sincere expression of service), he produced the vials as he asked the questions of consent. "Do you desire to receive medically assisted death? Is your suffering intolerable? Do you understand that your life will stop? Do you request this of your own free will?"

"Yes, yes, yes! Do it!" Kevin exclaimed. His head fell back; his body arched in pain. Then the nurse closed the door, blocking my view and muffling the cries. So quickly, the wails were silenced. So suddenly, there was… nothing. No sounds. No sobs. It was so… strange. A suffocating weight pressed upon my ears as if the air had become dense with death. And then they emerged – the doctor first, quietly acknowledging the staff and then sitting to write his report. Then the nurse, her face streaked with sorrow, moved quickly to the lunch room where she could collapse on the couch. I lifted my body from the nursing desk and entered to absorb the grief. Michael sat by the bed, his head upon Kevin's chest, sobbing. The man so tortured a moment ago now lay still.

It is critical to remain silent. It is essential to hold the space of lament with profound respect. One must not abandon any aspect of sorrow or guide it prematurely to anything other than its dark truth: Kevin was not only dead but died in anguish before Michael's eyes. He died in the worst possible way, refusing to listen, insisting on being independent, and rejecting the staff's advice when they told him sedation would be wise. This all could have gone so much smoother. Worse, we've seen this before; it's not uncommon. Why do they hesitate? Is it fear of the leap? Is it that primal instinct for life to be lived just a bit longer? Or is it not realizing the danger that allowing the disease to progress without using meds to stay ahead of the pain will be cataclysmic? Palliative sedation is another option, but many refuse to go that route. It lacks the finality of MAiD. It leaves too much room for limbo to loom without limits. Kevin was the oldest patient we've had who postponed MAiD after approval. Of all of them, I thought he would have understood the significance of better medication. But then, he might have lost the ability to consent.

"Why?" Michael wailed. "Why'd you have to do it this way?" His fist slammed the bed as he heaved, body twisting as if grief was being wrung out of him. His eyes rose to meet mine. He sought no answers, only the safety to disintegrate. "Kevin wouldn't listen. I knew he was dying. I tried to get him to talk about it. He shut me out. He shut down. Then, he just decided that one day, this would be how it is. This is how it is. Kind of how it's always been… this has not been an easy relationship. I didn't have a say in the matter. He would just have a good day until he couldn't."

I sighed, my breath heavy with the ache of it. In my own small way, I shared his distress. I had seen Kevin at times cavalier about cancer and casual about dying. I heard his outbursts with nurses, his cursing and seething. I wondered, did MAiD help him avoid the work of vulnerability, avoid sharing his feelings through any other filter than bravado or rage? It certainly seemed to be a theme of their relationship. This I learned a week earlier from Michael as we walked the halls, sat in my office, stared into coffee. He had been at Kevin's side through chemo and delirium, diarrhea and driving back and forth for radiation. Kevin became hostile, even violent at times, determined to engage cancer his way, on his terms. "I guess that's not so surprising," Michael said. "He's always been difficult." And then another wave of grief came over him. He sobbed with gulps of air as if swallowing his still-beating heart while Kevin's lay mute within his chest.

Sitting in my office at the end of the day, I ran the case through my head. What could we have done differently? Well, we respected this man's autonomy and self-determination to the point of not challenging him to open up. And I didn't dig deeper into the patterns of his past, into his fear and grief. Could the doctor have pressed harder on what death would look like? Did we adequately cover palliative sedation? I soon realized I was fuming, wringing my hands, pacing the floor. I wanted to scream. I wanted to hit something. I wanted to hit him. I wanted to hit everything.

Take a breath. Take another. When one feels like this, the best way forward is to slow down. Because you don't want to take this home with you, you want to leave it at the office. You want to push it out and shove it down and rip it all to shreds because this... this...

Is this what he felt? Is this what death does to you when you're cornered? Is this the energy of helplessness and futility? Is this the unacceptable truth against which one can do nothing but scream and curse and grab cancer by the throat and shove it up against the wall and spit in its face? "You f***ing shit! You think you'll take me down?" Is this what he felt, swallowing his days whole, lapping down every drop on his terms until the pain burst the door wide open and he could wail without reserve? Is this what it feels like to let loose the fury and agony and grief and defiance until the needle is shoved in… Kevin's way of giving death the finger. Was this what he felt?

I cried. I locked the door and quietly cried, gazing out at the ocean, sunlight blazing off its surface. My eyes hurt. My heart hurt. Breathe. Breathe again. Think it through. I was not his therapist. It was not my job to help him heal a lifetime of choices, whatever they were through his six decades. From what Michael shared, I suspected there was a lot of unfinished business. But it was not my job to help him cram for the exam. He barely let me into his story, compared to other patients. He barely let any of us in. I was his chaplain, there to incarnate compassion, bear witness to pain, and be available. It all felt so… passive. So pointless.

I couldn't stew in this, so I went to the lunch room and found Kevin's nurse quietly talking with two others. In that shared sorrow was healing as we laid the offerings of our pain upon the table, gifts of love and support to Kevin's spirit, to Michael, and to ourselves.

We die the way we live, true to form. As much as I want people to understand how MAiD is the ultimate act of ego self-preservation in the face of the process which naturally deconstructs it, as much as I want you to trust that you are wired with the wisdom to leave this world without rushing to life's end… as much as I don't want to do this again… I must acknowledge that it is not my homework. But it is our homework. As a culture, it is our responsibility. I can only hope that, as a society and a healthcare system, as families and individuals, we can help each other do it well.

If only Kevin had been open to counselling. Would it have changed the outcome? Probably not. But it would have addressed the distress that ended up shattering him, with the shrapnel of dignity and self-determination now embedded in all who accompanied him. Counselling could have identified his fear for what it was and helped him process it in ways wiser than he imagined. Could the assessor identify it? Was it noted in the assessment form? Again, probably not. The assessment form for Nova Scotia, where I live, is a two-page checklist that serves as a starting point for conversations that follow, which can span from minutes to hours. They are carried out with respect and great kindness. However, assessors are not briefed on the inner dimensions of existential distress driving most requests or how they can be processed. They are not skilled in engaging that distress as a functional process in dying. They're not even aware of that framework. They are simply asked to identify if distress is there. This gaping hole is identified well by William Rosa and researchers:

> "The existential experience is typically underemphasized or entirely absent as a clinical priority. If included at all, medical and nursing curricula commonly address existential care under the umbrella of broader psychosocial phenomena without distinct attention to developing literacies in understanding and specifically addressing the existential experience. However – by way of contract – existential issues are innately personal and fundamental to the cancer experience, hence underscoring a moral obligation that they are acknowledged and addressed."[213]

And they can be. Interventions designed to enhance meaning and purpose have been empirically shown to decrease anxiety, depression, demoralization, and a desire for hastened death for patients with cancer-related existential suffering.[214] But, in most hospitals, a counsellor will likely be unavailable, and the patient can refuse. I certainly understand the refusal of a chaplain – we are commonly lumped into the category of religious professionals who strain souls through the sieve of dogma and doctrine.

---

[213] Rosa, W.E. et al. "Attending to the Existential Experience in Oncology: Dignity and Meaning Amid Awareness of Death." *JCO Global Oncology* no. 8 (March 14, 2022). Published online March 14, 2022. https://ascopubs.org/doi/full/10.1200/GO.22.00038 Accessed March 16, 2022.

[214] Breitbart W, S. Poppito, B. Rosenfeld, et al: "Pilot randomized controlled trial of individual meaning-centered psychotherapy for patients with advanced cancer." *Journal of Clinical Oncology* 30 (2012): pp. 1304–1309.

We really do need a new PR campaign! Psychologists and psychiatrists may seem better positioned to provide this support. Still, few of them will be adept or comfortable with the spiritual dimensions of ego deconstruction and the dark night of the soul that precedes transformation.

Why wouldn't a patient considering MAiD take advantage of this? Well, once the assessments have been completed, most patients I've spoken with feel the steps have been taken. They've been approved, and in that relief, they experience a significant reduction in existential distress. They can breathe knowing their last breath will be on their terms when they're ready. Feeling so much better, why have a counsellor come in and stir it all up? Well, because the desire to hasten death is not constant. It is a normal and *temporary* aspect of mortality. The will to live can fluctuate over intervals as short as twelve hours, with some patients demonstrating extremely wide fluctuations within twelve to twenty-four hours; and even more over seven- to thirty-day intervals. Additionally, in a study of over 200 people near the end of life, those who reported a moderate to extreme loss of dignity only comprised 7 percent of all subjects, and none reported that loss of dignity was experienced all the time.[215] With this in mind, MAiD becomes a permanent solution to a temporary problem.

Let's imagine an ideal setting where all three factors in accessing counselling are optimal: the assessor identifies the critical aspects of distress, the patient is willing to receive support to process it, and somebody is available and qualified to do so. What would that counselling look like?

First, it must be provided by a professional who has already done their own existential homework. Otherwise, they will be unaware of the forces of distress as they subtly present themselves, and unable to resonate at the core with the patient's suffering. The patient will sense this through body language, tone of voice, choice of words, micro-expressions, and eye contact. They will not "click" with the therapist, making a true therapeutic connection impossible. But let's assume we have someone wise in the

[215] Chochinov, Harvey Max, et al. "Will to live in the terminally ill." *The Lancet* 354.9181 (1999): pp. 816–819.

ways of suffering. How does one treat the existential distress driving the MAiD request?

Several approaches are at our disposal, such as dignity therapy, reframing, logotherapy, rituals, and meditation. And then there is the deep dive into what could be described as a magic pill: psychedelics. We'll take that trip in the next chapter.

The quality of the therapist's presence with themself will determine the quality of their encounter with the dying. Facilitating this process, of course, is active listening, life review, imagery, finding meaning through storytelling, letting go through gratitude and forgiveness, touch, symbolism, prayer, silence, dreamwork, and contemplation. Let's explore the main approaches in more detail, along with resources, in case you want to dive deeper.

All therapies are explored here specifically in the context of existential distress at the end of life: meaninglessness, hopelessness, and despair. From this lens, symptoms will be understood both literally and symbolically. Whatever approach is used, intuition and first-hand experience with existential distress and genuine compassion will be needed for any connection to be effective – there is no algorithm at play here, no single method that will "work." But there is the fact that existential distress is driving requests – clinicians recognize that, but feel unease at its implications. Dr. Madeline Li, a psychiatrist who developed the MAiD program at University Health Network in Toronto, states it plainly: "There needs to be clarification that the suffering needs to be medical suffering directly related to the medical condition… sources of suffering indirectly related to the medical condition don't qualify."[216]

Too late. From day one, existential distress has been the driving factor, not physical pain. Let's remember what we're up against here: death phobia, ingrained in our culture. It is written into the framework and fabric of practically everyone. We're terrified, and we don't know how to die wisely, so we settle for dying on our terms by a professional's hand. Fortunately,

[216] Gillmore, Meagan. "Have Assisted Dying Laws Gone Too Far?" *The Walrus* (May 30, 2023). https://thewalrus.ca/assisted-dying/. Accessed June 8, 2023.

death has its own wisdom from which we cannot run. It is in our soul's genetics because it is written there by nature. She brought us into this world, and she knows how to take us out. In the end, we will be stripped of our illusions of control and self and be reduced to what is essential, what is fundamental. Let's acknowledge that while counselling can guide us to the edge of mortality as far as the mind experiences it, the rest of the way is a matter of surrender to a process the mind cannot comprehend. So let's walk to the edge by exploring the support that will help us unpack for the journey and at least give us some sense of being truly seen and held as we descend to the shattering of all illusions by grace.

DIGNITY THERAPY

Dignity is a term claimed by MAiD advocates as a core principle the procedure preserves. You stay in control. You die your way. You avoid the offence of prolonged suffering, dependency, and frailty. For many, dignity is clearly worth dying for. However, this is a distortion of the term. Dignity is inherent to the person and lived out in relationships. The challenge is not staking a claim on something you already have but in society stepping up to meet the dignity of those who suffer, and it is in this that dignity therapy excels.

This begs the question: What is the difference between a person whose dignity is robust and intact near the end of life, compared to those in whom it is fractured and unacceptably compromised? Well, it first boils down to the body – what researchers called *intimate dependencies of care*: bathing, dressing, toileting, and physical appearance. So, though dignity is defined as an intrinsic quality of being worthy of honour, respect, and esteem, independent of appearance and functioning, as a lived experience, it is very much dependent on the compassion and respect a person receives from their care providers. This greatly affects how the person perceives themselves as being seen. Is dignity being upheld? Consider this example:

> Mr. J. was a sixty-seven-year-old man with an end-stage gastrointestinal malignancy. Having decided he no longer

> wished to go on living, he had gone on a hunger strike, precipitating an admission to an inpatient tertiary palliative care unit. He reported that, aside from some minor discomforts, his symptom management was quite reasonable. Psychiatric consultation was initiated to determine if depression might be a factor influencing his wish to die. While he was not overtly suicidal and, in fact seemed ambivalent about his wish to die, he did state, "If I were in a European country where I could 'press the button now,' I would." After careful evaluation, it was determined that rather than depression, the driving force behind his desire for death was a sense that life no longer held purpose, meaning, or hope. While he spoke of a lingering wish to participate in various life activities, he bemoaned the fact that his body was simply too weak and too ill to allow him to do so. That being the case, he expressed the conviction that living had become redundant, his life had no worth, and there was little reason for him to carry on.[217]

What Mr. J. appears to want is a hastened death. What he needs is intrinsic dignity to be strengthened through appropriate palliation and creative, loving expressions of care from family and the community, along with his experience and life story to be honoured. Sharing your story may sound simple, but it is an ancient custom through which communities are formed, treaties are forged, and meaning is found. Stories become burdens if left untold, so sharing your life story is a liberating and revelatory experience. It requires vulnerability and courage, trust and respect. Yet how it happens in the hospital can be so casual, such as when housekeeping staff express brief, sincere words of compassion, acknowledgment, and encouragement, or formally, through intentional therapy that processes the patient's experience.

---

[217] Chochinov, Harvey Max. "Dignity and the eye of the beholder." *Journal of Clinical Oncology* 22.7, (2004): pp. 1336–1340.

Systematically providing such care is the goal of dignity therapy, a brief, individualized intervention designed to engender a sense of meaning and purpose among patients with a terminal illness. Developed by Dr. Harvey Chochinov, a Canadian psychiatrist specializing in palliative care, it offers patients an opportunity to speak about issues that matter to them most, as well as about aspects of their lives they wish to be remembered. It engages an effective tool, the Patient Dignity Inventory, to assess existential distress through twenty-five items that not only help the patient identify and come to understand their distress, but often lead to a profound conversation on the meaning of life, self-worth, and other issues related to the dying process.[218] These conversations are often recorded, with written transcripts reviewed by the patient for accuracy. This becomes a legacy document for the family, a process which, by design, restores dignity. This is attention to the person, not just to the patient. Existential distress has been found to fade in the face of such compassionate and meaningful encounters,[219] and it is this that needs to be the standard for those leaving this world. It builds belonging by creating the experience of being seen, heard, and connected.[220] Best of all, dignity therapy is simple. The instrument lays out the conversation, to which you only need to bring your compassion and time (there are no better investments!).

It begins with the ABCDs of dignity conserving care: the attitude, behaviour, compassion, and ensuing dialogue between the patient and the healthcare provider. Here we begin with the quality of the counsellor's presence with themselves, with their capacity for vulnerable presence. That's refreshing, as it focuses on the therapist first, not the patient. It is not some formula or algorithm that is paramount, but the therapeutic relationship

[218] "The Patient Dignity Inventory." Dignity in Care. https://www.dignityincare.ca/wp-content/uploads/2010/05/The_Patient_Dignity_Inventory.pdf Accessed Nov. 8, 2021.

[219] Martínez, Marina, et al. " 'Dignity therapy', a promising intervention in palliative care: A comprehensive systematic literature review." *Palliative Medicine* 31.6 (2017): pp. 492–509.

[220] Chochinov, Harvey Max, et al. "Effect of dignity therapy on distress and end-of-life experience in terminally ill patients: a randomised controlled trial." *The Lancet Oncology* 12.8 (2011): pp. 753–762.

itself. This resonates with a startling assertion by Anne Harrington, professor of the History of Science at Harvard University: that in one hundred years of psychotherapy, the only consistent factor in patient success was not the method used or the theory employed but the compassion of the therapist.[221]

The **Attitude** of the healthcare provider greatly influences the patient's experience of dignity. This is about self-awareness during difficult conversations and fostered through basic questions: How would I feel if I were dying? How does my attitude affect the patient? How do past experiences, anxieties, and fears influence it? Does my role as the healthcare professional help or hinder my ability to develop an empathic professional relationship? These are questions to explore *before* and *after* seeing the patient and to be discussed with colleagues.

Behaviour looks to how the healthcare provider demonstrates care to build the common ground on which therapy can begin. It's displayed through tone of voice, eye contact, body language (sitting down as opposed to looming over the bed or near the door) and the gift of taking time to truly connect. Behaviour honours privacy by respecting personal space and the patient's modesty, demonstrating empathy, and respecting the patient's energy. It's also about maintaining kind and respectful contact even though medical interventions have stopped.

Compassion is clarified as the ability to suffer with another and to be comfortable with your vulnerability. You're getting in touch with the patient's experience and honouring them as a person, not just someone with an illness. An understanding look, a gentle touch on the arm, a simple nod or simply silence and presence form a deeper connection than words can provide.

More than clinical engagement, such a profoundly human encounter preserves the dying person's **dignity** since it identifies them as so much more than their disease. It empowers them with simple questions, such as "What do I need to know about you as a person to provide the best care

---

[221] Harrington, Anne. *Mind Fixers: Psychiatry's Troubled Search for the Biology of Mental Illness.* WW Norton & Company, 2019.

that I can?" or "What concerns you most?" Dignity is upheld through the clinician's interest in humanity itself, for the secret behind the care *of* the patient is care *for* the patient.[222] It is the practice of what Carl Rogers called unconditional positive regard.

With the ABCDs of dignity therapy in place, the clinician interviews the patient through the Patient Dignity Inventory. All this is recorded, transcribed, distilled to a paragraph, reviewed for accuracy by the patient… and placed in their chart. The results model best practice in patient-centred care. All patients said it was valuable. All reported it was accurate and wanted it on their chart as it would be important for their health provider to know. For healthcare staff, it increased respect and empathy by shifting their relationship with a patient to one with the person. The first person enrolled in a study on dignity therapy said, "If I could push the button and end it, I would." After commencing dignity therapy, he was asked if he felt the same. "No," he replied. "There's actually more I would like to do now."[223]

A wonderful benefit of dignity therapy is that it also deepens the life and awareness of the healthcare provider. Many reported they were emotionally affected by the experience, which increased empathy, respect, and connectedness. It may sound fundamental as you read this, but this type of engagement is often in short supply in hospitals, where staff are stressed, worn out, or disengaged because dying is… dare we admit it… too familiar. Having the Patient Dignity Inventory at hand brings the staff and the patient to their better selves.

REFRAMING

You don't need to believe everything you think. That's a healthy reality check on an average day when wrestling with the critical voice within, and a lifesaver when we're engaging overwhelming anxiety.

[222] "The A,B,C,D's of Dignity Conserving Care." https://dignityincare.ca/en/the-abcds-of-dignity-in-care.html. Accessed Nov. 20, 2022.

[223] Chochinov, Harvey Max, et al. "Effect of dignity therapy." *The Lancet Oncology* 12.8 (2011): pp. 753–762.

Reframing is an initial approach that replaces catastrophic thoughts with realistic, supportive ones. It's a way of saying, "I'm safe right now. It could be worse, but it isn't." And we've been training in this effort all our lives. From infancy to adolescence to infirmity, our imagination has tended to be more painful than our reality. That's even more so with death. Our fears of dying orbit around not knowing when we will die and how it will feel as it happens. This is precisely why MAiD significantly reduces or eliminates death anxiety. You have the time and place, the means and, one imagines, the mettle to do it. You're able to take the tragedy and make it safe. You can even make it beautiful. But let's take a more dangerous path. Let's engage the anxiety without a remedy.

Reframing is a cognitive practice that alters our perception of stressors, so it requires sufficient emotional stability (Figure 4). That's difficult, to say the least, when contemplating your death or being swallowed by fear, so the first thing to do is breathe slowly and deeply. (In fact, do that with all of these approaches!) It's a fundamental step in resetting the fight-or-flight response. Also, though reframing is cognitive therapy, when one engages the heart as well as the head, it can still be a powerful tool in activating gratitude. That's because the nature of death anxiety is primal, visceral, and spiritual. A cognitive approach will only go so far, but a soulful approach will hit the core. After all, the spiritual goal is not to quell the distress but engage it to move deeper through the deconstruction of ego-identity without resistance to support the emergence of an identity more intimately connected to the Ground of Being, with all of life. Reframing is an excellent first step in that endeavour.

After taking those calming breaths, the process begins: identify your thoughts, examine if they are true (and what they represent), then balance them with a realistic statement. Even more, we want to identify how suffering awakens us to the gift of ordinary moments and the extraordinary love around us. Let's look at some examples specific to contemplating medically assisted death. I offer these not to be directive – only you can sense what your heart desires – but to help you imagine new possibilities in a landscape that appears barren of them.

Thoughts and Feelings	Examination	Reframing
I'm a burden to my family and to the medical staff.	It's true that I am increasingly dependent on others. I find this difficult, but it is part of the dying process. It reveals how I see myself and want to be seen by others.	I can use my frailty as a way to help them practise compassion and love. My vulnerability is part of my final lessons in how to die connected and grateful for them. This may be the most important gift I can give them.
I'm scared of pain.	I'm scared of what pain may come. Am I in pain now? Can I accurately share that? I have pain meds on hand, and can take them regularly to stay ahead of the pain.	Fear of pain is natural, and something I can talk to my nurse/doctor about. If the pain goes up, I can have breakthrough medication. This is also about losing control, which invites me to trust my care team.
There's no point in suffering.	I'm scared of future suffering. I feel the toll this takes on my loved ones. This is the hardest thing I've ever faced. Can suffering open me to the compassionate care I'm receiving?	My suffering enables my loved ones to step forward in compassion, and this shapes who they are. I am grateful for their care, and that of my medical team. I appreciate the simple things like never before.
I have no purpose.	It's true that I can no longer work or contribute to my family. My purpose has always been defined by my ability, but now that shifts from action to presence. This is the heart of relationships. My role is now to shape my soul, and theirs.	I can use my dying to teach and help my family in loving deeply. I am about to experience my transformation into mystery. My task is to give myself to that with hope and hard questions. I can still grow and learn from this ultimate event.

Figure 4: Reframing

Notice how reframing reshapes dying as an opportunity to delve into the heart of life and the depths of love. It animates our ultimate homework, as all of these approaches can. It redefines the problem of death as a challenge to practise a deeper humanity. Such a redefinition is a radical and empowering shift in perspective, for while a problem is a wall, a challenge is a way. Finding that way will require some deep conversations and courageous vulnerability. It's a hard thing to say to family members, "I feel like a burden." Their instinct may be to correct you, to reassure you. Not helpful! Hopefully, someone will simply sit at your side and say, "That sounds really hard. That's a heavy feeling. Can you tell me more about what it's like for you?" Only after a lot of listening can our words have any power to register in the heart. Only in compassionately receiving their pain can we animate imagination for something better beyond that barrier. Grief and gratitude can live side by side, and what emerges as they dance is truly beautiful. The expression of existential pain is the invitation to dance. Take the hand, trust the music, and feel the way forward. As much as anxiety is an avoidance of what is within, it is also an indication that something wants to be born.

We tend not to be so good at this in daily life, let alone when leaving life. One reason is negative bias. That's our tendency to register and hold to negative stimuli and messages. You could go through a whole day of praises and affirmations, but you know the one negative comment has more staying power than all the rest. And we are the ones who give it that power! We replay the critical voice within instead of defaulting to an affirmation of self-worth. Studies even show that we tend to believe negative news is more truthful. And, since it draws more attention, it gets reinforced. So, in reflecting on our life and considering our demise, we tend to focus on how we have fallen short, how we have not loved well or been well loved. We wonder what difference we have made... if any. The decades have flown by, and we are suddenly here at the end. Our reality cheque has bounced.

That's understandable. Negativity bias has given humans an evolutionary advantage, ensuring the survival of those most alert to danger.[224]

---

[224] Cacioppo JT, S. Cacioppo, and JK Gollan. "The negativity bias: Conceptualization, quantification, and individual differences." *Behavioral and Brain Sciences* 37(3) (2014): pp. 309–310. doi:10.1017/s0140525x13002537

This hardwiring even shows up in infancy, before the first year of life is complete.[225] Fortunately, there's a greater force within that has helped you reach for another day, rise above the situations that beat you down, and shine as a gift in this world, a unique expression of life itself. That mystery, that tenacity or stubbornness or whatever you want to call it… that force has brought you here, to this bed, to this book, to this moment, and to the elusive meaning behind it all. But I'm getting ahead of myself (and want you to enjoy the anticipation).

LOGOTHERAPY

While reframing might seem like positive thinking, it's about changing your relationship to suffering, not about improving outcomes. Even when facing death, this approach can be transformative. I say this confidently as we're drawing from an expert in that: Viktor Frankl. This man endured astonishing suffering as a Holocaust survivor, an experience that led to one of the greatest contributions to the field of psychology: logotherapy. Grounded in the wisdom of spiritual traditions, it encompasses three core principles:

1. **Will to Meaning:** Everyone has an inherent drive to find meaning and purpose in life.
2. **Meaning in Suffering:** Suffering can have meaning if we approach it with the right attitude.
3. **Freedom of Will:** We have the freedom to choose our attitudes and responses, even in the face of unavoidable suffering.

As with all therapeutic practices, we start with compassion. Frankl observed that those in the concentration camp who practiced compassion for others, even though they were suffering, maintained their humanity and a sense of purpose, which supported resilience in the face of their

[225] Hamlin JK, K. Wynn, and P. Bloom. "3-month-olds show a negativity bias in their social evaluations." *Developmental Science* 13(6) (2010): pp. 923–929. doi:10.1111/j.1467-7687.2010.00951.x

own suffering. This resonates with the heart of sacrificial suffering, in which one enters their suffering on behalf of others. Sharing food rations, assisting another as they labor, or intervening when it might harm you are acts of solidarity with those suffering. Building on this compassionate foundation, logotherapy employs three key techniques to change one's relationship to their suffering:

1. **Dereflection:** Shifting focus away from oneself and onto others or tasks to alleviate excessive self-reflection and anxiety.
2. **Paradoxical Intention:** Encouraging individuals to engage in or embrace their fears to diminish their power.
3. **Socratic Dialogue:** Using guided questions to help individuals uncover and articulate their own beliefs and meanings.

Logotherapy focuses on addressing the existential vacuum, the void felt when life seems meaningless, rather than merely reconciling self-conflicts or societal adjustments, for we are not destroyed by suffering, but by suffering without meaning.[226] Regardless of the situation, we can reframe our attitude toward an unchangeable fate, like dying.

How can a person swallowed in suffering possibly find a "why" to live? What sudden purpose could infuse their day when the slow disintegration of purpose and autonomy has eroded them to a shell of what was? Logotherapy is bold in asserting that meaning can be found even when the imagination cannot grasp it. How? By reaching in, not back. Here's how Frankl put it:

> An active life serves the purpose of giving man the opportunity to realize values in creative work, while a passive life of enjoyment afford him the opportunity to obtain fulfillment in experiencing beauty, art, or nature. But there is also purpose in that life which is almost barren of both creation and enjoyment, and which admits of but one possibility of high

[226] Frankl, Viktor E. *Man's Search for Meaning.* Simon & Schuster, 1985, pp. 67–68.

> moral behaviour: namely, in man's attitude to his existence, an existence restricted by eternal forces. A creative life and a life of enjoyment are banned to him. But not only creativity and enjoyment are meaningful. If there is a meaning in life at all, then there must be a meaning in suffering. Suffering is an ineradicable part of life, even as fate and death. Without suffering and death human life cannot be complete.[227]

Frankl identified that meaning is foundational to human consciousness, central to our functioning and existence. He posited that meaning is often discovered through creative, experiential, and attitudinal values, driven by self-transcendence rather than self-interest. For someone contemplating assisted death, their motivations – often rooted in fear of pain, loss of dignity, or perceived purposelessness – can be viewed as reflections of self-preservation and ego-centric concerns. However, Frankl would argue that these fears, while significant, offer an opportunity for the noetic (the defiant power of the human spirit) to transcend such concerns. The search for meaning often involves confronting and moving beyond these fears, finding purpose not just in enduring but in transforming one's experience through relationships, creative expressions, and spiritual connections. In essence, meaning is forged through struggle and adversity, rather than found casually. It emerges through profound wrestling and release, through a complete reorientation to one's physical, psychological, emotional, and spiritual pain. Frankl asserts that this is the fuel for transformation and can be discovered even up to the last moments of life. This process requires a deep engagement with one's own existential questions and challenges, which can ultimately reveal a more profound sense of purpose. In fact, as we will explore, meaning shifts into overdrive in those last moments. It becomes our awakening to wonder through the final surrender that integrates all dimensions of the person at end of life.

Those familiar with Frankl's writings may perceive a tension in applying logotherapy to MAiD cases, particularly given his assertion that

[227] Ibid

"man's freedom of choice concerns the freedom to choose not only one's own way of living, but even one's own way of dying."[228] While Frankl underscores the importance of freedom of will and the avoidance of unnecessary suffering, this does not undermine the relevance of logotherapy for individuals contemplating MAiD. The stark reality is that the vast majority of those opting for MAiD do so without engaging in profound therapeutic dialogue to address the existential fears propelling their decision.

Let's remember that Frankl's logotherapy was forged in the crucible of the Holocaust, a response to the deepest forms of human suffering, and developed at a time when medical treatments for terminal illnesses were rudimentary. Today, with significant advancements in palliative care and pain management, the process of dying can be made more manageable and dignified. Yet, despite these advancements, many choose MAiD without ever confronting their fears of dying, their need for control, or their lack of understanding about the dying process with a therapist.

This widespread bypassing of deep existential exploration reveals a profound spiritual poverty in our culture, underscoring a lack of integrative care and insufficient psychosocial resources. In the rush to respect autonomy and alleviate suffering, we are missing an unparalleled opportunity for personal insight, spiritual growth, and the discovery of meaning at life's ultimate juncture – its end. The modern tendency to recoil from death has led to a culture where the sacred, transformative potential of the dying process is often overlooked.

Frankl's logotherapy offers a crucial framework for navigating this existential terrain. It encourages us to confront our deepest fears, find meaning in our suffering, and embrace the dying process as a final stage of personal and spiritual development. To choose euthanasia without this exploration is to forfeit a significant moment for profound personal and spiritual awakening. It is not merely a matter of dignity and choice; it is about ensuring that these choices are informed by a deep, reflective understanding of what it means to live and die with meaning.

---

[228] Frankl, Viktor E. *Man's search for meaning*. Simon and Schuster, 1985. p. 123

DEPRESSION AND GRIEF

Finding meaning in suffering through directly engaging it in self-reflection is a difficult sell in this age of distraction, comfort and pleasure, which is why Frankl called our modern period one marked by an existential vacuum, devoid of deep meaning. What our culture offers – possessions, privilege, power – only reinforces the myth of the individual separate from others, and normalizes our use and control of nature, resources, and even populations. This goes to the heart of capitalist culture. And it hollows out our soul. No wonder depression afflicts at least 5 percent of the global population[229] and is higher in cancer patients.[230]

Depression is marked by a loss of pleasure or interest in activities for weeks on end, poor concentration, feelings of excessive guilt or low self-worth, hopelessness, disrupted sleep, changes in appetite or weight, and feeling especially tired or lacking in energy, all this along with the existential distress. When one's world is reduced to the size of the body in the bed for weeks or months on end, depression is understandable. No longer able to work or contribute to the household, no longer able to participate in life, it's a natural question to ask, "What am I here for? Who am I now?" Without a robust spirituality, an ability to source meaning from within, or the opportunity to explore this with others, the questions will reverberate in the echo chamber of the mind, accelerating the descent into meaningless. This, on top of the tragic reality that suicide is the second leading cause of death for young adults in North America and the tenth leading cause overall.[231] That risk is four times higher for cancer patients.[232]

While suicidal thoughts are common among the terminally ill, they are often temporary. Therefore, the desire to hasten death should not be

---

[229] "Depressive disorder (depression)." World Health Organization. https://www.who.int/news-room/fact-sheets/detail/depression. Accessed Nov. 6, 2021.

[230] McFarland, D et. al. "Suicide in Patients With Cancer: Identifying the Risk Factors." https://www.cancernetwork.com/view/suicide-patients-cancer-identifying-risk-factors. Accessed Nov. 6, 2021.

[231] "Suicide." National Institute of Mental Health. https://www.nimh.nih.gov/health/statistics/suicide#part_2556. Accessed Oct. 30, 2021.

[232] Zaorsky, Nicholas G., et al. "Suicide among cancer patients." *Nature Communications* 10.1 (2019): pp. 1–7.

equated with a request to hasten death. A request for MAiD does not necessarily mean that someone wants to be killed, but rather that they are expressing a loss of identity and purpose. It indicates that they are in distress, not that they have a desire to die. This should never be taken literally, especially considering that the desire for hastened death is a common symptom of depression. That is why the Hospital Anxiety and Depression Scale should be used as an automatic assessment tool for all MAiD requests. Psychiatrists are typically cautious about diagnosing depression based on just one session with a patient, and medical doctors are even more reluctant to do so. However, now that assisted dying is legalized, the desire for hastened death is recognized, normalized, and approved through two assessment conversations based on its surface meaning: *I want out!* But beneath those words lies the true plea for help: *I'm scared. I'm overwhelmed. I'm powerless. I've lost who I want to be in the world.*

The research is clear on this. Combing through six medical databases reveals that the request to hasten death "is a response to overwhelming emotional distress and has differing meanings, which do not necessarily imply a genuine wish to hasten one's death."[233] The distress was consistent among over one hundred cases: loss of self, fear of dying, MAiD as an escape from final deterioration, and control (often described as an ace up one's sleeve). It is spiritual distress, which only increased as they imagined their demise. This aspect is well illustrated in a German study with twelve patients exploring their sense of suffering at the end of life. "The interviews provided a rich visual imagery of the experience of time and agony… dominated by expressive language and superlatives. Nearly all patients described very vivid pictures about anticipated situations which they tried to avoid."[234] And what they wanted to avoid was the suffering they imagined ahead. This suffocates one's ability to sit with ambiguity,

---

[233] Monforte-Royo, Cristina, et al. "What lies behind the wish to hasten death? A systematic review and meta-ethnography from the perspective of patients." *PLoS One* 7.5 (2012): e37117.

[234] Pestinger, Martina, et al. "The desire to hasten death: using Grounded Theory for a better understanding 'When perception of time tends to be a slippery slope.'" *Palliative Medicine* 29.8 (2015): pp. 711–719.

with that state of being so unlike any experience before. What is seen is misery made all the more real by the imagining. So, while depression is a dominant factor in MAiD requests, for most, it is a temporary state on the path of ego deconstruction.[235] The researchers also found that the purpose of talking about hastened death was not to have medical staff carry that out but instead to process their experience and have it respected. Among the conclusions were that the desire to hasten death "is an extreme coping strategy for intrusive emotional and cognitive experiences" and that "patients expressing a desire to hasten death are in need of more information about the dying process. Medical staff providing this information can be supportive in managing the distressing anticipated images of agony."[236]

These thoughts are entirely understandable, especially when death takes its sweet time. "I've said my goodbyes, I've taken care of my affairs, I've accepted my death, and now I lie here. Why is this taking so long?" It's a complaint I've heard many times, clearly indicating the dominance of a frustrated ego-identity in the face of a stubborn and all-too-resilient body. This "delay" marks the waiting period in which we are challenged to a deeper level of stillness, contemplation, opening, and final ego erosion. It is astonishingly difficult, increasing existential agitation that's taken out on family and the healthcare team.[237]

Let's explore this by first affirming that depression is different from grief (Figure 5). Grief is the natural process of letting go of this world, while depression is a process of withdrawing from the world. Anticipatory grief is that of the family and loved ones. Preparatory grief is that of the patient. Here's a simple overview of the differences:

---

[235] Emanuel, Ezekiel J., DL Fairclough, and LL Emanuel. "Attitudes and desires related to euthanasia and physician-assisted suicide among terminally ill patients and their caregivers." *Jama* 284.19 (2000): pp. 2460–2468 https://jamanetwork.com/journals/jama/fullarticle/193281. Accessed Oct. 31, 2021.

[236] Ibid

[237] To help with this, I'm producing some videos to assist with contemplation. They will be available online at davidmaginey.com, along with other resources to help you and your loved ones face this ultimate moment of life.

Anticipatory Grief	**Preparatory Grief**	**Depression**
Mood fluctuates	Mood fluctuates	Decreased pleasure in all aspects of life
Helplessness to change the situation	Self-esteem generally intact	Decreased self-esteem
Can feel surreal	Enjoys company but also withdraws	Hopelessness
Can strengthen sibling bonds	Able to look forward to special occasions	Guilt
Intensifies attachment to the one dying	Temporary agitation	Suicidal thoughts
Increased concern for the person's comfort	Increased concern for the family's well-being	Apathy

Figure 5: Grief vs Depression

Though we prepare to say goodbye to the individual dying, they prepare to say goodbye to reality, to everything they've ever known, to everything they think they are. As overwhelming as that sounds, most can do so quite well without professional counselling.[238] That's because, of course, grief is not a mental illness. It is a natural, even noble quality that testifies to a person's character and ability to love. When experienced without too much complication, grief is healthy because it is an expression of your humanity, good heart, and ability to feel love and connection. After all, the problem is not dying so much as leaving. The sorrow accompanying farewell is edged with a poignant beauty, for it indicates goodness at the ground of our being. It flows from the best of our humanity. This sadness is all the more an invitation to draw people close to say those final words, to express that heartfelt gratitude, to ask for reconciliation where relationships are in need of repair, and to say goodbye. The four most important statements through which we conclude our journey, explored so well by

[238] Bonanno, George A. *The Other Side of Sadness: What the New Science of Bereavement Tells Us About Life After Loss*. New York: Basic Books, 2009.

palliative physician and author Dr. Ira Byock in his book, *Four Things That Matter Most*, are *I love you, thank you, I forgive you, and forgive me* (then, of course, goodbye). Of note is when the dying experience the mystical shift in consciousness known as nearing-death awareness, fear of death evaporates, grief is supplanted by expectation, and one is filled with profound peace and connection to all. Thankfully, you don't need to die in order to experience this. You just need to show up.

EXERCISE 18: FOUR THINGS THAT MATTER

The exercise is designed to assist individuals in reflecting on important aspects of their lives and relationships as they prepare to leave this world. It is based on the principles outlined in Dr. Ira Byock's book, The Four Things That Matter Most. *The exercise focuses on four questions that encompass love, gratitude, forgiveness, and saying goodbye. The aim is to foster emotional healing, closure, and meaningful connections with loved ones.*

Instructions:

1. *Find a quiet and comfortable space where you can reflect without distractions. Have a journal or a piece of paper and a pen ready.*
2. *Take a few deep breaths, allowing yourself to relax and be present in the moment.*
3. *Begin with the first question: "Who do I love?" Take some time to contemplate the people in your life who hold a special place in your heart. Consider family members, friends, partners, or anyone else who has played a significant role in your life. Reflect on the love you feel for them and the impact they have had on your journey.*
    - *Write down the names of the individuals you love and reflect on the qualities and experiences that make your love for them meaningful.*
4. *Move on to the second question: "Who am I grateful for, and what am I thankful for?" Think about the people, experiences, or aspects of your life that you are grateful for. Consider the support, love, kindness, or lessons you have received from others.*
    - *Write down the names or specific things you are grateful for and reflect on the reasons behind your gratitude. Consider expressing your gratitude directly to those individuals.*
5. *Shift to the third question: "Whom do I need to forgive, and who do I seek forgiveness from?" Reflect on any unresolved conflicts,*

resentments, or hurts you may have towards others and any actions or behaviours you regret.

- *Write down the names of the individuals you need to forgive or seek forgiveness from, and consider the reasons behind these feelings. Reflect on what forgiveness means to you and how it can bring emotional healing and closure.*
- *Reflect on how you need to forgive yourself. This existential assignment is the hardest for most people, so it's helpful to notice any judgemental statements or messages you give yourself. Allow them by noticing where they stem from. What event in your past planted this seed of self-judgement? Can you return to that memory with lovingkindness, with compassion for your younger self?*

6. *Finally, address the fourth question: "What would I like to say in my goodbyes?" Contemplate what you want to express to your loved ones and the world as you prepare to depart. Consider the messages of love, gratitude, forgiveness, and closure you want to leave behind.*
    - *Write down your thoughts, messages, or final words, expressing your feelings and intentions as you say goodbye.*
7. *Take a moment to reflect on your answers and emotions. Allow yourself to experience the thoughts and feelings that arise.*
8. *Consider sharing your reflections and messages with trusted loved ones, as it can contribute to meaningful conversations and connections.*

Remember that this exercise is a personal journey, and there are no right or wrong answers. The goal is to engage in self-reflection, promote emotional well-being, and cultivate a sense of peace and closure as you prepare for the next phase of your journey.

Chapter 19

MEDITATION

You are the sky. The rest is just the weather.

– Pema Chödrön

On a telephone pole at the corner of a major intersection on my way to work is a promise: a poster that seems to float above the mosaic of rusty staples, concert advertisements, and info sessions on newly legalized marijuana. Against its soft yellow and green background is a smiling man, eyes gentle and peaceful, head bald and smooth as a freshly peeled egg. The script reads, "Learn meditation, find inner peace. Free sessions."

"Oh boy," I thought. "There's trouble." Meditation is definitely not the way to go if you want inner peace. Better to have a now-legal toke and go to one of those concerts, especially the jazz trio on the waterfront. Why? Because meditation is a war zone. It is raw engagement with the monkey mind, the cacophony of thoughts and distractions stirred up by naked awareness. No, I'll take smooth grooves and a joint over meditation any day. (Confession: I'm a drug virgin – never used weed, dragged on a cigarette, or even been drunk. I'm taking a literary license here to make a point.)

The promise on the poster was typical of popular spirituality, which sells something traditional spirituality couldn't care less about – achieving your potential, personal fulfillment, and finding your purpose. Or inner peace. I say this because these aspirations predominantly stem from our desire to feel better, get "it" right, and grow. Healthy spirituality, in contrast, is that in which the *I* who desires diminishes, as does desire itself.

Healthy spirituality, ironically, is never about you, for there is no *you*. There is only the *one*, not the *other*.

All the same, there's no denying the benefits of daily meditation, and it's wonderful that so many are turning to meditation to feel better. But this is not about liking your experience. It's about noticing your experience, allowing it, being authentic with it, and with how you are. There was some truth in that poster – the only way to happiness or well-being is through the inner path. This is about developing the capacity to feel the unpleasant aspects of your humanity, which, I would assert, are even more critical than the pleasant ones, for it is in our emotional pain that we most effectively learn the heart lessons of life: forgiveness, reconciliation, release of what cannot be, acceptance of what can, and seriously imagining that we can be at peace with death, that we can trust the mystery to come by fully feeling your experience without too much resistance. In fact, some resistance needs to remain. One does not become a master automatically! In allowing the resistance to be fully present at this moment, you are deepening your skill of awareness. We want to develop the ability to feel difficult emotions, including resistance to them, without acting on them. This is about sitting down and doing the opposite of what we are doing. This is about *being* – a state increasingly forced upon you as you die.

Meditation is tough. Let me state that upfront. If reframing is the introductory course to facing mortality, and logotherapy is the undergraduate level, then meditation is the master's degree. And that's when you're feeling well! If you're facing the end of your life, well... surprise, it could actually be easier at first in that your material will likely leap up for engagement. Additionally, for those who've never practised meditation, it can have surprising effectiveness precisely because you are a novice; when you don't know what to expect, that alone can facilitate a fantastic first session. The second one, though, will likely be relatively shallow in comparison precisely because you may desire an encore. Never happens.

Meditation is not calming the mind. That's not going to happen, either. The mind is designed to think, and the more one tries to stop that process, the more intense thinking will become. Instead, meditation is opening up to all the noise in the outer environment and all the noise within. We are attempting to be fully present with this moment and all it contains. All your feelings, all your thoughts, all your aches and pains. All the unfinished, unintegrated matters of the heart. It takes great courage to open up to all that.

No wonder we spend so much energy avoiding ourselves! But think of it this way: you've been taking treatment to fight for more moments of life but likely have avoided the moment you have because it's hard. It's thick with unfinished love stories, unsaid words, and the unknown aspects of yourself that are aching for integration. It's overwhelming! But the goal here is not to stay cool and calm and in control. The goal is to be authentic. If you're considering MAiD, this is the opportunity to dive deep and listen to the stirrings of fear, anxiety, grief, and distress that drive your desire for a more straightforward exit. Listen to the loss of what was, what you were, and the mystery of all that lies within. And be kind with it. This is not something that needs to be fixed. It needs to be loved. With practice, one becomes accustomed to this noise and allows it without resistance. This is the art of interoception: being aware of how you are aware – watching your thoughts, watching your own experience – returning to the centre of stillness and pure awareness. Can you allow yourself to be impaled upon this present moment?

Ken Wilber comments on this ability. "To the extent that you actually realize that you are not, for example, your anxieties, then your anxieties no longer threaten you. Even if anxiety is present, it no longer overwhelms you because you are no longer exclusively tied to it. You are no longer courting it, fighting it, resisting it, or running from it. In the most radical fashion, anxiety is thoroughly accepted and allowed to move as it will. You have nothing to lose, nothing to gain, by its presence or absence, for you are simply watching it pass by."[239]

The very act of watching your distress means part of you has no distress. Even more, that which observes pain is painless, that which observes

---

[239] Wilber, Ken. *No Boundary: Eastern and Western Approaches to Personal Growth.* Shambhala Publications, 2001.

fear is fearless. And that which observes dying is deathless. To witness a state is to transcend it. They no longer seize you from behind because you look at them from the front. There comes, with practice, a point of stillness in which the Ground of Being reveals itself, like moonlight reflected on calm water. Opening to this, the Presence pours into the self, which we experience as an integration, opening, enfoldment, and expansion. Powerful psycho-spiritual processes are at play here. Identification with the personal self dissolves, and the mind is healed of its exhausting habits and illusions of separation and defence. It is the deepest level of healing and restoration. This is a pivotal point at which a person transitions to the next level of conscious development.

Recalling Kathleen Dowling Singh's insights, spiritual transformation begins when we heal the rift between our subconscious shadow and the persona, the perceived self. We literally expand in being, accessing the deeper dimensions of the repressed self to reach greater authenticity. No longer suppressing our material, we are in a state of heightened vitality. This is optimal in healing the next rift, that of mind and body.

Our ego, in this practice, is not destroyed but healed and integrated. And so much of our ego is entwined with our physical ability, appearance, and processes – especially as we die. This is a powerful dynamic in the request for assisted death, as the body becomes frail and foul, as its functioning is severely compromised. Meditation, at this point, helps us be kind and grateful for our fleshly form, allowing it to be as it is. No longer "my body," there becomes only experience itself of "being," not "being in form."

Integration and expansion continue as the constant inner dialogue, so persistent over the decades, dissolves. In this unravelling, there is no fortress of self to defend, no solid ground on which to stand. One simply is. And this is where it all blows up. Anxiety erupts as primal repression becomes frail in the presence of the Ground of Being. The fundamental level of fear has been laid bare – the level at which we have always identified as a self separate from that from which we emanate and by which we are sustained. Call it God, or consciousness, or the quantum field, or life itself. Its name does not matter, for here is the last defence of ego against the mystery, the void, the wonder. As we give ourselves to the experience of surrender and not-knowing, joy, peace, ecstasy, and light burst forth. A secret abundance becomes that which you are.

Now, if you think this is too exceptional and you're no good at meditation, I'll remind you that you already know how to do it. You've been doing it sporadically throughout life, and your best practice was when you were very young. As an infant, you were a master, but the skill became shrouded by layers of distraction and unfocused attention in a world filled with dangers and pretty shiny things. But it never left. Mindful awareness is as wired into you as tears and laughter. It's as simple as dust motes in the air or the sun upon your face. It's all there. As thought is awareness in motion, we need to slip underneath that current to the still waters waiting in the depths.

Letting yourself sink into that will be challenging. This is simple, but it is not easy. This focused awareness cuts through and dissolves the boundaries of persona and shadow, animate and inanimate, body and mind, self and other. Remember, those are the lines by which ego draws its existence. Do you think there won't be resistance when erasing them?

GAINING FOCUS

I AM AN AVID PHOTOGRAPHER. ONE OF THE GREATEST PLEASURES AND challenges with this hobby is astrophotography: capturing images of galaxies and nebula. I recall heading out one clear night with a gorgeous moon, which is something you don't want! Reflected light from that orb washes out the stars. I was frustrated, but you work with what you've got. I pointed the camera at its cratered surface, yet even with a good lens, my photograph wasn't as clear and sharp as I wanted. Multiple factors were at play, including automatic camera settings, atmospheric distortion, and electronic noise on the camera sensor. I would have to overcome all of them to get the image I needed. Simply pointing the camera and clicking the shutter would not be enough.

The first step was to switch to manual focus and exposure; I had to override the camera's programming and focus on infinity, then tell it to underexpose; otherwise, the bright moon would be washed out against the black sky. Second, I set the camera to record RAW files containing all the image data instead of JPEGs, which compress the data. This would give me more control in fine-tuning the image. Third, I used stacking, taking multiple images of the moon and digitally combining them. Stacking software averages the differences to refine features and improve the signal-to-noise ratio. Finally, I carefully adjusted contrast, luminance, and clarity in post-production. The result revealed fine details that would be impossible to render with a single, unprocessed shot.

A similar process also improves meditation, especially in our distracted age. The first step is taking manual control of our thoughts, so they don't automatically focus on whatever wanders onto the mental landscape. We can also reduce exposure to social media and virtual environments, which have severely compromised our ability to stay focused, and clouded our consciousness with internal noise. All the more with meditation, where this noise appears in the form of a short attention span, attachment to outcome, the voice of the ego, fear, and doubt. Most of us ignore all this and compress it into the subconscious (like a JPEG file). Yet that information is critical in achieving the highest state of coherent consciousness. Training and guidance can help us work wisely with these distortions and engage that RAW material in such a way as to improve our clarity and resolution while the noise drops. And you know what they say: shoot for the moon. Even if you miss, you'll land among the stars.

Another analogy that may help also involves light. If we were to shine a powerful flashlight down a dark road, the beam would fade as it would not be focused enough to avoid being scattered by dust particles. On the other hand, a laser is a coherent light, a narrow beam that, even with little power, can pierce the darkness and mark a spot a kilometre away (and even one on the moon if it's powerful enough). Such is meditation. This is coherent awareness, a focused consciousness that cuts through the noise of the ego, mind, and environment to illuminate deeper dimensions of self.

Meditation can be understood as a rehearsal for dying since it is an intentional deconstruction of the ego. As such, it is not an intellectual process. This is not something you "understand" or a method or "spiritual technology." It is a letting go of what is. In the beginning, it is controlling awareness, but quickly the need for control dissolves as one approaches the still-point. Here even the self disappears as the Ground of Being emerges from the fog of perception. As one goes further, there is a union, a merging in which one "arrives" at what has always been: this moment. Authenticity, congruency, integrity, abundance, openness, relaxation, and profound interconnectivity all mark this state of being.

COMMITTING TO THE CHAOS

KEN WILBER, ONE OF THE WORLD'S MOST PROLIFIC THINKERS AND LEADERS in transpersonal psychology, states: 'Ultimately, a person in meditation must face having no recourse, no way out, no forward or backward; [one] is reduced to the simplicity of the moment.... [One's] boundaries collapse, and, as St. Augustine put it, one "arrives at That Which Is."'[240]

"That Which Is" is all you'll be after death. To take the pressure off, if this seems like a lofty goal, it's reassuring to note that few people have progressed beyond the level of ego-identity, and if they have, they find they cannot maintain that state, for in maintaining itself emerges the effort of control once again. Even as we die, the ego instinctively activates strategies that bury subconscious material, reinforcing the perceived separation from others, objects, and the environment. It will strive to *prevent* the perception of reality *as it is*, for in that distortion, the ego establishes itself, and through that distortion, we experience the human journey. No wonder there's such resistance to the ego's deconstruction when it's time to leave! And no wonder MAiD is attractive to the modern mind, which is a stranger to the wisdom of spiritual traditions and a skeptic of mystical and non-ordinary states of being, which often come through suffering. The ego sees suffering as something to avoid at all costs – even the cost of experiencing transformation. Ironic that surrender is not a weakness in this situation, but wisdom, for vulnerability is transcended due to its acceptance. In light of this, MAiD becomes the ultimate act of the ego to preserve its locus of control, a manoeuvre of regression to the early stages

[240] Wilber, Ken. *The Spectrum of Consciousness*. Quest Books, 1993, p. 283

of ego development in which safety was paramount. So, the great tragedy is not that we suffer from our darkness but our shallowness. This is why I assert that the orientation to death from which MAiD stems serves only to preserve the self. It is the resistance to being apprehended by that which we are incapable of understanding.

Kathleen Dowling Singh reminds us that the rituals and practices of any robust spiritual tradition (and specifically meditation) are meant to help this by breaking down the separation of the self from the Sacred. This is exponentially so at death. These "skillful means" reveal the path home. The process by which they work is… annoying.

> "Any skillful means frustrate the identity of the level of consciousness that is being offered for transformation. The practice of skillful means puts enabling energy into the system of the self, allowing expansion of consciousness. In the act of frustrating the present level of identification, a skillful means forces the destabilized consciousness through the transformative fields of experience [toward the Ground of Being]."[241]

In other words, it's good stress. Through life, this purposeful pressure is called *eustress*, but in death, it's felt as misery at the level of mind by which you are functioning. Dying forces you (as there is no reverse gear) into the wilderness of not knowing, not controlling… it is a surrender to the transformative process, in which we disentangle ourselves from the present experience and move to a state of self-abidance. This state is the essence of prayer or meditation. It is simple awareness without interpretation. It is being, not doing. It is the return to the Ground of Being, in which you no longer say "I don't like this," or even "I am dying," but simply "I am."

As cliché as it is, this is the story of the dragonfly, beautifully written by Doris Stickney to explain death to children.[242] It tells a tale of an

---

[241] Singh, Kathleen Dowling. *The Grace in Dying: How We Are Transformed Spiritually as We Die*. New York: HarperSanFrancisco, 1998, p. 114.

[242] Stickney, Doris. *Water Bugs and Dragonflies: Explaining Death to Young Children*. Pilgrim Press, 1987.

instinctive knowing that transformation will come. A dragonfly larva is *driven* to emerge from the water. It is *compelled* to create the chrysalis and enter unconsciousness. It *must* emerge as an entirely new creature. Resisting this process is not an option for any animal on earth, save one. We are so developed that we can see demise approaching and so deluded that we mistake our minds and thoughts for ourselves, all about to end. So, we resist our deconstruction and increase our suffering through that resistance. I've repeatedly seen this in people who are swimming in despair, uttering what sounds like a surprise. "I'm dying. I'm actually dying."

Frustrating present levels of identity. In Zen practice, this is the job of the spiritual teacher: to insult you. To offend the ego's identity in order that it is seen for what it is: a projection of fear, of alienation from the Ground of Being. That's our state through much of life, what the Christian tradition calls "original sin" (a word that means separation). We are cut off from aspects of ourselves, others, and the Spirit.

Most of us don't have a Zen teacher sitting at our side to slap awakening into us. Well, existential distress is up to the task. That is its function. That's what illness, suffering, and dying do as movement toward something greater. You can see why I assert that MAiD is the ultimate act of ego self-preservation in the face of the very process that deconstructs it for our transformation. We are grabbing control back, and it feels good. Empowering. Self-actualizing. But, unknowingly and instinctively, this is a refusal to allow the final stage of human development.

I sat with one man who was sick and tired of dying. He was consumed with frustration bordering, at times, on manic-depressive episodes. He had mentally accepted his impending death, but had not yet experienced the full physical dimension of it, nor the psycho-spiritual opening to it. Those were stages he dreaded exploring! His children were concerned because he seemed so withdrawn, but I knew this as evidence of his cognitive acceptance. Pulling away from relationships, shutting down, no longer gazing at the sunlight sparkling on the water; he was saying goodbye to the world and thought he was ready to leave. "When can I die? Let's get this over with!" Each morning he woke with a sigh. "Still here, still here."

Those receiving MAiD avoid the chrysalis and think this is the better choice, as they don't have to linger longer than they want. The procedure preserves the autonomy, identity, and integrity of the mental ego. It avoids the incubation found only in solitude, frailty, and periods of unconsciousness before death. When mortality is breathing down our necks, we become aware that our disconnection from everything will become permanent, for we will leave all we have known and move into nothing we have ever experienced. No "other." No "self." Oblivion or transformation can feel the same for the soul that has not yet allowed the chrysalis to form. Both are states we cannot comprehend because they are beyond apprehension yet are inevitable. One man, so gregarious and successful through life, summed it up with a sigh, then tears as he confessed, *My God, I feel so alone. . . .*

Sitting kindly with this, practising self-compassion, and presenting instead of projecting your distress through accurately stating how it feels, what it's like, and how you don't want it, is how one discovers that you can allow it. And then identifying what does bring meaning, what is your story… this is what processes the experience. Here it is essential to no longer confuse the storyteller with the story. This requires you *not knowing how it will go,* not understanding any of it, but allowing it. This is why we meditate: practising deep, compassionate presence with our experience, not abandoning any part of ourselves on the road of deconstruction. It's not about peaceful relaxation, as promised on the poster stapled to the telephone pole. Peaceful relaxation is a state to arrive at to *begin* the practice.

I have a confession. Observing the mind's noise as inconsequential as the sound of traffic in the distance or the soft murmur of voices in a cozy café on a winter afternoon while you enjoy that perfect Americano… I mean, green tea… is the state I most often achieve in meditation. Nothing spectacular (there's that ego again, judging the experience!). Only once did I awaken to that state of consciousness Ken Wilber is talking about, to arrive at *That Which Is*: when I died.

I'll recount that in Chapter 26, but here I'll mention that the greatest gift of my near-death experience is that this orientation of being and identity lives in me to this day. I need only pause and return my awareness to the event for it to become animated with the same intensity, depth, wonder, abundance, and fullness of being as it had for those brief fifteen minutes thirty years ago. It is a living memory. This is consistent with research that shows the emotional intensity and detail of recall for experiencers never fades, unlike everyday memories.[243] But it leaves us forever homesick for that land which lies within. This is not a condition or way of being; it is that which apprehends me. I am the object, not the subject, in this experience. There is no "I" at all in it. And yet the "me" that I experience as the self, seemingly separate from this keyboard and computer in "front" of me, seemingly something, someone "other" than the trees outside my window, from you, the reader holding this book, from the world spinning ever more in this insanity of perceived separation… all this individuation and objectification breaks down as one is opened to the Ground of Being.

Michael Washburn, professor of Philosophy at Indiana University, called this egoic evaporation in the face of the transpersonal dimensions of being "regression in the service of transcendence," which leads to "regeneration in spirit."[244] One is emptied of self (most unpleasant!) to be filled with everything and made whole (the meaning of the word "salvation"). All I know is that I long to disappear once again in that beauty, that love (which is not an emotion but the highest state of consciousness). And I can, when I slow down, observe, accept, and surrender to that Living Presence. Because this is that from which reality emanates; you can too.

In the Buddhist tradition, this is *samadhi*, a state of profound and utterly absorptive contemplation of the Absolute that is undisturbed by desire, anger, or any other ego-generated thought or emotion. It is a state of joyful calm, or even of rapture and beatitude, in which one maintains one's full mental alertness and acuity. It is a state of grace.

---

[243] Thonnard, Marie, et al. "Characteristics of near-death experiences memories as compared to real and imagined events memories." *PloS One* 8.3 (2013): e57620.

[244] Washburn, Michael. *The Ego and the Dynamic Ground: A Transpersonal Theory of Human Development*. SUNY Press, 1988.

In the Christian tradition, it is to be "in Christ," which is not his last name, but a term for "the everything."[245] So encompassing is this connection that St. Paul states, "you are a new creation in Christ."[246] So absolute our reintegration that Jesus claims we can be one with God.[247]

When I do meditate on this, when I recall my transcendent experience… I cry. I weep. It's so much. But I have to function in this world, so I can't stay there too long. A brief five minutes is enough to recalibrate me to compassion, remind me that I don't need to believe everything I think, and recharge my faith in God's love so I can meet the next moment, person, or crisis with my love. It reminds me of the saying, "Before enlightenment, chop wood and haul water. After enlightenment, chop wood and haul water." I am not claiming to be enlightened. In fact, the perspective from within is that my awareness remains so abysmally erratic, ridiculously inconsistent, and astonishingly inefficient that I can claim to be little more than a clever primate.

This brings us to a central aspect of the "successful" meditative practice: a sense of humour with yourself. Humour allows you to be curious and compassionately detached from your own experience. It enables you to realize that you are not your thoughts, feelings, body, or life story. You are the actor on a stage, and the people you touch become the living documents of your life.

BEING KIND TO YOURSELF

Meditation insists that you be kind to yourself. Buddhists call this *matri*. One greets all that arises within… all the chaos, anger, frustration, indignity, powerlessness, self-pity, regret, denial, and longing… with a gentle smile. A sincere embrace. With compassion. And yes, one can meet even the desire for assisted death in the same way.

---

[245] Rohr, Richard. *The Universal Christ: How a Forgotten Reality Can Change Everything We See, Hope For, and Believe*. Convergent Books, 2019. See also his excellent presentation, "Richard Rohr on the Universal Christ." YouTube video. Sept 16, 2018. Uploaded by the Center for Action and Contemplation. www.youtube.com/watch?v=KD7B3wr3xeY. Accessed April 13, 2020.

[246] 2 Corinthians 5:17

[247] John 17:21

Meditation is lovely in that it fosters compassion and tenderness for your suffering. Engaging our frailty and distress with softness is not instinctive; the ego represses it, controls it, and judges it as we strive to "get our shit together." So tough. All spiritual work is a matter of shedding, of letting go. In meditation, the mind is the noise-maker, the creator of persona, of the imagined sense of who and what we are in the world. What are we shedding? Anything other than what is essential and perennial to your being. In the spiritual traditions, this is, again, ego deconstruction to merge with the Ground of Being, the fundamental consciousness that is all there is.

It sounds very fluffy, I know, but the call to loving-kindness for yourself is the opening to something wondrous. It can be summarized in one word that instantly liberates you. And yet, that word often triggers negative feelings; it instills guilt. It can make one feel unworthy. It can make one feel depraved. That word is mercy, heard weekly by churchgoers in the prayerful petition, "Lord, have mercy!" Have mercy and don't punish me; have mercy and give me your undeserved grace and favour; have mercy on me, a poor sinner. In centuries past, the pious would flog themselves while crying this out to the heavens. The penitent would bow their heads with hands bound before their executioner and whisper this wish. It is uttered by the unworthy. Well, let's put that aside as it's already God's nature to be that way – to be completely understanding, kind, compassionate, and gracious beyond measure. The problem is not that we need to ask it of God, but of ourselves.

We are ruthless critics. We tear ourselves and each other apart with instinctive cruelty. To practise mercy for ourselves and those who injure us is to see behind the veil. It is to honour and elevate the divine, the good, and the beauty in everyone, even when they don't honour it in themselves. We do not define them by the pain they are projecting. That is what it is to be a bodhisattva, a warrior of compassion.

More problematic still is practising this for ourselves when we are afraid. Fear amplifies suffering. We are habituated to it, the critical inner voice. We are used to it, much more comfortable equating our essence to how we have fallen short than to our magnificence. Now that we are dying, this assignment is cranked up: to be compassionate with your sorrow, to soften into your grief, to be gentle with your unfinished life.

I sat with Kathy, a ninety-six-year-old who was swallowed in lament for her unfinished life "cut short." I thought that was ridiculous. Ninety-six years! And yet, what appeared before me as we opened to her grief was a young woman, a teenager, who lived as large as ever within the tumour-laden wrinkled form before me. "I love life! I love the sky and the flowers and the stars. I'm not done yet! Why is God doing this to me? What did I do to deserve this? What did I do?"

She did love the flowers. Paintings she had done years earlier were hung on the walls; her stories of sitting in those mountain meadows back in Germany evoked the breeze in the trees and warm sunshine upon her face. Those were the good old days in which she had loved well: a wonderful marriage, a loving daughter, and many friends. Her husband died thirty years earlier, yet she had found purpose and new dimensions of herself in the years that followed. Even more than this, she had seen the horrors of war as a child. That suffering was fuel for this enthusiasm, this appreciation for life. The flowers, the mountains, the sky… the freedom. The exhilaration of being free and alive. Cancer had crudely interrupted it all with a grotesque tumour on the side of her neck. It threatened to collapse her airway. She contemplated slow suffocation. Her tears seemed inconsolable.

Moving tenderly into this awareness didn't "fix" her; it opened her to how beautiful her soul had become. What a lovely human being to be so awake to the gift of life! Yet, as clear as that was to me, she burst into even greater wailing. "But I want more!" This is the greatest sorrow. And we all have it – unfinished business, clinging to what we know, resisting the opening to come.

She was with us for months, and, fortunately, the tumour did not grow toward her trachea, but it did spread into her chest and back. Medication kept pain under control, and movement was maintained as long as possible with the help of physiotherapy. But it was the kindness that touched her the deepest. Daily she was dipped in the waters of compassion. Slowly she was washed of her wailing. I sat with her and listened to the story of her days. We identified what she was most proud of (her daughter), what was most important (to be seen as the young woman within, a person of vitality and energy), and what was to come (seeing her husband again).

Death anxiety diminished, and eventually, now lying in her bed, she was able to say the words, "I am dying." She was able to contemplate her life with gratitude. And she could imagine there would be flowers where she was headed.

I did not find out if she saw them, for like so many patients, Kathy died in the night, her nurse and daughter at her side. Surrounded by love, secure in good pain management, and with her husband's embrace just beyond the veil. That was more than enough. I say this confidently as others I have supported related exactly that, modelling grace in dying and allowing their ego deconstruction in a way that is nothing less than sublime. Here, through the connection to the Ground of Being, all fear of death evaporated and was replaced with a deep peace beyond understanding. This is a complete recalibration of consciousness, a reorientation to the present moment that occurs as one moves through the transitional and transformative stages of chaos, despair, and struggle.

People eligible for MAiD, especially those in a hospital, are ideally positioned to experience this. With good pain management and compassionate care, we are well set up to be shocked by how safe death is. And the more we trust mercy, grace, and loving-kindness, the wiser our work with anxiety will be as we approach that final moment. Phenomenal insight is available, but on our deathbed, our concentration will be thin. Pain medication will cloud perception. Weakness will suppress self-awareness. We should practise before we die to develop trust in going beyond who we have been. We do this by stepping out of the familiar role of self and observing what we imagine ourselves to be. We practise by trusting our default state of simple awareness, a state that is constant throughout life but clouded by thoughts, experiences, and desires. We practise realizing we are the condensation of a mystery, lightly dusted with form to animate the Ground of Being on the material level of existence. We practise to return to our original nature. This is why meditation is a rehearsal for death, helping us consider how we have identified the self with thoughts, feelings, body, persona, and ego instead of simple awareness. Not even with experience, but with awareness, for awareness precedes experience. Enlightenment is, then, waking up to this authenticity.

JUST A PINCH

How about a simple test to experience these principles? Let's use an unpleasant sensation, pain, but do so in a way that keeps you in complete control. I choose pain because it's the one thing people dread most: unbearable suffering of the body. We hate our pain; we run from it, medicate it, and have nightmares about it. So, let's work with that one and make it manageable. (This, of course, applies only to a certain level of pain. If you are suffering significant or extreme pain, drop the book now and take appropriate medication. Remember those drugs are meant to stay ahead of the pain, not to chase it. Please don't be stubborn about that. OK, back to practice.)

Pinch yourself. Use the fleshy part of your thumb where it meets your palm. Apply moderate pressure with the nail of your other thumb, not so hard that it damages the skin but certainly feels uncomfortable. Notice the sensation of pain, how it pulses, how it shifts. Notice the sharpness and how localized that is. Explore with your observation how the pain sits within your hand and the other sensations that arise in your body. Does your breath change, your vision shift, or your head feel different? As you keep the pressure constant, you may find the pain dulling. You're adapting to the sensation, or the area may become numb. If so, increase the pressure. Amplify the pain and your observation of it. Breathe into it. Breathe deeply. Try to discern the sensation in the pinching thumb compared to the one being pinched. Tell yourself, "I am in control. This is a sensation I want to learn how to observe my own experience." We can also reframe our relationship to the pain. Pain is, after all, a good thing, wired to help alert us to danger. If we accidentally touch a hot oven, pain kicks in before our brain even registers the contact, initiating a muscle reflex to pull the hand away before too much damage is done. We can be grateful for the pain, as it ensures our survival. (Of course, when dying, pain indicates advancing disease. Your healthcare team is there to help you manage that!)

You've been pinching your thumb for some time now, so release. Feel the sensation of blood returning to the pressure point, the sting that remains, and the possible pulsing in the muscle. Move the thumb, feeling not only the dissipating pain but being aware of how the mind relaxes, knowing the pain has stopped.

Can we relate to existential distress in the same way as to that physical pain? That it is there to tell us something important? How about with grief? Both your own and your family's? Can we do so with our fear? I appreciate that fear is overwhelming at times. But think of it: can a thunderstorm overwhelm the sky? The fear, as real as it seems, is your reaction to an experience that threatens the integrity of your identity. Yet, if you observe the fear, with the curiosity of meeting a stranger, your relationship to it will be quite different than if you allow it to swallow you. Of course, we don't want to be afraid. Of course we want to avoid the suffering and sinking into death's embrace. Yet to die without fear, we must first learn to live with fear. We must become familiar with its form and not place a bandage on any part of the experience. Rather, we learn to observe the experience. This holds a great surprise for us: awareness cannot experience fear. The mind certainly can, and it's very good at it! But awareness, the neutral and infinite state of that which is you, cannot. It is challenging to interrupt your response before it happens, yet it can be done so in a moment. It only takes a moment.

Can we do this when we know we are going to die? I've said before that grief is the price we pay for love, for love connects our consciousness to others. When we realize death is approaching, we enter the initial stages of preparatory grief – saying goodbye to everyone we've known, to reality itself. We are who we are through our relationships – to self, others, the world, and our life story. All of that will be deconstructed through suffering and dying. On that level, as shattering as it is, we can be thankful for our grief, just as we could be thankful for our pain a moment ago, because our grief indicates our connection, our interrelationship to all that is. It is a noble aspect of our humanity. One who grieves the unfinished love stories is both broken and beautiful. I would aspire to be so fully human at the end of life.

Let's also acknowledge, though, that grief can be powerfully fuelled by fear. It can be grasping and holding onto our attachments – to others, our role in the world, our persona and perceived independence, control, and self-determination. Resisting the release of these aspects of ego is understandable. Still, we need to be aware that resistance compromises our well-being and significantly increases our suffering as we die. Indeed, resistance to this type of suffering is the motivating factor in most MAiD requests.

Thankfully, meditation increases your ability to experience difficult emotions (equanimity) and even rewire the brain, (specifically the anterior cingulate cortex).[248] This regulates the more primitive signals from the amygdala – such as fight, flight, or freeze response when considering one's death – with the higher regulatory function of the neocortex. So one can not only tolerate the instinct to flee but override it. This is a game-changer for someone considering MAiD to escape the imagined suffering ahead. But what if you're new to the practice? Fortunately, meditating for as little as ten seconds has been found to benefit emotional regulation and even initiate neuronal growth in the brain. Still, it must be ten seconds several times an hour. That's manageable and far less daunting than thirty minutes straight.

Pema Chödrön said it was torture the first time she did it. She sat with others in a meditation room, cross-legged on a cushion. Very uncomfortable! They were instructed to focus on their breath and observe their experience for thirty minutes. Then the gong sounded. Those were the most difficult thirty minutes she could imagine. Her thoughts were constantly running off, interrupting, demanding attention, and insisting they were real. They were what she was all about. All this, of course, was not overt, but the dynamic underlying all our collective delusion – that we *are* our thoughts, we *are* our feelings. This is why we see the world as we are, not as the world is. What a refreshing realization: that we are so much more than that. I have my thoughts; I have my feelings. They do not have me. That truth may work on a good day, but when you're dying, the challenge is exponential. And here is where it is critical for you to do something that sounds abysmally innocuous: be kind to yourself. Be gentle with that scared part of you and engage, if only slightly, with self-compassion. It's helpful to use reframing within your meditation practice, especially when you're struggling. Here are some examples of how a person facing the end of life might experience this (Figure 6).

[248] Taren, Adrienne A., J. David Creswell, and Peter J. Gianaros. "Dispositional mindfulness co-varies with smaller amygdala and caudate volumes in community adults." *PloS One* 8.5 (2013): e64574.

Avoidance	Engagement
Distract, don't think about it. I'll sleep, I'll feel nothing, or push my sadness, anger, resentment, regret, and grief away. I'll avoid deep conversations.	Notice what it feels like to resist these emotions. How are the feelings held in my body? What are these feelings? I will try to "hold the space" of my own experience.
Difficult thoughts and feelings arise, and I label them as bad, because they are unpleasant. "I don't like this." "This is awful."	I can describe, instead of judge, my thoughts and feelings. I can engage them with curiosity. As difficult as thoughts and feelings are, I have them, they don't have me.
As feelings intensify, I react and resist. "I can't do this!" "What if it gets worse?" "I'm overwhelmed." I cry, my stomach feels tight, my head feels dizzy. I want to curl into a ball. I'm scared.	I can bring my attention to the present moment. I can notice that I am handling it now. This moment is hard, but I am here, and these emotions and thoughts are temporary. They come and go.
My critical voice says, "I shouldn't feel this way. I need to be strong and calm. I'm falling apart."	I do feel this way, but I can choose how to respond and act on my feelings. They are saying something important about my life.
My thoughts and behaviour change so rapidly – panic, escape, shut down, lash out… I'm overwhelmed.	Curiosity helps me name, describe, and explore my feelings. If I am panicking, I can use my breath to reset, and rely on others to help me feel safe in this moment.
I'm scared of the pain. I'm scared dying will be awful.	Am I in pain now? I can ask for more medication. My team will ensure I am comfortable as I die. Their compassion and the love of my family can enfold me. "I do not know what it is like to die, but this is the universal human experience. I am supported, I am not alone."

Figure 6: Avoidance and Engagement

Reframing and meditation are best practised early (as in now) before you are overwhelmed. Test them in the shallow waters before venturing into the deep. Practise while the surface is relatively calm before the storm hits. You'll discover that, in the end, the goal is not to calm the waves but to learn how to surf. And then, when death comes, to discover you didn't need the board at all.

Pema Chödrön echoes the Buddhist concept of "the second arrow," in that our relationship to our body's pain causes a second injury: mental suffering. The two then dance in a feedback loop of distress, amplifying each other. So embedded is this pattern in the human animal that the body believes even the memory of pain is as real as the original experience and sends out an identical cascade of neural signals and stress hormones. Ironically, the solution to this spiral of pain and suffering is so counterintuitive that the ego mind instinctively recoils in anticipated anxiety. It is also so effective that I've had patients exclaim in astonishment that it worked at all. It is simple but slippery. It is profoundly challenging yet persistently available. It is… surrender – giving yourself entirely to the experience. It is the skill of becoming embedded in that intolerable moment. As intentional and terrifying as that is, this is achieved by not doing but simply being.

EXERCISE 19: REHEARSAL

Let's try this out with a simulation. I invite you to imagine your death. (After all, meditation is simply rehearsing the end of your ego through not identifying with it.) While I've recorded this at davidmaginley.com, you could do this meditation with a loved one present. That person would read the meditation to you, taking significant time, about twenty to thirty seconds, between each phrase. If you are that support person, your assignment is to be fully present with whatever arises in your loved one and yourself. If they become emotional, you should not make them feel better or stop the session, but only pause and let your voice remain soft. Words too quickly seek to understand, to contain, to assert connection. Trust that you both have that at a much deeper level. Give yourself to the rehearsal from the heart, not the head. From the body, not the mind. From the soul, the mystery, the grace and the sorrow.

This may be very emotional. It will be awkward at best and heartbreaking at worst. Let it be what it will be. It's only a rehearsal, a safe way to open up to the experience we all dread, but I have found it to be the most transformative event in the human journey. So, let's begin.

Lie down. Breathe...

Let your eyes drink in the surroundings. Observe. Note the quality of light in the room... bright or dim... sharp shadows or soft... notice the colours... the lines and shapes of objects, of forms...

Breathe.

Now close your eyes. Feel the weight of eyelids on pupils... note the shifting afterimage of light and colour upon your inner field of vision...

Breathe.

Shift awareness to sound. Listen to the noise in your environment... those that are far... the sounds outside your room... your home... perhaps traffic or people speaking... listen to the sounds in your room... a fan, a creak... your breath...

Breathe. Feel the flow of air through your nose or mouth... feel the air flow down into your lungs... feel your chest or stomach rise and fall... relax your diaphragm, your belly as you are able... allow the air to flow as deep and relaxed as you can... whatever its quality, observe your breathing...

Shift awareness to your body... feel the weight of it supported by your bed... Open to any sensations your body may have... as you move your attention to your feet... feel your toes, your heel on the mattress... move your awareness up your calves, to your knees, your thighs... notice any sensations and allow them, even if unpleasant...

Breathe. Notice how your hips feel... your lower back... stomach... middle back... chest... upper back... move your awareness gently up to your neck... your scalp... your face... your lips... your tongue... feel your physicality... your embodiment... feel the weight of your body supported by the bed...

Your body has changed so much over the decades... Some cells have lived for years; others are replaced every hour... So, your body, with which you have identified all your life, is not essential to who and what you are... Breathe gratitude to your body for providing you with a physical experience of life... it is truly unique, though now it feels frail... allow the feeling of weakness... allow the aches and pains... notice how those sensations shift... they do not remain still... notice any pulsing, any movement...

Breathe. Notice your thoughts... allow whatever thoughts there are to flow... to be... no judgment, no filtering... step back and observe your thoughts... Most of us have a thought every three to five seconds... the mind is a noise highway... no need to understand, no need to analyze, no need to fix... let it flow... for these thoughts are not essential to who you are.

Breathe. Notice your feelings... sense where you hold feelings in your body... try to identify their texture, their edges... the feelings may be intense... overwhelming... breathe into them... allow them... observe them... they do not sit still; they flow... they change... they are not essential to what you are...

Breathe... you have this body but are not this body... you have these thoughts, but are not these thoughts... move back with your awareness even further... watch your experience... notice how even that is always in motion... constantly changing... even your experience is not essential to who you are... to what you are...

Breathe... notice... that you are awareness... you are awareness... you are awareness having an experience... sense the space of this... sense the expansive unknown... it is independent of the sounds... the body... the thoughts...

the feelings... the experience... it is neither in the past nor future... for there is only now... only now...

Be. Let the rest go... and be.

For an extended guided experience of this meditation, go to https://soundcloud.com/david-maginley/rehearsal

Chapter 20

A MIRACLE PILL?

What we call reality is in fact nothing more than a culturally sanctioned and linguistically reinforced hallucination.

– Terence Mckenna

If only we could have given Kevin, who died in agony from acute leukemia (as discussed in Chapter 19), something to soothe his anxiety around dying long before those physical symptoms became torturous. We know he requested assisted death because he wanted to stay in control, even more so as we said his natural end would be sudden. We did not, however, emphasize that it would be so severe. Palliative sedation was offered, but this man was a risk taker who went all-out on anything he did. He did not even realize the terror of the existential wave deep within until it became a tsunami upon the more shallow shores of self-awareness. Our pain medications have some power to mitigate that, but they only mask distress or sedate it into submission.

There is another approach, though, that has grabbed the interest of the public and medical professionals. It's being touted as the next best thing due to its surprising effectiveness in eliminating death anxiety and inducing an expanded state of consciousness. With a single dose, many report an experience of pure love and unity. Unfortunately, this type of drug is being stripped from its cultural heritage and employed for purposes it was never intended for.

Most know psychedelics by their notable reputation for altering sensory perceptions, thought processes, energy levels… the list goes on. Study in psychedelics was lively from the late 1950s to the early 1970s, exploring their use in psychotherapy. Over a thousand scientific papers were published, with more than forty thousand research subjects, showing its effectiveness in treating various conditions, including alcoholism and mental health disorders. They were also legal and easy to obtain.

When one is exploring the psychological and spiritual states induced by a drug, it helps to have first-hand experience. After all, these are subjective experiences. (BTW, I offer this information as someone with no first-hand and very little second-hand knowledge on the subject. Everything I present is from the rabbit hole of research I've done for this book, so please forgive the generalizations.) Psychologist Bill Richards, a leading researcher in the field, realized diving into the deep end was a necessary step in studying the substance. His experience with LSD is evocative not so much of the Beatle's "Lucy in the Sky with Diamonds" as of the visions of mystics from various Indigenous spiritual traditions. On ingesting the drug, he was transported.

"I felt immersed in this incredibly detailed imagery that looked like Islamic architecture, with Arabic script, about which I knew nothing. And then I somehow *became* these exquisitely intricate patterns, losing my usual identity. And all I can say is that the eternal brilliance of mystical consciousness manifested itself. My awareness flooded with love, beauty, and peace beyond anything I had ever known or imagined possible. 'Awe,' 'glory,' and 'gratitude' were the only words that remained relevant."[249]

That kind of experience is enough to evoke folklore fervour that the remedy to all our ills has been found in the ancient temples of Peru, but the historical narrative around psychedelics is far from complete. In fact, anthropologists have very little to go on when compiling evidence to demonstrate the most popular story, that their use goes back thousands of years and may be the origins of religion.[250] That certainly makes sense

[249] Pollan, Michael. *How To Change Your Mind: What the New Science Of Psychedelics Teaches Us About Consciousness, Dying, Addiction, Depression, and Transcendence.* Penguin, 2019, p. 53

[250] Singh, Manvir. "Psychedelics Weren't as Common in Ancient Cultures as We Think." Vice.com. Dec. 10, 2020. www.vice.com/en/article/4adngq/psychedelic-drug-use-in-ancient-indigenous-cultures. Accessed May 6, 2023.

and is an attractive assumption, but humanity and history are far more complex. Despite our tendency to simplify and romanticize cultural matters, one aspect of psychedelics does emerge: they were never intended for recreational use and were never just for the individual's benefit. These are regarded as sacred substances to be employed under guidance from a shaman and within specific customs and rituals for the sake of the community.

Maria Magdalena Garcia, a Mazatec *curandera,* or shaman, describes her role in facilitating the wisdom imparted through these substances:

> There is a world beyond ours, a world that is far away, nearby, and invisible. And there it is where God lives, where the dead live, the spirits and the saints, a world where everything has already happened and everything is known. That world talks. It has a language of its own. I report what it says. The sacred mushroom takes me by the hand and brings me to the world where everything is known. It is they, the sacred mushrooms, that speak in a way that I can understand. I ask them, and they answer me. When I return from the trip that I have taken with them, I tell what they have told me and what they have shown me.[251]

Note how the mushrooms are regarded as having their own consciousness and intelligence. And while modern researchers do not hold this perspective, they still apply their own rituals: systematic protocols and standard methodologies to assess the participant's mental and existential state. This is critical as the drugs can amplify aspects of a person's self-identity. If that's dominated by shame or narcissistic distortion, the trip can be rough.

A peaceful environment is intentionally created, resembling a living room more than a clinic, with plants, soft music, and pleasant, calming decor. It's like a spa in a hospital setting. "Set and setting," a term made popular by Timothy Leary, emphasizes that this is not a journey to be taken in sterile clinic rooms (though that is where much research has happened)

[251] R. Gordon Wasson, "Seeking the Magic Mushroom," Life, May 13, 1957, 100-120.

but in an environment conducive to supporting the existential transformation about to occur.

The therapist stays with the individual throughout their experience, guiding them toward manifestations that may appear scary but are also doorways to deeper dimensions of being. Curiosity, compassion, and forgiveness for the self play a central role here, as they do with any spiritual practice. And here is the challenge psychedelics present to traditional psychotherapy. By blurring the boundaries between religion and science, sickness and health, and between the healer and sufferer, the psychedelic model entered the realm of applied mysticism.

Finally, the therapist debriefs and supports the patient as they reflect and contemplate the experience. These sessions continue weekly after the psychedelic experience. They even use a standardized evaluation tool, the Mystical Experiences Questionnaire, to assist with processing the experience.[252] Of course, in our modern age, there is also the option for an immersive cultural experience with the Indigenous traditions in which psychedelics have their therapeutic origin. That was much more challenging for the early experimenters. They just had to dive into this unknown land themselves.

SPIRITUAL ROOTS

Psychedelics are seriously being considered to treat death anxiety, in no small part because no other drugs work. In a review of research papers to assess the effectiveness of drug therapy (excluding Schedule 1 drugs or psychedelics) for treating anxiety symptoms in adults in their last year of life, none were effective.[253] This is partly why clinical guidelines from the major health organizations recommend non-drug therapy treatments for anxiety in palliative care patients – that would be psychosocial

---

[252] "The Mystical Experiences Questionnaire (30 Questions)." Psychology Tools, https://psychology-tools.com/test/meq-30. Accessed March 17, 2022.

[253] Candy, Bridget, et al. "Drug therapy for symptoms associated with anxiety in adult palliative care patients." *Cochrane Database of Systematic Reviews* 10 (2012). https://www.cochranelibrary.com/cdsr/doi/10.1002/14651858.CD004596.pub2/abstract. Accessed Aug. 13, 2021.

and spiritual care.[254] This also means not providing counselling for those requesting medically assisted death is serious negligence in the standard of care. All the more so as MAiD assessors are mandated to inform their patients of services that can address existential distress. However, while spiritual care focuses on precisely that, many healthcare providers and most patients do not understand that as our scope of practice. It will take a cultural shift for people to realize spiritual care is not about religious practice, but helping people engage a life crisis to deepen their humanity and awaken to the deeper dimensions of love, awareness, and, at the end of life, their true nature.

Psychedelic journeys have traditionally been the path to such awakening, accessed to gain insight as part of a healing journey and to bring wisdom and growth primarily for the community, not the individual. They were also part of an entire cosmological framework of reality shared by the community. Their use was not meant to indulge in your curiosity, personal knowledge, entertainment, or pleasure. And their use was not to treat death anxiety near the end of life. They were not meant for what we call palliative care, they were meant for the health of the living, who then provided all dimensions of care for the dying.

Leaders and shamans had extensive training in using these sacred substances, often extending to decades of mentorship. This intentionality, however, hasn't fully translated into modern society, where social and recreational use of psychedelics is widespread. That they transitioned from the temple to clinical therapy is no surprise, but their use divorced from an understanding of spirituality is devastating. At least they are referred to as *entheogens*, medicines that engender an experience of the sacred. (This is, admittedly, a rebranding of the word "psychedelic," meaning "inspiring fullness of the divine.") Also of concern is how scientific insights and clinical applications have not been shared with or led by the Indigenous communities from which they originate. These people gain no benefit from their sacred plant's scrutiny under the microscope of science or

[254] National Institute for Health and Care Excellence. *Improving supportive and palliative care for adults with cancer: The Manual.* Cancer Service Guideline (CSG4), 2004. www.nice.org.uk/guidance/csg4. Accessed Aug. 13, 2021.

commercialization by the pharmaceutical industry. They have, instead, had their cultures destroyed. From an Indigenous perspective, psilocybin research and drug development tells a story of extraction, cultural appropriation, bioprospecting, and colonization.[255] Despite the United Nations Declaration on the Rights of Indigenous Peoples and several other international statements, no pharmaceutical developers have reached any legitimate or reciprocal agreements with the Mazatecs, or any other Indigenous communities.[256]

Among the many psychedelic substances known throughout the world, psilocybin is most promising for the dying. It's a component derived from a small brown mushroom the Aztecs used to call the "flesh of the gods." I don't like mushrooms. Being more a sweet than savoury fellow, their earthiness is a foreign sensation on my palate. So, I have severed myself from a world of flavours, nuances, and culinary pleasures, much like we are severed from the mystical realm so commonly reported by those who ingest psilocybin, the active ingredient in these tiny, potent fungi.[257]

Perhaps it's better that the dry communion wafer we call the Body of Christ does not have the same effect as the flesh of the gods. One can't have Sunday worship become a "trip." Direct experience of God is fine for the saints of old, but mainline churches, interestingly, tend to frown upon mystical experience, while charismatic ones encourage it: speaking in tongues, being slain in the spirit, or simply discerning the voice of God within one's heart… all within specific doctrinal constraints, of course, and definitely without the aid of any drugs.

An ironic contrast, as the most commonly reported effect of psychedelics is a life-changing sense of the sacred marked by a remarkable connection

---

[255] Gerber, Konstantin, et al. "Ethical concerns about psilocybin intellectual property." *ACS Pharmacology & Translational Science* 4.2 (2021): pp. 573–577.

[256] Gerber, Konstantin, Inti García Flores, Angela Christina Ruiz, Ismail Ali, Natalie Lyla Ginsberg, and Eduardo E. Schenberg. "Ethical concerns about psilocybin intellectual property." ACS Pharmacology & Translational Science 4, no. 2 (2021): 573-577.

[257] Griffiths, Roland R., et al. "Psilocybin produces substantial and sustained decreases in depression and anxiety in patients with life-threatening cancer: A randomized double-blind trial." *Journal of Psychopharmacology* 30.12 (2016): pp. 1181–1197. https://www.ncbi.nlm.nih.gov/pmc/articles/PMC5367557/. Accessed Aug. 12, 2021.

to all of life and interoceptive clarity – an acute awareness of how you are aware. It's been described as "unsanity," a state beyond the ego's control. Recall that suffering and dying calibrate us for transformation by deconstructing the ego. Well, perhaps one need not wait for those difficult days to experience some sense of this.

As foreign as the clinical setting is from the traditional use of mushrooms, and as destructive as their casual use is to the heart of the spiritual encounter, one cannot deny that the therapeutic effects of psilocybin are remarkable. In a double-blind, placebo-controlled study involving patients with cancer-related anxiety and depression, twenty-nine were randomly assigned and received treatment with single-dose psilocybin (0.2 mg/kg) or niacin, both in conjunction with psychotherapy. The researchers were pleasantly surprised to find immediate, substantial, and sustained improvements in anxiety and depression and, most significantly for MAiD, massive decreases in cancer-related demoralization and hopelessness, improved spiritual well-being, and increased quality of life. And the effects endured until the patient's death.[258]

This excited Thomas Hartle, a fifty-three-year-old father of two from Saskatoon and a drug virgin. He was dying of colon cancer and heard about the study. The experience was profound. "My views on death have really changed tremendously," he says. "Before, life after death was a sort of academic, intellectual concept, whereas now it feels tangible. I've physically experienced states of consciousness that have nothing to do with this life or anything that I would identify with 'Thomas.' "[259]

As promising as this sounds, it should not replace comprehensive palliative care. That is the approach shown to decrease existential distress as well as physical suffering. Until then, the least we can do is ensure people receive the best evidence-based care, and the best evidence shows spiritual

[258] Grob, Charles S., et al. "Pilot study of psilocybin treatment for anxiety in patients with advanced-stage cancer." *Archives of General Psychiatry* 68.1 (2011): 71–78.

[259] Perry, Kevin " 'I've experienced states of consciousness beyond this life': The people turning to psychedelics on their deathbeds." *Independent* (Nov. 1, 2021). https://www.independent.co.uk/life-style/health-and-families/psychadelic-drugs-cancer-terminal-deathbed-b1946466.html. Accessed Feb. 27, 2022.

care should be front and centre. The contributions chaplains can give to the use of psychedelics are significant. We are trained in non-anxious presence, the ability to abide with equanimity, mindful awareness, "evenly suspended attention," and "doing by non-doing." We have experience with altered states of consciousness due to working so closely and consistently with the dying, and we have contemplative practice at the core of our work. This gives us a strongly developed interoceptive capacity – we are aware of how we are aware.

The nature of our work necessitates profound trust, vulnerability and authenticity, spiritual intelligence, and ethical integrity. Some of us are proficient in complementary techniques, including energy medicine and meditation. Perhaps most importantly, all of us are trained in relational processing, trauma resolution, spiritual mentoring, and meaning-making, especially in the community and transpersonal dimensions of being. Our ethics are embedded in respect for Indigenous traditions and a person's spirituality, and we are proficient in navigating the spiritual crisis. We liaise with spiritual and cultural communities and are well-trained in ritual, sacraments, ceremonies, and sacred space. And, we are with the dying regularly, helping them and their loved ones navigate grief and sorrow, witnessing them manifest love and deep life. Spiritual care providers are ideally suited to facilitate psychedelic therapies.

Yet there are significant gaps that hinder our involvement: our profession does not explore psychedelics, we are not standardized as a college in most provinces, there is poor understanding of our role in health care both by hospitals and the public, and professional spiritual care practitioners are thin on the ground, even more so as some provinces have cut our service altogether in the interest of saving pennies and the ignorance of realizing the depth of counselling we provide for staff and the organizations, let alone patients and families.

Fortunately, there is some movement toward certifying chaplains to counsel patients through psychedelic sessions alongside psychologists and doctors.[260] Policies are being examined to have chaplains take a more active role. Organizations are advocating for spirituality to return to the centre of the process, led by the Indigenous communities from which psychedelics came. I hope that initiative is fruitful, for as much as I am disheartened by the pharmaceutical industry devouring and profiting from the cultural heritage of Indigenous peoples, I cannot help but reflect on the cases where it could have made a profound difference.

260 "Psychedelics | Relief of Spiritual and Existential Suffering | Master Clinician Case Review." Center to Advance Palliative Care. Mar. 18, 2022. www.capc.org/events/case-reviews/how-psychedelics-can-be-used-for-relief-of-spiritual-and-existential-suffering. Accessed July 26, 2023.

EXERCISE 20: SURRENDER

Releasing the ego-mind and dropping attachments of identity is about surrendering fully to the present moment. Because psychedelics are not legal in Canada, I offer here two alternatives: one through guided visualization and the second through floatation. The first is free and available to everyone; the second will cost, depending on the length of the float, and is available, of course, only where there is a floatation centre.

Floating helps with deep relaxation, reducing chronic pain and stress-like symptoms. By floating in a solution of water and several hundred pounds of Epsom salt dissolved in it, you reset your body and mind by removing all outside stimulants. This is an effective way to allow yourself to be vulnerable, to truly surrender, as you are naked, giving yourself to the water as a teacher to help you give yourself to the moment. This environment is designed to help you lose yourself and ego-identity, observe your thoughts and feelings, and move into an open, effortless presence. In one study, people reported more relaxation with floating than with any other stress management technique, including medication, counselling, or meditation.[261]

This guided visualization also aims to assist you in cultivating surrender and letting go of control. It encourages a shift in perspective, fostering a sense of peace, acceptance, and trust in the process of life. You can listen to it at https://soundcloud.com/david-maginley/surender

Instructions:

1. *Find a quiet and comfortable space where you can relax without distractions. Sit in a comfortable position, close your eyes, and take a few deep breaths to centre yourself.*
2. *Bring your attention to the present moment. Notice any thoughts, worries, or attachments that may be weighing on your mind. Acknowledge them without judgement and set the intention to temporarily release them.*

[261] Feinstein, Justin S., et al. "Examining the Short-term Anxiolytic and Antidepressant Effect of Floatation-REST." *PLoS ONE*, vol. 13, no. 2 (Feb. 2018): p. e0190292. https://doi.org/10.1371/journal.pone.0190292.

3. *Focus on your breath. Feel the sensations of the breath as it enters and leaves your body. Allow the breath to guide you into a state of relaxation and openness.*

4. *Begin to reflect on the concept of surrender. Visualize a gentle river flowing before you, representing the flow of life. See yourself standing at the edge of the river, ready to surrender and let go.*

5. *Repeat the following affirmations silently or aloud, allowing the words to sink deeply into your being:*

    - *"I surrender to what is, embracing the present moment."*
    - *"I release my need for control and trust in the unfolding of life."*
    - *"I let go of attachments and allow life to guide me."*
    - *"I find peace in surrendering to the natural rhythm of the universe."*

6. *As you continue to breathe, imagine yourself gently stepping into the river. Feel the cool water embracing your body, symbolizing the act of surrender. Allow the river to carry you effortlessly, trusting that it will guide you to where you need to be.*

7. *Notice any resistance or tension that arises within you as you surrender. Observe these feelings without judgement, and with each exhale, release them into the flow of the river. Allow yourself to fully surrender and let go.*

8. *Stay in this visualization for a few moments, allowing yourself to be fully immersed in the experience of surrender. Notice any sensations, emotions, or thoughts that arise as you let go.*

9. *When you feel ready, bring your attention back to the present moment. Take a few deep breaths, grounding yourself in your physical body. Recognize that surrender is a continuous practice, and you can revisit this meditation whenever you need to reconnect with its essence.*

10. *As you go about your day, carry the spirit of surrender with you. Whenever you encounter challenges or moments of resistance, remind yourself to surrender and trust in the natural flow of life.*

Remember, surrender is not about giving up or resigning yourself to fate, but, rather, giving yourself to the present moment. You are opening to find peace and acceptance in the face of uncertainty and change. With practice, surrender can become a powerful tool for cultivating inner peace, resilience, and a greater comfort with not knowing what will future moments will hold.

Chapter 21

THE SOUL'S WOUND

The love we fail to give in life becomes the pain we carry through it.
– Unknown

He was a giant in their eyes, six-foot-three with piercing blue eyes. His muscular form had won him instant respect from friends and co-workers. But it was Frank's smile, his character, that brought people close. He radiated warmth and kindness. In his company, one could feel safe. How he longed to feel that now, as he lay curled in the hospital bed. Frank had been diagnosed with cancer months earlier but had declined treatment and told no one. Even more, now he had requested MAiD. Well, more than just requested it – he adamantly asked for it. A red flag – Frank was running from something. MAiD was his out. His gentle light had a dark shadow. Now, facing cancer, that darkness consumed him and was expressed in a theological statement:

"This is my punishment." Those four words contained a lifetime of pain.

We talked. For days, we talked. He named all the common reasons people request MAiD – loss of autonomy, could see nothing good in suffering, and, most of all, his children's grief. "I can't put them through this. They have enough challenges. What's the point?"

"The point," I prematurely offered, "is that your children love you and can love you to the end of your days. Grief ennobles them as they stay by your side while you lose consciousness, as your breath gently fades. It's the hardest thing in the world, yet it makes us better people and prepares us for our own eventual death. By allowing them this, you let them in. You could be giving them the last great teaching a parent can impart."

The sermon had no effect. Frank wept like a child and curled even tighter. Then shut it down. He would not allow emotional disintegration, for that would be a release. No, something in him wanted to own this pain and hold it tightly. Punishment.

"What happened?" I asked. "Where does this sorrow come from?" Given the astonishing statistics around violence in the home, I knew this pain probably began when he was small.

"Take me back. Take me to the beginning. Was your childhood safe?"

The tears flowed again. The typical tragedy came out of hiding. His father drank, his parents yelled, and someone got hit… a lot. Frank could only whisper the details due to his rapidly fading vitality. I realized there was little time for me to help grace repair decades of pain. He turned his eyes away, leaned back on the pillow, and shook his head.

"OK. So, it was a lousy start to your life story. Did it get any better? Did you build a home of love?"

His breath became soft. We paused while he whispered, "Yes. My wife. My wife."

"Mmmm." There was gratitude and regret in those words. "How did you meet?"

"In the grocery store," he softly said. A smile began – in the corners of the mouth, then the eyes.

"You can see it clearly, in your memory?"

"Yes." The smile was complete.

"And was this marriage better than that of your parents?"

Another pause, then the tears, and the smile dissolved. He would not answer. I could feel his energy fold back on itself, swallowed again in sorrow.

"This is my punishment. I've broken the commandments. This is why I have cancer. I just want it to end."

Commandments. We were approaching the core. His confession was close to expression.

"Punishment. You feel cancer is God's punishment for something you've done."

"Yes, yes."

The pieces of the broken man were strewn through our conversations, but with this statement, they all began to make sense. Frank had lived on his own for seventeen years. Divorce, money problems, drinking. He had sold his house and now was renting his own basement. Just after his diagnosis, but before his hospital admission, a pipe burst, and the basement flooded. No matter. The ultimate problem had supplanted all others. Cancer had come. His days were done. Declining treatment, he moved into our palliative care unit and walked away from the mess of his life. He had not told his friends of the disease. He ignored his buzzing phone and declined encouragement to come out of his room. He only recently told his children, who rearranged their lives to pour love into their father. Now Frank had begun to reveal the sin, the singular pain with which he defined himself: irredeemable. Unlovable. What weight could become reason enough to die?

"Broken the commandments," I said. "Well, there's something we hold in common. Most men have broken a few of them by this time. We cheat, we steal, we lie and lust, we snap and snarl at our wives. We forget the love and hide in anger or fear. But you're talking about something more, aren't you? What happened, Frank? What are you dragging behind as you die?"

He would not speak.

What could I offer this man except for compassion? How could I help him feel safe enough to be completely vulnerable and real, no longer hiding from any aspect of himself? Well, I knew he had faith. I knew he believed.

"God loves you, man. God loves you more than you could ever imagine. You will soon be transformed through death into wonder. There's no need to carry such a heavy load to the other side. You don't need to wait for that forgiveness. We could pray; I could offer you absolution. You could be free."

"I don't deserve it," he whispered with vacant eyes. Their striking light blue seemed to have faded to grey. His skin was ashen.

At the heart of it was some sin so deep that this man defined himself by it. There was no question God would forgive him. But he would not allow it – an ironic twist in the prison of pride. One would think hubris could only make you arrogant, but pride can also engulf one in misplaced humility, far beyond the reach of love, even if that's divine love. We certainly don't feel it as pride – it's more a prison of recycled pain we can't seem to shake. Perhaps to believe we are unredeemable in the face of the infinite speaks of the power of shame to distort us, to even protect us from the freedom of love. He was not unique in this; we all identify more comfortably with our darkness than our glory. Frank had taken the helm of his ship and was determined to smash it into the rocks.

Here was the unfinished love story, yet again. We are afflicted by how we have not been loved well, then project that which prevents us from loving well. And, here was the grace, longing to be known, so close. So close. God never condemns us to hell; we're the experts in that judgment. And this is why my stomach was twisting as I worried he would not only die this way but do it earlier by our hand, that he would take his existential pain with him. Who knows what that would do? And what could I do?

I gazed at the trail of tears on his sunken cheeks. And I prayed, softly speaking the grace. I prayed Frank would know that God completely understood his pain, had compassion for his heart, and abundant forgiveness for whatever sins he committed. I prayed God would fill him with peace and that Frank would be free. As I opened my eyes, I saw his were closed. A squeeze of his hand seemed to pull him back, but he faded again moments later, exhausted. I would have to resume this when he had more strength. There were nine days left before the second and final assessment for MAiD. Frank also had to be able to give consent just before the injection that would stop his heart. I hoped he would die before that. Speaking with his doctor after the visit, she confirmed that would likely be the case; she estimated he had only a few days left. Would he have time to forgive himself for whatever he had done?

I got the news three days later, sooner than I expected. Frank had been approved for an accelerated second assessment, as he would lose capacity before the waiting period expired. He had insisted that his suffering was intolerable and demonstrated complete competency. Then they carried out the procedure. The doctor said he seemed very much at peace with his children and the duty chaplain at his side.

I sat and wept. If only there had been more time. If only we could have gone further. His intolerable suffering was of the soul, not the body. We used a medical procedure to treat spiritual pain. And Frank had used it to avoid the homework of his heart. As far as I knew, he left this world as trapped as ever. We… I… had not done enough.

I know, I know. I showed up. I did what I could. I went further into his darkness than anyone on the team. I provided compassionate care. I prayed. And I continue to pray that in God's presence, Frank is indeed free. But… shit. We can do better than this.

FORGIVENESS

THE WRITER NORMAN COUSINS ONCE SAID LIFE IS AN ADVENTURE IN FORgiveness. Heaven knows the world needs more of that kind of grace, a restoration we really don't understand until we experience its power upon our own broken souls. Surprisingly, that does not mean we need to forgive ourselves. It may even mean we are incapable of doing so, and in this is an ironic twist: your freedom from shame and guilt is not dependent on your ability to declare absolution for yourself. As a pastor, I need to explain why I'm bucking the trend on this one.

Our culture tells us self-forgiveness is not only a category of forgiveness but the most important one. Writing in *Psychology Today*, psychotherapist Beverly Engel says, "I believe that self-forgiveness is the most powerful step you can take to rid yourself of debilitating shame."[262] Yet there is no example of this in the Bible, the Quran, in the teachings of Buddhism or Hinduism. Yes, there is a strong emphasis on compassion, even self-compassion, but this is a different dynamic than forgiveness. It may be an even more powerful dynamic, the only restorative effort we actually can engage for the shame that isolates us from others and our own wholeness.

---

[262] Engle, Beverly. "Healing Your Shame and Guilt through Self-Forgiveness." *Psychology Today* (June 1, 2017). www.psychologytoday.com/us/blog/the-compassion-chronicles/201706/healing-your-shame-and-guilt-through-self-forgiveness.

Self-compassion goes beyond attempts to forgive yourself by animating self-kindness and allowing your brokenness to be part of our common humanity. Your pain and any mess you've made are used for greater wisdom and compassion for others in the same boat. Self-compassion is a powerful medicine for any distress we may have, especially as we die; there's no need to carry unnecessary baggage to the great beyond. But it is not self-forgiveness. You cannot be both the transgressor, jury, and judge to enact freedom (as much as the ego would like to wear every hat).

There are only two biblical categories of forgiveness: horizontal and vertical. The first comes from others, the second from God. Seeking forgiveness is mandatory for Christians, as St. Paul states in Colossians 3:12–13. "Put on then, as God's chosen ones, holy and beloved, compassionate hearts, kindness, humility, meekness, and patience, bearing with one another and, if one has a complaint against another, forgiving each other; as the Lord has forgiven you, so you also must forgive." This release is always relational, a dynamic received from others, not from oneself. The compassion we practise for ourselves afterwards, though, is in many ways more powerful, for here we engage an ongoing affirmation of a new identity as one free from the pain, wiser for it, and connected by it to the rest of humanity. It leaves one humble, grateful, and authentic.

Frank's transgression required relationships strong enough to bear the weight of its truth and loving enough not to define him by it. But, like so many, he did not have such a community. And the resources within him were not adequate to lift his head above the storm of existential pain and lament. If only Frank could have been supported earlier.

Can we consider that psychosocial and spiritual care should be automatically activated when a patient expresses a desire to die? This care requires time, personal investment, patience, creativity, community, and the capacity to suffer with others instead of fixing their suffering. This calls on healthcare providers to invest themselves in meaning-making conversations and relationships of depth and significance. These can transform the daunting steps of the dying process into moments of profound connection, self-awareness, and gratitude. Grief can be grounded in its noble power to forge deep human relationships. Existential suffering can be engaged wisely, tenderly, and courageously. Each step on the stairway to heaven can resonate with the music of love itself, each rest on the scale a sacred silence, as important as any other note.

THE EFFECT ON MAiD PROVIDERS

IT'S NOT ONLY FOR THE PATIENT'S BENEFIT; PHYSICIANS NEED THESE COMpassionate conversations for themselves as well. One survey revealed that up to 24 percent of family doctors had received a request for assisted death. This rises to 57 percent for oncologists.[263] And following through with those requests does not, indeed cannot, leave a person unaffected. When you stop a person's life, it shifts your relationship to your own humanity in ways many MAiD providers sense but don't share – part of that culture of resiliency and competency among your medical colleagues. And, as critical as it is for them to recognize the nature of the distress driving MAiD requests, training in how to have a therapeutic discussion on the subject with patients is sorely lacking. Physicians know this; a study on doctors' beliefs about assisted dying found that 60 percent disagreed with the statement that physicians who are not psychiatrists are adequately trained to screen for depression in patients seeking assisted dying, and 60 percent disagreed with the idea that physicians can predict with certainty whether a patient seeking euthanasia has six months or less to live.[264]

Despite MAiD providing a specific deadline and a structured opportunity for patients to explore why they feel their life no longer has meaning, the assessment of existential distress remains shallow. The context of that distress, such as the passage through the dark night of the soul, remains absent from the discussion. Supporting and even challenging the patient to move through, rather than around, that distress in order to ultimately

---

[263] Back, Anthony L., et al. "Clinician-patient interactions about requests for physician-assisted suicide: a patient and family view." *Archives of Internal Medicine* 162, no. 11 (2002): pp. 1257–1265.

[264] Hetzler, Peter T., et al. "A Report of Physicians' Beliefs about Physician-Assisted Suicide: A National Study." *The Yale Journal of Biology and Medicine* 92, no. 4 (2019): p. 575.

discover a state of grace and forgiveness is still not considered. This illustrates the spiritual poverty in both MAiD and our culture. While returning the mind to peace and feeling one with everything may be nice, it should not be the goal of clinical care.

Furthermore, addressing the problem of existential suffering is not a part of medical education. The program is already saturated with the volumes of information that need to be imparted to young minds, some of whom crack under the pressure. Weighty philosophical and humanistic endeavours are inadvertently obtained, especially in the trenches of the hospital corridor, as they progress from resident to fellow, attending physician, and specialist. This results in a rapid rush to the limits of one's resilience. Many physicians I know became assessors or MAiD practitioners out of a deep and sincere desire to help those seeking MAiD, to alleviate the backlog of patients requesting it, and to make a real difference. However, they soon discover that the service compromises their private lives, happiness, and well-being.

You can't swim through suffering without getting wet. And without regular self-care, healthcare providers will become waterlogged. This soaking progresses steadily not because of individual cases – although there are always some that stand out as watershed events – but because there is no time to process, grieve, or release between cases. The cases just keep coming, one after the other, day after day, year after year. This leads to compassion fatigue and vicarious trauma. The body recognizes it well before the mind dares to acknowledge it. Symptoms such as becoming grumpy and irritable, developing migraines and stomach cramps, experiencing nightmares, and falling into addictions may start to arise.

Others will notice it before you do. "You look tired." And the response is usually dismissive. "Yeah, we're all tired. I'm fine." (By the way, in this case fine means Flustered, Insecure, Neurotic, and Emotional.) We carry on because it's our job. Because there's always another patient. And, subliminally, because focusing on the patient enables us to avoid focusing on ourselves. We use the patient as a buffer between ourselves and our own experience. In the long run, this suffocates our joy, drains our demeanour, and compromises our care because we can no longer care for ourselves.[265] It's important to explore this in the context of assisted death because the act is such an empowering alternative for those struggling with compassion fatigue. You are ending a person's suffering; you are honouring their wishes. You are doing something that feels so much more compassionate and active than witnessing the final deterioration and fading away. Most subliminally, death is no longer a failure. You and your patient meet it on the patient's terms, not those of biological and existential disintegration.

So, what is it like for the assessors and the one administering the injections? That depends on the person. Research shows a wide range of emotions and a singular blind spot that is quite understandable, given the profession. One doctor shared with me at the nursing desk on a palliative care floor that she felt quite close to her patients, that MAiD discussions increased that emotional connection. "It opens up conversations on their life, their values, their hopes and what's important to them." I had no doubt her conversations were very comforting, given her gentle nature and excellent bedside manner.

Another found his connections more casual. "I'm not the physician caring for them on a day-to-day basis. I come in and do the assessment, and my questions are fairly standard to ensure they have competency and are requesting this of their own volition. We do talk about their values, but it's around the burden they feel upon their family and avoiding the suffering to come. It feels very kind when I do the procedure, considering what they're dealing with." Without the ongoing connection and a history of caring for the patient, this response makes sense – a more surface-level assessment in which distress is recognized but honoured as confirmation for the procedure, not as an invitation to go deeper.

Research supports that the depth of the conversation depends mainly on that connection in the assessment. For some physicians, this is a brief

[265] An excellent resource for your self-care is the Figley Institute Basics of Compassion Fatigue, http://www.figleyinstitute.com/documents/Workbook_AMEDD_SanAntonio_2012July20_RevAugust2013.pdf
See also Mathieu, Françoise. *The Compassion Fatigue Workbook: Creative Tools for Transforming Compassion Fatigue and Vicarious Traumatization*. Routledge, 2012.

process; for others, it can extend much longer. All the assessors I've spoken with recognize that when a person asks about assisted death, they're opening the door to discussions on symptom care and what it's like to die naturally from their disease. They're asking for a road map, and informed consent cannot be complete without those more difficult conversations. Good questions include, "Why is this coming up right now? How well is your pain being managed?" Then, go deeper: "What's been going on at home? What are you afraid of? How do you think the end of your life will look?" These conversations are more therapeutic when the family is present, as long as they're not trying to console or reassure the patient but to participate in the experience of grief, worry, and saying goodbye. However, assessors, as a group, are not well-skilled in exploring existential distress and suffering at the end of life. Writing lethal prescriptions does not address these deficiencies in practice or training. It's a professionally dangerous thing to do, creating a situation ripe for moral distress.

I draw upon an excellent study exploring these difficult conversations: "Discussing physician-assisted dying: physicians' experiences in the United States and the Netherlands," in *The Gerontologist*. The compassion of the doctors shines through in these conversations, especially from those who feel one should not perform the procedure unless you have an established relationship with the patient. (In reality, that is often *not* the case – there are too many people requesting euthanasia.)

One doctor commented on the significance of knowing her patient. "That was... why she asked me to do the euthanasia because... I knew her. I knew... she suffered that much already... and I knew so much about her life story that I knew that this was too much for her to bear."[266]

Many MAiD practitioners say these conversations deepen their relationship with the patient and family.

"I probably had the most intense relationship with this patient than any other patient because you are really taking time to discuss with him... you

---

[266] Voorhees, Jennifer R., et al. "Discussing physician-assisted dying: physicians' experiences in the United States and the Netherlands." *The Gerontologist* 54.5, (2014): pp. 808–817.

go much deeper into his feelings and his ideas. So, this was actually quite intense. I think, from both sides, it felt good."[267]

This confirms what I have observed – doctors and nurse practitioners performing MAiD feel strongly that it is a service to the patient. It is an act of compassion that honours the individual. But when the assessment for MAiD is not supportive, it can end the relationship.

"The conversation with him was brief and kind of brutal – brutal coming from his side, because I continued to try and make contact . . . That was right at the beginning… while I was doing the history and physical . . . As soon as I told him I couldn't do PAD [physician assisted death], he broke communication with me, wanted nothing to do with me, was barely civil for the rest of the time he was under my care."[268]

When your entire career has been focused on helping people live, the heart of the Hippocratic oath can live in you as a core ethical principle, enriching your humanity and your care. No wonder some physicians viscerally wrestle with assisted death. No wonder they are swallowed by yet another dimension of distress when they say "no" to ending a person's life.

"[I]t was really hard [when the patient brought up PAD]… it was like a knife in the heart… I think I was shocked."[269]

"In our hospital, once you are actively involved in a euthanasia question, for the rest of the year you think, 'Well, please let someone else do this question.' "[270]

"He and his wife asked me to help them. Literally, I felt as though the blood had frozen in my veins. I just felt just totally cold all over. I had no idea of what to do. I realized there was no help I could get from anywhere."[271]

"I was busy all the time with the question, 'Is it possible, and is it morally defendable, and is it a good decision?'… making pluses and minuses

---

[267] Ibid, p. 812

[268] Ibid

[269] Ibid

[270] Ibid

[271] Ibid, p. 813

about it... but... what's it doing to me? I'm going to kill someone tonight." [respondent began to cry].[272]

In a 2020 survey from the British Medical Association, respondents who were supportive of euthanasia were mainly retired doctors, medical students and those in specialties which involve little or no contact with terminally or otherwise incurably ill patients, while only 5% of palliative care doctors were in favour.[273] It seems that the more doctors are involved in caring for dying patients, the greater the likelihood that they will oppose a change in British law.[274]

Of course, many physicians have no moral distress about providing MAiD. They feel it is a compassionate service, that they are ending a person's suffering and respecting their patient's autonomy. Dr. Stephanie Greene, author of *This Is Assisted Dying,* spends 90 percent of her day helping people leave this world. "They can stop thinking and worrying about what exactly is going to happen at the end of their life. They can really grab onto those final days or weeks or months that they have left and really focus on living them intently and with purpose," she said. Clearly, she experiences MAiD as profoundly merciful. "I'm giving them a gift."[275]

Her comments raise a critical question: What is the effect of killing upon the mind of the one administering the injection? Even for those comfortable with the procedure, there is an emotional numbing. That's not a criticism; it's an observation of what research shows consistently: repeated exposure to traumatic incidents triggers adaptive strategies to support functioning. In other words, we find a way to endure. And we get

---

[272] Ibid

[273] Kantar Public Division. "BMA Survey on Physician-Assisted Dying, British Medical Association." 2020. https://www.bma.org.uk/media/3367/bma-physician-assisted-dying-survey-report-oct-2020.pdf. Accessed April 30, 2024.

[274] Twycross, Robert. "Assisted Dying: Principles, Possibilities, and Practicalities. An English Physician's Perspective." BMC Palliative Care 23, no. 1 (April 13, 2024). Accessed April 30, 2024. https://doi.org/10.1186/s12904-024-01422-6. Accessed April 30, 2024

[275] Favaro, Avis. "A rare look at Canada's growing demand for medical assistance in dying." *W5*. CTV News. https://www.ctvnews.ca/mobile/w5/a-rare-look-at-canada-s-growing-demand-for-medical-assistance-in-dying-1.5854612. Accessed April 12, 2022.

used to it; this is true for all of health care. For those who experience moral distress, though, the cost is high – it can drive professionals out of their careers, compromise well-being, and induce significant PTSD.[276] This is on top of the already high rates of burnout and suicide among physicians. A 2019 survey of over 15,000 doctors found that 44 percent reported burnout, and a shocking 20 percent thought about suicide.[277] For burnout, the main factor identified was not compassion fatigue but bureaucratic fatigue: paperwork. However, when exploring depression and suicide, cumulative exposure to suffering and extraordinary demands on time and personal energy was significant. Of course, most healthcare providers adapt to the difficult environment of illness and death in part by becoming used to it. Now they can adapt by taking control of it.

What was distressing at first becomes manageable, as health care is a deeply satisfying experience for one who has the tools and knowledge to remedy, or at least manage, illness. There are MAiD providers who feel exactly this way about the procedure. However, a critical edge of their humanity becomes dulled through repeated participation. That edge is a blurring of the line between non-maleficence and beneficence, the balance of acting in a manner that cultivates benefit for another and simultaneously protects that person from harm. Recall the insight of Dr. Rachel Naomi Remen: "When you help, you see life as weak. When you fix, you see life as broken. When you serve, you see life as whole."

MAiD seeks to fix suffering by ending the life of the sufferer, and, in this way, it is the latest example of our divorce from death. We've sterilized this ultimate moment, reducing it to the individual's autonomy and control over the most significant spiritual event that can ever happen in life. And this has been done by those who, for the most part, are not regularly at the bedside of the dying. Perhaps some involved in forming this legislation have seen a loved one die. Certainly, the dying and their

[276] MacNair, Rachel M. "Psychology of nonkilling," in JE Pim (ed) *Toward a nonkilling paradigm.* Honolulu, Hawaii. Center for Global Nonkilling, 2009, pp. 327–347.

[277] Kane, L. *Medscape National Physician Burnout, Depression & Suicide Report 2019* https://www.medscape.com/slideshow/2019-lifestyle-burnout-depression-6011056?faf=1#1. Accessed March 31, 2022.

families were consulted. But experts in the *lived* experience of dying (I know how odd that sounds) were not central to the conversations, which remained, in the end, predominantly legal and ethical. Chaplains, nurses, and hospice workers, more than any other healthcare providers, and certainly more than any doctors (even palliative care physicians), are the ones at the bedside at the moment of death. They are the ones who support the patient as they daily wrestle with grief and mortality. They are the ones who walk through the weeks of suffering on the patient's side. They are the ones who witness the subtle shifts in consciousness, the giving of breath to body, the mystical nearing-death awareness, the final exhalation, and the moments of sacred silence that infuse the room afterwards. They are the ones who are grazed by immanent grace and find themselves brushed in glory and sadness, if only for a moment, before moving on to the next patient and doing it again, and again, and again, hundreds of times a year.

EXERCISE 21: SELF-CARE

The cost of caring is high for healthcare professionals. Stress accumulates gradually until it registers in the body. It starts as burnout, then builds to compassion fatigue, and then vicarious trauma. The longer it's ignored, the deeper it becomes embedded in the body.

Find a quiet and comfortable space where you can reflect without distractions. Have a pen and paper or a journal ready.

Instructions:

Take a few deep breaths to centre yourself and bring your focus to the present moment.

Reflect on the following questions and write down your responses:

1. *If you have provided MAiD, reflect on how you felt after performing your first procedure. Did you take time to care for yourself and reflect? Did you even have time?*
2. *Does concern for burnout prevent you from 'suffering with' your patients even more than you do already?*
3. *Check the table to identify what physical, emotional and affective signs indicate you may be experiencing compassion fatigue.*

Physical	**Behavioural**	**Affective**
Exhaustion	Irritability	Emotional numbness
Chronic fatigue	Anger and resentment	Hypersensitivity
Headache, backpain	Guilt or self-blame	Cynicism
GI problems	Relationship difficulties	Apathy
Sleep disturbances	Rigid thinking	Helplessness
Muscular tension	Depersonalization	Over-identification
Vulnerability to illness	Self-righteousness	Reduced personal accomplishment
Lingering illness	Addictions	Depression

Cardiovascular changes	Problems with intimacy	Failure to nurture non-work-related aspects of life
Changes in appetite	Inability to tolerate strong feelings	Difficulty separating personal and professional life
Changes in weight	Heightened anxiety	Mood swings

Figure 7: Signs of Compassion Fatigue

4. *What are the specific challenges and stressors you encounter in providing MAiD?*
5. *Consider the ethical dilemmas, emotional intensity, personal beliefs, and societal perspectives that may contribute to your experience. What self-care practices or strategies have you found helpful in managing compassion fatigue?*
6. *Identify any activities or techniques that have helped you recharge, relax, or find emotional balance.*
7. *Once you have completed your reflections, take a moment to review your responses.*

   Identify one or two specific self-care practices or strategies that resonate with you and that you believe could help you manage compassion fatigue more effectively.
8. *Develop an actionable plan:*
   a. *Define how and when you will incorporate these self-care practices into your daily or weekly routine.*
   b. *Consider any adjustments or boundaries you may need to set to prioritize your well-being.*
   c. *Determine how you will hold yourself accountable and track your progress.*

Take a few more deep breaths, acknowledging the importance of self-care and compassion for yourself as a healthcare provider.

Remember, this exercise is a starting point for self-reflection and self-care. It is essential to seek support from colleagues, mentors, or mental health professionals when needed, as they can provide additional guidance and resources specific to your situation. Prioritizing your own well-being ensures you can continue providing care to those in need. In fact, you have an ethical obligation to care for yourself, otherwise, you compromise your ability to care for others. These resources will help:

Professional Quality of Life Scale (ProQOL) https://proqol.org/proqol-measure

Finley Institute Compassion Fatigue Workbook bit.ly/3Iy8ydu

https://compassionfatigue.ca/

PART 4

MAiD AND SPIRIT

Chapter 22

INTEGRAL SPIRITUALITY

Authentic spirituality is revolutionary.
It does not legitimate the world, it breaks the world;
it does not console the world, it shatters it.
And it does not render the self content, it renders it undone.

– Ken Wilber

"In the night in which he was betrayed, our Lord Jesus took bread, gave thanks, broke it, and gave it to his disciples, saying: 'Take and eat; this is my body, given for you.'"

I'm standing at the altar, presiding over an ancient ritual that is now rote after 500+ Sundays. The liturgy, vestments, and music were originally intended to help people see beyond the ordinary world and connect with the sacred, allowing their consciousness to open up and resonate with the Spirit of Life. It was meant to energize them as members of the mystical Body of Christ, even to embody that connection through the Eucharist: bread and wine, body and blood, life force of reality. However, even in this setting, the ego's sense of separateness prevails. We find comfort in keeping God as something "other," distant in a realm called "heaven," rather than realizing that God is immanent and dwells within. We feel safer lifting our petitions to an external God, since it reinforces the separation of self from Source, instead of participating in the consciousness of God, which obliterates such distinction. True spiritual growth entails awakening to this greater reality and, in turn, discovering our greater identity. However, religion has been stagnant for centuries, out of sync with the modern mind. Is there a way to convey the wisdom of world religions that can effectively bring about cultural transformation?

Here's that more intelligent model I promised: integral spirituality. I want to explore this before examining religion's position on MAiD, as I hope it can offer a high-level view into how these spiritual traditions function. In fact, the insights of integral spirituality give me great hope that we are seeing the dawn of a new stage of spiritual growth… as long as we make it through the turbulent terrain immediately ahead. Climate change, pandemics, and national tensions threaten to collapse the modern world. It's taken 300,000 years for Homo sapiens to explore the depths of space and perfect deep-fried donuts. We have access to the world's knowledge through our phones, yet are addicted to social media. We are a species of extremes, both utterly brilliant and abysmally immature. Our rational intelligence is exceptional, but our spiritual intelligence is in the basement. This does not bode well when discussing MAiD! Yet, when looking at the long game, perhaps MAiD can be seen as a temporary development in the human story. There is much to hope for as long as, spiritually, we are able to wake up as well as grow up.

I must forewarn you that this chapter will cover weighty subjects. We will delve into topics such as human and cultural development, the structures of consciousness, stages of spiritual growth, and how MAiD fits into this framework. If this is not of interest to you, feel free to skip ahead to Chapter 23, where we will explore the argument of the sanctity of life.

Integral theory, a model of human development that incorporates all aspects of the world's spiritual traditions and psychological theories, illustrates the problem before us well. This approach informed Kathleen Dowling Singh's work and is based on the central insight that there are both *structures* and *states* of consciousness.

Structures of consciousness pertain to our process of growing up or maturing. Progressing through cultural and human development, growth occurs across six levels: archaic, magical, mythic, rational, pluralistic, and integral. It is crucial to recognize that the latter levels do not supersede the earlier ones but rather encompass and build upon them. All stages must be present for the holistic development of human consciousness as they continue to shape experiences and identity to varying degrees.

States of consciousness, on the other hand, refer to our capacity to wake up. It involves a movement towards more expansive states of awareness, from the material or gross state to the subtle, causal, and ultimately, the non-dual state. While structures of consciousness reflect psychological development, states of consciousness reflect spiritual development.[278]

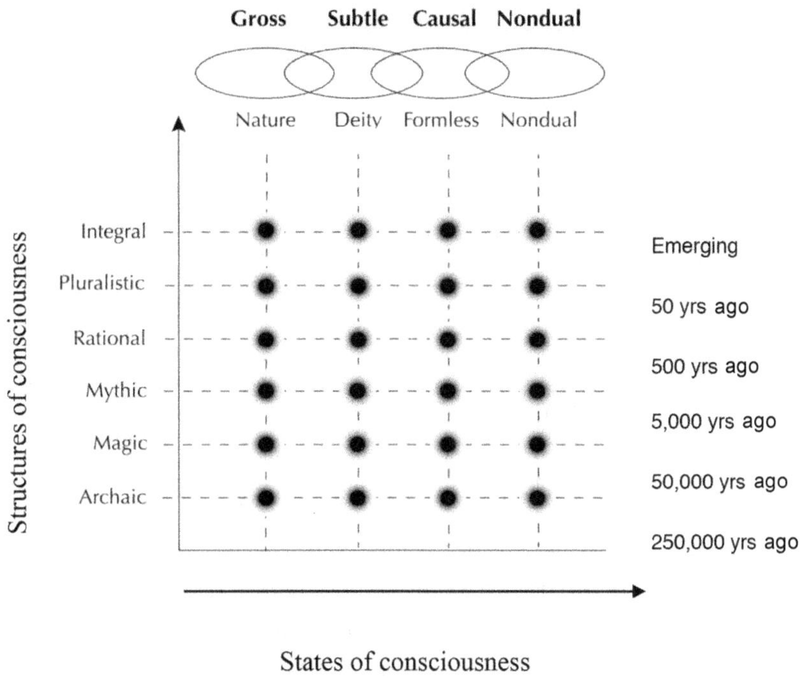

Figure 8: Wilber-Combs Lattice (modified)[279]

[278] Esbjorn-Hargens, S. "An overview of integral theory: An all-inclusive framework for the twenty-first century." *Integral Theory in action: Applied, theoretical, and constructive perspectives on the AQAL model.* State University of New York Press, 2009, pp. 33–61.

[279] Combs, Allan. *Consciousness Explained Better: Towards an Integral Understanding of the Multifaceted Nature of Consciousness.* Minnesota: Paragon House, 2009, p. 101.

GROWING UP

First, let's consider how our consciousness and culture grow up through structures of consciousness, and then explore how they wake up through states of consciousness and the implications this has for MAiD. Understanding this is pivotal in comprehending how our present spiritual and moral development intersects with euthanasia.

Western spirituality still grapples with transitioning from a dualistic model of reality, which reinforces the notion of two separate realms - physical and spiritual, to a non-dual model where everything exists solely within consciousness. The division between the self and others, and the distinction between objects and time, all manifest within the realm of consciousness.

A dualistic model that separates the physical and spiritual realms results in a belief that emphasizes an external God – religion, as opposed to a practice that develops the direct experience of God – mysticism. It also results in the notion that I have a life (which is mine and which I will lose at the end) rather than I *am* a life (a unique expression of the Ground of Being manifest in this form).

Integral spirituality asserts that not only will everyone have a direct experience of Spirit at the end of life, since dropping the body moves you automatically to the non-dual state, but that we all will also have it, if only momentarily, throughout life. This is because we dwell in a seemingly separate physical state that, nonetheless, arises from a realm of pure consciousness.[280] You cannot help but catch a glimpse of this truth at some point in your journey. So sublime and transitory are these encounters with the Ground of Being that we savour them but for a moment and speak of them simply as pleasant, though some are perplexing, even provocative. Occasionally, they are also shattering.

The power of these encounters calibrates us to joy, awe, profound stillness, and overflowing gratitude. Many will not think of these as sacred;

---

[280] Closer to Truth, "What is Consciousness?" YouTube video, 29:54, posted by Donald Hoffman, November 22, 2020, https://www.youtube.com/watch?v=ynTqCFBhRmw. Accessed Dec. 18, 2022

they are simply wonderful. Yet, their spiritual essence is nonetheless revealed in how they rapidly dissolve the self, the ego, fully connecting you to *this* moment, to something greater.

Perplexing events seem like strange coincidences, synchronicities, and alignments that manifest despite astonishing odds that anything else should occur. Hints of a pattern to life's ups and downs are laid bare, then evaporate like dew. Numbers, dates, names, objects and experiences resonate with precise calibration at impossibly perfect moments.

Provocative encounters startle you as revelations from the Ground of Being that manifest so abruptly like a bark from beyond, waking you in the dark of night when the presence of a deceased loved one is felt pressing upon the bed or the clear guiding voice within the mind so unlike your internal dialogue or imagination.

Shattering encounters… well, that would be death. That would be what we're exploring here. Yet even these are safe, for all of them seek not our destruction but our awakening.

STRUCTURES OF CONSCIOUSNESS

1. **The archaic structure** of consciousness was experienced by our species throughout the eons of early development up to about 250,000 years ago. It is also our state in the last few weeks before birth and in the first months of life. There is no ego development or conscious self, but a unitive and symbiotic relationship with one's environment. One can think of many life forms that live continually in this state of unity, such as trees and fungi. We awaken to this state at the end of life, but now with a developed identity. It can also be revisited through mystical experiences and psychedelics. Death and life are not reflected upon in this stage – one simply is, in this moment, with this experience.

2. **The magic structure** is a model that appeared in human development from the middle Paleolithic period until about 50,000

years ago, when there was a marked increase in the diversity of artifacts found associated with modern human remains. Here is the first contraction of consciousness on the road to forming ego-identity, experienced in early childhood. It's an inherently egocentric time, through which the toddler believes the outside world revolves around the self. It's also an enchanting time in which her magical beliefs reveal that she cannot clearly distinguish between her own emerging mental images or symbols and the external world.

3. **The mythic structure** emerged roughly 5,000 years ago. In human growth, we reach pre-adolescence when a child's ego development is framed by "behaving properly." It is also the stage in which much of religion has remained, with a God above, rulers and priests between, and the common people below. God is related to as a parental authority and a means to fulfill the child's narcissistic wants, very much like the Christmas song that chimes, "He knows if you've been bad or good, so be good for goodness sake." This stage struggles to engage suffering through allowing, ambiguity, waiting, or vulnerable openness.

4. **The rational structure** emerged in our species 500 years ago with the Enlightenment and the emergence of the scientific method. The map of reality that religions offered came into question here and, for an increasing portion of people today, has become irrelevant. So, too, in human development, we reach a rebellious state: adolescence. Maturity requires questioning and testing to emerge as an adult with an integrated value system. Consciousness is becoming more "awake," even more so on a cultural level. In the rational structure, suffering and death are engaged as problems. MAiD becomes a practical response to mortality and struggle, as one's purpose and identity in this world are no longer experienced as satisfying, much less sustaining.

5. **The pluralistic structure** burst on the scene in the 1960s with the countercultural revolution, psychedelics, and the women's liberation movement. The established patriarchy, of course, resisted these critical developments (an ongoing issue – racism is only one example of the resistance to moving into a pluralistic structure of consciousness). Death in this stage is engaged with more profound compassion and consideration of everyone's unique life story. It's no surprise that MAiD has emerged when our culture has been pluralistic for several decades, with a rational structure still dominating the medical and legal systems.
6. **The integral structure**, emerging now, reflects a truly Gaia or cosmos-centred identity as citizens of the planet. This structure of consciousness is desperately needed as we face the realities of climate change, rampant exploitation, and greed. Integration of all previous stages ensures compassionate engagement with others in their development and a setting aside of the self on national and individual levels. The integral structure emerges from the symbiotic nature of all life forms. This structure is overtly spiritual, though this can be expressed through secular or non-theistic terminology.

You may notice that the structures of consciousness are appearing at an increasingly rapid pace. The first step in growth took hundreds of thousands of years, then tens of thousands, then 500, and eventually just fifty. This gives hope that the current generation will reach a level of integral saturation that can not only steer human progress away from danger but also propel it into new stages of development. We cannot yet envision these stages in specific detail, but it is likely that they will be shaped by spiritual intelligence. Given the exponential rate of awakening, it is possible that the rising trend of exploring spirituality through conscious evolution, rather than traditional religious practices, represents the leading edge of a second reformation.

This brings us to the second factor of consciousness: waking up, or the states of consciousness.

STATES OF CONSCIOUSNESS

STRUCTURES OF CONSCIOUSNESS ARE LEVELS OF GROWTH AND MATURITY, while states refer to experiences of contracted or expanded consciousness – one's connection to everything that exists. Structures are linked to psychological development, while states are associated with spiritual growth. In other words, structures are the lens through which we perceive the world, while states become our reality. Structures relate to growing up, while states relate to waking up. States can be thought of as spheres or dimensions of existence that become denser as you expand from the physical level to the mind, and then progress towards unity with the Ground of Being.

Although we originate from a sublime realm, most of us tend to identify primarily with the densest realm – our physical bodies. As a result, leaving our bodies behind can be quite problematic. We experience various states of consciousness, ranging from common ones like waking, sleeping, and dreaming, to more spiritual states such as meditative witnessing, peak experiences, and mystical awareness. For example, one patient who claimed not to be religious described her process of dying as a journey that opened her up, like a lotus flower blossoming. The ordinary moments before her seemed unlike anything she had previously experienced. Even if her awareness was limited to the confines of the hospital room, she felt increasingly connected to Spirit, to the Ground of Being from which she emanated in every moment.

While Abrahamic religions, such as Christianity and Islam, offer guidance on developing more expansive states of consciousness through contemplative practices and rituals, they tend to focus predominantly on an external God and a divine plan for individual salvation and the restoration of creation for humanity. This emphasis on an external deity and the performance of rituals often maintains a primarily magical and mythical approach in their widespread practice. Nonetheless, the rituals and core principles of these religions can still lead to a direct experience of the divine

– what is commonly referred to as awakening or enlightenment.States of consciousness are closely linked to ego deconstruction and the opening up to the Ground of Being. This connection is fundamental to overall well-being, especially as one approaches death. The more an individual clings to their ego-identity in the face of suffering, the more they will inevitably suffer. However, by opening to mindful awareness rather than seeking understanding, a dying person can embrace their suffering as part of the transformative process. This practice is spiritual in nature and does not depend on belief, but rather on self-compassion. Psychological models do not address the purpose of spirituality in helping individuals awaken to these deeper, more profound realms and the corresponding states of consciousness that accompany this awakening. And, while spiritual teachings explore this in depth, many religious leaders will not use such terminology to describe the process. (I do hope my phrasing and framing is helping to translate these deep concepts in a way that makes sense!)

It is important to recognize that states of consciousness are not limited by culture or historical time periods. These experiences of heightened awareness are universally accessible to all individuals. Each state of consciousness interacts with and overlaps with the next. Much like different worlds or realities, each of these realms is governed by its own set of laws, with the principles of resonance, attraction, and compassion playing a role in the subtle realm, similar to how gravity, entropy, and magnetism operate in the material realm.

The process of waking up always starts at the material or gross level, which represents the natural world and our existence as physical beings. This level of awareness can be so convincing that we may mistakenly believe it is the only reality, particularly if we have rejected religious traditions. The modern paradigm of material reductionism and atheism further reinforces the notion that "what you see is what you get." This perspective emerged during the Renaissance and the advent of the scientific method. In addition to encompassing the external world, this state of consciousness also includes our thoughts, feelings, and the internal world of our personal story or identity.

When a person's belief system is entirely in the gross form, there is no reaching for an afterlife, so how one dies may as well be as controlled as possible. Most requesting MAiD, though, have some hope in the hereafter and are curious and expectant of the relief they will experience there, even as their existential state remains very much in this world, in this body, and with the story of their life, which disintegrates as they move ever closer to its end. Unless, of course, they experience an expansion of consciousness to the next state.

Waking up to the *subtle* realm of reality is described by many as a mystical experience. Here are non-material forms of life energy: chakras, intuitive wisdom, and vivid dreams, but it can also include the infilling of transcendent presence, if only for a moment. This is the encounter with a personal God, a religious experience that feels very much like waking up to a healed, restored state of being, being saved, filled with the spirit, born again. Yet it can have a dark side, for here we can also encounter the shadow aspect of consciousness, all that is suppressed and hidden from the ego. This is why using psychedelics to open one's consciousness is best done under the guidance of a therapist. Those chemicals suppress a mechanism in the brain called the default-mode network, resulting in amplified communication pathways between brain structures that are experienced as mystical and mystifying manifestations of what has been suppressed. No wonder navigating the subtle realms can be disorienting, even terrifying. This is similar to the *bardo*, or liminal stage of consciousness between incarnations, spoken of in the Buddhist tradition. You are confronted with your homework, and this suppressed inner reality has the danger of becoming the environment in which you can become trapped. Turning toward whatever fearful apparitions await with curiosity and acceptance shifts them from consuming you to catapulting you to the causal state. Of course, you don't need drugs for this! Meditation is always your best route to rarified awareness.

The *causal* state is the posture of the witness to everything. It has been reported by meditators and those who have near-death or mystical experiences. While there often is very much a sense of the divine, it is all-encompassing, no longer a personal God but all that is. There is an infinite expanse of potentiality, of ultimate possibility. Physics may represent this through the concept of the quantum field, from which our reality arises. The dying may dwell in this state beneath words, forms, and ideas. Think of it as an incubation, an abiding with the drama without any attachment to it.

Finally, the *non-dual* state of consciousness is that in which there is no sense of *other*. In this respect, it brings us full circle to the archaic structure of complete interconnectedness, but now with a fully formed and integrated identity. One's experience is that of the universe. Interestingly, Eastern spiritual traditions express this as a complete void, while Western traditions describe it as fullness or oneness with everything. So, as ultimate as this state is, it can only be inadequately expressed through the individual's language, culture, and existential framework.

How to describe this? Let's have a look at an ancient example. Dionysius the Areopagite was a first-century judge in the city-state of Athens. His description of the non-dual state, expressed in a letter to his friend Timothy, is laden with superlatives that still fall short of his experience:

> Timothy, in the diligent exercise of mystical contemplation, leave behind the senses and the operations of the intellect, and all things sensible and intellectual, and all things in the world of being and non-being, that you may arise by unknowing towards the union, as far as is attainable, with it that transcends all being and all knowledge. For by the unceasing and absolute renunciation of yourself and of all things, you may be borne on high, through pure and entire self-abnegation, into the superessential Radiance of the Divine Darkness.[281]

This is a common theme in the writings of the mystics: one is stripped of ego-identity and apprehended by that which is beyond description. A great surprise in this understanding is that at the non-dual level there is, of

[281] Rorem, Paul. *The Dionysian Mystical Theology*. Augsburg Fortress Publishers, 2015.

course, no opposite. Everything is of one consciousness. What we call God shifts from "a Being" to the Ground of All Being. And, since no "other" is experienced in this state, you become that.

So, while on our level, there is "this" and "that," there is "right" and "wrong," those labels and forms are functional *for that level of existence.* They are not absolute. That's a very challenging concept, for it asserts that all the suffering, all the evil, all the pain, and all the death, along with MAiD, is part of the Holy, the Sacred. Nothing is profane. This is why, in near-death experiences with a life review, nothing is judged as "wrong," only assessed as to whether it helped the soul and others wake up to love.

On our level, though, this judgment and determination of right and wrong, healthy or unhealthy, moral or immoral, are necessary, for these are the boundaries that guide us to a complete humanity on the physical plane. The key is to employ them with compassion as the guide, justice as the fuel, and forgiveness as the inner orientation determined to honour the sacred in all things, in all people… even when they do not honour it in themselves. Perhaps, in the span of eternity, all things, including MAiD, can be used to help us wake up.

Even more hopeful is that dying accelerates our spiritual awakening by shifting us quickly (though it feels like an eternity when you're dying) through the gross state of awareness to the subtle and causal states. Nearing-death awareness is the hallmark of this transformation. Countless palliative and hospice nurses have observed that most people move into these more profound dimensions of consciousness as they die. This can be marked by deep contemplation, yet such silence and full presence can make us quite uncomfortable. No wonder; rapid acceleration to spiritual states of being is unfamiliar to most in the modern world. One may touch on this again and again in the dying process through dreams and visions or the infilling of peace and light. This eliminates the fear of death and dying. And this, more than at any other time, is where a spiritual care professional can guide the person to that deep dimension through meditation, visualization, ritual, self-awareness, and authentic vulnerability. Without such support, the dying sink into the dark night of the soul without navigation.

So few realize this is a functional stage, even a required one, the prelude to illumination. So many simply want it to end.

MAiD is the ultimate expression of this desire to escape—a way out instead of sinking further into the quicksand of not knowing, not doing, and the disintegration of the self. How ironic, for we only sink faster with every effort of struggle. Becoming still, we get our bearings in this liminal landscape in which we are unfolded for the shift to a transpersonal state of being. As bold as it is to say, I believe MAiD interrupts that process of waking to this deeper dimension of consciousness. This is the final stage of human development while we are here in physical form, but is compromised because of the ego's control over the process which requires its deconstruction, and at the optimal time in which that occurs.

Does this mean that those who receive MAiD do not experience any of this mystery? No. I have supported several individuals who were approved for MAiD and, in the following weeks or days, had lucid dreams and mystical visions. However, they still went through with it because they did not wish to enter the final stage of unconsciousness. They did not want their family to wait for their last breath, nor did they realize the profound lessons on life, love, and presence that this would teach those who were present. Before MAiD, there was no choice but to be captured by that arduous grace. Now, the allure of choice is increasingly compelling for those who are departing from this world. This option empowers the ego to grasp onto deception and issue commands. Its voice is all too familiar. "You don't want to suffer, do you? It will only get worse, and you don't want that. We can't put the family through this, can we?"

The ego's grip on identity is so strong that it is not uncommon for it to persist until the very end, processing experiences through the rational mind rather than allowing them to be fully experienced through one's entire being. Sometimes even the lucid dreams that rise as one falls are questioned with doubt and uncertainty. We are not accustomed to such a level of life energy, something that may seem feeble and diminished on the surface yet possesses a resounding authority of NOW – this very moment, this particular place.

Integral dying necessitates the application of spiritual intelligence in consciously preparing for one's death by gracefully relating to all the physical and mental aspects that will occur during the dying process. Astounding spiritual opportunities will arise during this time, moments that facilitate the integration of unfinished aspects of one's self, conversations that help awaken others to their true nature, and, most importantly, the ability to release the ego's narrative of self with grace. This is experienced as an anticipatory, expectant, yet unhurried wonder. Here's how the great mystic, theologian, and activist Thomas Merton expressed it:

> For the world and time are the dance of the Lord in emptiness. The silence of the spheres is the music of a wedding feast. The more we persist in misunderstanding the phenomena of life, the more we analyze them out into strange finalities and complex purposes of our own, the more we involve ourselves in sadness, absurdity and despair. But it does not matter much, because no despair of ours can alter the reality of things; or stain the joy of the cosmic dance which is always there. Indeed, we are in the midst of it, and it is in the midst of us, for it beats in our very blood, whether we want it to or not... the fact remains that we are invited to forget ourselves on purpose, cast our awful solemnity to the winds and join in the general dance.[282]

[282] Merton, Thomas. *New Seeds of Contemplation*. Shambhala, 2003, pp. 302–303.

EXERCISE 22: OBSERVING THE SELF

Time for another guided meditation. This one is going to be brief, specifically because surrendering the ego will trigger the ego's defence mechanisms for self-preservation. To avoid that, I'm going to use some lighthearted humour. You can listen to this meditation at https://soundcloud.com/david-maginley/Exercise22. (Hopefully, your ego isn't listening in!)

Find a comfortable spot where you won't be disturbed, and take a few deep breaths. Imagine yourself in a peaceful and serene location – maybe a beach, a forest, or a luxurious hammock.

As you relax, you might notice your mind wants to distract you with thoughts about the past or future. Just acknowledge those thoughts and gently bring your attention back to the present moment. Remember, your mind can be like a squirrel on caffeine – constantly darting from one thing to the next!

Now, imagine a bright light shining down from above, enveloping you in a warm, loving hug. This light represents your true self, your essence, the part of you that isn't bogged down by your ego or pesky thoughts.

As you bask in the glow of this light, imagine yourself observing your thoughts and emotions from a distance – like you're watching a soap opera or a sitcom. Notice any patterns or tendencies, and try not to get too caught up in the drama. Remember, your thoughts and emotions can be like divas – always craving attention and the spotlight.

Now, imagine the bright light within you beginning to dissolve any barriers or obstacles that stand in the way of your true self. Allow yourself to surrender your ego, your sense of self-importance, and any limiting beliefs or judgments that hold you back. It's like taking off a heavy backpack after a long hike.

As you let go of your ego, you may feel a sense of peace and liberation, like a bird finally released from its cage. Allow yourself to enjoy this feeling, and know that you can always come back to this moment of observation and surrender.

When you're ready, take a few more deep breaths and open your eyes. Congratulations, you've just given your ego a much-needed vacation!

CHAPTER 23

THE SANCTITY OF LIFE

The shrugging acceptance of war, famine, epidemic,
pain, and lifelong, grinding poverty show us that,
whatever we tell ourselves, we've made only
the most feeble of efforts to really treat human life as sacred.

– CAITLIN MORAN

IT WAS 2 A.M. WHEN MY PAGER JARRED ME AWAKE. I GROPED AROUND the nightstand to silence it, checked the number, and pulled myself up. It's never good news when it goes off, but at this hour, I knew it must be really bad. I called in.

"We've got a patient in ICU," the nurse said calmly. "Car accident, pretty bad. The family's here, Roman Catholic. They'd like prayers and support before we remove life support. Can you come in?"

"No problem, be there in ten minutes." Living close to the hospital helps at times like these. The short walk in the fresh night air blew the cobwebs from my mind and helped me connect with that strange mixture of adrenaline and calm awareness. You become very focused in these moments, with a heightened observation of human behaviour as you dive into the catastrophe and help others drowning in sorrow.

My badge quickly gained me access to the unit to find the nurse ready at the desk. She was precise and professional in relaying the essentials. The patient was young, twenty-nine, her body shattered beneath the bedsheets, her face swollen and bruised. It was a drunk driver, it was sudden, and they did all they could do to make her comfortable. What remained was bereavement support, the prayers and blessing, and commending her to the great beyond. Three family members were gathered round the bed: parents and a brother. The nurse introduced us, then drew the curtain as she left.

"This is Myia," her mother said softly. "This is our Myia."

"Myia. Beautiful name."

"Yes, it means 'gift from God.' "

I swallowed hard. I stepped up to the bed. I glanced at the respirator sustaining her life, the forest of tubes anchoring her to this earth. "She is that, I'm sure. But I can't imagine giving her back… not this way."

He mother cried, nodded. "Exactly. Exactly." She leaned over and kissed her daughter. "But we understand there's nothing more to do. She's only suffering here, like this."

I pulled up chairs so we could sit in the sacred sorrow, and asked what I always ask before life support is removed. "Tell me about her. Tell me so that I may appreciate who I am praying for."

The stories flowed of a young, independent kid who loved music, loved to dance, and was returning from a party where moments before she was having such fun. Stubborn, brilliant, caring… all the ingredients to make this all the more a tragedy. We talked for almost an hour, until the lull in the conversation indicated we need not talk anymore.

"Let's come together around her," I invited. Let's pour in the love." We rose, held hands, bowed heads, breathed deep. "Loving God…" my prayer began, and then stalled. I felt the hand holding mine squeeze slightly, the sound of the respirator seemed sharp and loud. "Loving God… we don't want this. We don't want this to happen." The best prayer says it like it is, states the truth of it without any quick affirmation of faith or hope or grace. "We don't know how to do this, how to let Myia go. It all feels so… so strange." Someone gently moaned while I paused yet again. "Loving God, may you enfold this family in your presence. May you shine through their broken hearts as the brokenness itself, for you are love. And here we are, commending her to you. May the wonder to which she awakens through death be more than paradise. May it be home, may it be safer than this world, may it be filled with adventures through which Myia can continue to grow and learn and laugh. And may this family sense that, in whatever ways to come. May they somehow know that Myia continues, and will greet them on the day of their transformation. Until then… bless her and keep her. Make your face shine upon her and be gracious to her. May you look upon her with favour and give her peace."

Why was this important? Why do people want a prayer, a blessing, an acknowledgment that something greater is at play beneath the finality of death? It is to affirm that life is sacred, that life possesses inherent value and should be regarded as inviolable and worthy of reverence. That remains an abstract concept until life is shattered, until life is about to end. Yet when it does, there is a deep knowing beyond words that resonates in the core of our being: that life is a mystery, that we do not understand it, and, therefore, we are a mystery, for we do not understand ourselves. Life is sacred because its nature is unknowable by the rational mind, and yet we are expressions of it. This sacred nature need not be linked to a deity – it can be understood as an inherent wisdom written into the fabric of reality itself, and that fabric is highly patterned. We access this pattern by being in an open state of awareness, not labelling experience, identifying or controlling it. This is the heart of the creative process, and yes, that process is not only present as we die, it is concentrated through death. Here is the metamorphosis, the universe shifting life from one state to another. As we give ourselves to this cycle of nature, we participate more fully in the underlying process by which the universe operates. We become connected to all that is. We live this mystery every moment, yet do so unconsciously until the end of our journey condenses the process so acutely that we are destabilized from our familiar state of ego-awareness, judgment, and control. Without a daily practice of opening consciousness, we will find ourselves cramming for the exam of being fully human. How strange.

Life support was removed from Myia. We watched her breath quickly fade, and it seemed as if she evaporated before our eyes. Marking this ultimate moment well meant reaching out to that mystery and inviting it to come near, to open us and receive this life that walked among us, as one of us. Now she had become something completely different, and we knew in her dying that we would die as well. So we hope, we pray, we imagine, and eventually surrender that the mystery will be... kind. That it will be safe. That it, and life, will be more.

As optimistic as I may sound that the dying process opens us to transcendence, I need to ensure that hope does not dilute your distress too quickly. The struggle itself, with all its agony and despair, is how we wrestle with mortality. It is the very process through which we are prepared for transformation. While many come to their death peacefully, dying is generally devastating. It is an awful undulation down to the basement of our being, where all the clutter of our unsorted self awaits. Most of us who die from illness or old age will experience durations of a painful, sometimes excruciating, almost always humiliating, breakdown of the body. How we face that is the ultimate test of our character, so everyone should be given plenty of slack if we stumble as we crumble. To face one's fate directly is to experience the final stage of our growth toward complete authenticity and ultimate integration.

On serious reflection, we must admit that the most challenging things we've gone through have triggered the most personal growth. That is exponentially so at the end of life. Dying matures the soul in ways living never could, but it's a bumpy way to grow up. Fortunately, the world's spiritual traditions have provided road maps, all of which explore the journey as a road to awakening to something the self is incapable of understanding while on this side of the veil.

THE SACRED GIFT

The most commonly cited spiritual argument against medically assisted death is that life is sacred. But what does that even mean? According to *Merriam-Webster*, it alludes to some connection to a divine source worthy of reverence and respect. Drilling deeper, it speaks of life as a *gift* or something irreplaceable imparted to us from the spiritual realm. That will be fine for the faithful but falls flat for those who don't believe in God, which is great! We need the challenge of updating spiritual language, so it's relevant and respectful to the modern mind.

That update is long overdue. Throughout history, theology mirrored cosmology; concepts of the gods reflected the culture and one's sense of place in the world. Yahweh was the god of ancient nomadic Israelites, a warrior and storm deity that dwelt in the desert. Their enemy, the Canaanites, were a coastal people who worshipped the storm and water deity Hadad (the gods often threw temper tantrums through the weather). But now, with our images of Earth as a pale blue dot in a universe grander than our wildest dreams, these archaic notions of the divine persist nonetheless in spiritual catchphrases that seek a higher purpose in terrestrial affairs (forces of nature are still referred to as "acts of God"). Our depiction of the divine reveals, as it did in ancient times, more of our cultural framework, worldview, sense of place, purpose, and perception than the actual spiritual realm. We will forever see the world as we are, not as the world is. And so it must be, for we are limited to the cognitive storehouse of our language, our existential framework, in describing the divine. The primitive and fearful view of an external, personal God that grants favour to some while cursing others continues for much of the human family. So many who I have counselled speak of God allowing, or, worse, causing cancer "for some reason." At least a divine plan feels safer than random chaos.

Further, in its unknowable wisdom, the deity withdraws the gift of life, "taking" their loved one in the end. This is no different from the god of the Bronze Age Israelites. Their image of the divine reflected their identity as a nomadic, tribal people, worshipping one god among many. When they ran up against the Hittites or Canaanites, it was all a matter of whose god was mightier. Their belief systems also reflected their understanding of their place in the cosmos, a realm shaped and controlled by unseen forces around which they developed their mythologies. This progressed at a pace that supported existential adaptation. Hundreds of years of slow change tend to lock ideas into a convincing cosmology. Still, while our understanding of our place in the universe has expanded exponentially, our concept of God has not expanded with it. Perhaps this lag is understandable when most of earth's citizens live in cities where entire generations can pass by without ever truly seeing the night sky. But it is abysmally inadequate when asking the tough questions about suffering, dignity, and dying.

The argument that life is sacred, despite its profundity, can feel shallow due to its inconsistency; to believe this, one has to filter their parameters to suit their comfort zone. If human life is so sacred, why not protest avoidable poverty, the genocide of First Nations children in residential schools with their thousands of unmarked graves, or the rampant opioid addiction sweeping North America? Why not work to end war or to protect children from sexual abuse or human trafficking, which destroys thousands of souls every year long before their bodies give out? The argument for the sanctity of life has little traction when exercised for a particular situation. So, why do people employ it?

Because we invest ourselves in what has emotional proximity to our identity, our story. You may know someone who has cancer. You may know someone who has died from it. And it is not unrealistic to consider that you may develop cancer someday too. The Indigenous communities in Canada that struggle to have safe drinking water may come to you only through the evening news. But cancer could be next door, could be in your family. Since we are who we are through our relationships, the closer to home an issue is, the more personal it becomes. And, in the end, we're all going to die, so even in the abstract sense, this topic hits home eventually. (On that note, a spiritually evolved person will resonate with all who suffer, no matter their proximity or path through life. And in this will be found a secret to transforming your own suffering, especially as you die. We'll get back to that later.)

As inconsistently as we apply the term, at its core, the sanctity of life asserts that this animating principle of our consciousness is imparted to us from God. As such, it is a mysterious gift manifesting from beyond this material realm, so when we end a life, we don't know what we're stopping. That's the bottom line in the religious argument against medically assisted death, even more so now, as MAiD can be used by those who are sick or disabled but not dying. And this goes against fundamental principles of life for the vast majority of believers.[283] Derek Ross, the executive director of Christian Legal Fellowship, states in an interfaith statement against MAiD, "We're now dealing with a legal system that is making more and more exceptions to the once exception-less principle that you cannot consent to the harm of having your life ended by another person and that all lives are inherently and equally full of worth and value of dignity. Instead of prioritizing supports to help people to live meaningful lives, we've prioritized ways to make death more accessible."[284]

The sanctity of life argument also reinforces the notion that God is above, somehow "outside" us, a deity that bestows life upon us and then watches, knows, and judges. No wonder *sanctity of life* is a term fraught with fear of punishment should a difficult life be treated as disposable. It is also a term that reveals the moral parameters of a person's identity, the compass by which they navigate life and death. Therefore, when the term is employed in discussing MAiD, a fruitful conversation will only be had once we share the same terms and map, especially since we share the same ship. Let's look at the world's main faiths; how they understand this term, *the sanctity of life*; and how they offer guidance as our ship takes its final voyage.[285]

---

[283] Rev. Allan, Bill, et al. "We Can and Must Do *Much* Better: Religious Leaders in Canada oppose Bill C-7." Evangelical Fellowship. https://files.evangelicalfellowship.ca/si/Euthanasia/MAiD_Religious-Leaders-oppose-Bill-C-7_Oct-2020.pdf

[284] Gillmore, Meagan. "After Physician-Assisted Suicide Bill, Canadian Evangelicals Reassess." Christianity Today. April 20, 2021. https://www.christianitytoday.com/news/2021/april/canada-MAiD-physician-suicide-law-evangelical-disability.html. Accessed April 17, 2022.

[285] For quotes from the various spiritual traditions, see "Religious Perspectives on Euthanasia and Medical Aid in Dying." Britannica ProCon.org. https://euthanasia.procon.org/religious-perspectives-on-euthanasia-and-physician-assisted-suicide-pas/

BUDDHISM

THERE ARE MANY EXPRESSIONS OF BUDDHISM, AS THERE ARE WITH Christianity. These arose from various cultures and teachers throughout time. Buddhists are not unanimous in their view of euthanasia, with some seeing it as an act of compassion. Most traditional Buddhist perspectives view intentional acts to end life as problematic due to the value placed on life and the intention behind actions. And while there was no equivalent term in ancient Buddhism for euthanasia, the Buddha did issue a precept for the monastic code, stating it was immoral "to embark on any course of action whose aim is to destroy human life, irrespective of the quality of the individual's motive."[286]

As with all matters of religious teaching, it gets complicated. There are cases within the Buddha's teachings that seem to condone suicide. One involves the actions of two monks who, at the end of a lengthy period of suffering, seemed to have achieved enlightenment.[287] This meant they had perfected their compassionate detachment from the physical form and had attained a state of complete release from the attraction, aversion, and delusion around life and death, indeed all of reality. Remaining incarnate no longer served their spiritual development. However, it's generally agreed that these cases are exceptional and do not provide a general endorsement of suicide in Buddhism. Additionally, the spiritual work of helping others wake up to their true nature begins when one becomes enlightened – it's why choosing to remain embodied for the sake of others is such a great act of compassion.

Suicide had also been used as a political weapon by Buddhist monks during the Vietnam war. However, it's crucial to note that these acts were seen as extreme forms of protest and not as endorsements of suicide or euthanasia. Additionally, we must remember that these were monks with a life devoted to spiritual disciplines for awakening. This enlightenment is quite different from feeling grateful and accepting as a person dies

[286] Keown, Damien. "End of life: The Buddhist view." *The Lancet* 366.9489 (2005): pp. 952–955.

[287] Keown, Damien. "Suicide, assisted suicide and euthanasia: A Buddhist perspective." *Journal of Law and Religion* 13.2 (1998): pp. 385–405.

through MAiD, which entails another facilitating your death – expressly forbidden in the Buddhist tradition, which understands that to be born human is an auspicious and fortunate experience to attain enlightenment. To intentionally cause death, even with the motive of reducing or ending a person's suffering, is to bond one's will with death and perpetuate the karmic process of reincarnation, or *samsara*.

Unlike other life forms, being human means experiencing the best conditions for spiritual growth. An enlightened person not only respects the difficulty of obtaining a human body, but also cherishes life in all its forms. Moreover, the idea of killing a living being as a solution to suffering perpetuates the Buddhist principle of *dukkha*, often translated as "suffering," "pain," "unsatisfactoriness," or "stress." However, its meaning is broader than just physical or emotional pain. Dukkha refers to the inherent dissatisfaction and discomfort that permeate human existence. Dukkha is one of the three marks of existence, along with *anatman* (not-self) and *anitya* (impermanence). Therefore, to live is to suffer when one experiences the illusion of being separate from others and the entire world. One is in it, but not of it, so nothing is guaranteed. Life is not safe.

An invaluable gift from the Buddhist tradition is its emphasis on gaining insight into one's suffering and cultivating compassion and respect for life in order to transform it. This process is outlined in the four truths of the noble ones (often called the Four Noble Truths), which provide a succinct reality check on suffering and the best approach to overcome it.

The first noble truth is that suffering is an integral part of life. This makes sense as the majority of humanity functions with the perceptual error of a dualistic mindset; that they are separate beings in a world of separate objects. Such mistaken perception exposes individuals to limitations, danger, and mortality, while underscoring the importance of realizing the impermanent and interconnected nature of all things. Reincarnation, in this context, provides countless opportunities for individuals to progress on the path to enlightenment by cultivating wisdom and compassion, ultimately helping others to awaken from the illusion of separateness.

The second noble truth is about *samudaya*, which states that suffering arises from our attachments, cravings, desires, and karma (the law of cause and effect). This attachment is known as *shenpa*, meaning "that which has its hooks in you," and includes identifying with aspects of our personal narrative that shape our identity. For instance, I am a chaplain, father, friend, author, and person of my culture. However, I am much more than these roles; they are merely the expressions of who I am in the world. Our relationships – with our body, environment, and roles within the family and community – contribute to who we think we are. Naturally, we protect and sometimes cling to these roles, ensuring our survival and, more importantly for the ego, safeguarding our identity. (And I don't want that to be dismantled through dying. The ego is the part of me I enjoy the most!) Therefore, when we lose our favorite possession, friend, job, home, marriage, or our perception of tomorrow, we grieve. We buy into the illusion that we are losing a part of ourselves. Consequently, when we die, we suffer because we still cling to the mistaken notion of a permanent self, and we experience the pain of losing all the things we are attached to, the story we've attached our identity to.

The third is the truth of *nirodha*, the ending of suffering through compassionate detachment from it all, even from our identity. By not clinging to what we want or even what we think we are, we are more fully embedded in the transitory nature of life and can accept what is… including the process of death. Awakening is, therefore, a relaxing into what always was the case: there is no separate self, not even mind. There is only the nondual nature of reality. What a wonderful and simple surprise!

Through mindfulness (in-the-moment awareness) and meditation (the long-term practice of awareness), one starts to disengage from craving and clinging to impermanent states and things like health, independence, agency, and the body with all its sufferings, even to thoughts and feelings. You no longer believe everything you think, are no longer controlled by everything you feel, and no longer identify with the ego or your experience. You move simply to awareness. From this centre, you remain stable while the storm around you (and within you) threatens to capsize everyone, everything. You engage this storm not with disinterest or apathy but with compassion. No desire or need to change it, correct it, feel better, or be anything other than what you are. It is a state completely free from preferences or bias. As innocuous as it may sound, this has the profound effect of dissolving suffering. Vulnerability is transcended as a consequence of its acceptance.

The fourth is the truth of *marga*, a practical guide to ethical and mental development with the goal of freeing individuals from suffering and ultimately attaining enlightenment. It consists of eight interconnected practices:

1. Right Understanding: Seeing the world clearly, understanding the nature of reality, and knowing that life involves challenges and change.
2. Right Thought: Cultivating positive intentions, such as kindness, compassion, and letting go of harmful desires.
3. Right Speech: Speaking truthfully and kindly, avoiding lies, hurtful words, and gossip.
4. Right Action: Behaving ethically by not harming others, stealing, or engaging in irresponsible behaviors.
5. Right Livelihood: Choosing a job or way of life that does not cause harm to others and aligns with ethical principles.
6. Right Effort: Putting effort into developing good qualities, such as patience and love, while avoiding harmful ones, like anger and jealousy.
7. Right Mindfulness: Being aware and present in each moment, paying attention to thoughts, feelings, and experiences without getting lost in them.
8. Right Concentration: Focusing the mind through practices like meditation, leading to deep mental clarity and inner peace.

Together, these eight practices form a comprehensive path that guides individuals toward the cessation of suffering and the realization of enlightenment, embodying the essence of the Buddhist way of life. These principles suggest that instead of seeking to end suffering through MAiD, one might focus on cultivating a compassionate and mindful approach to life's challenges, especially it's end. After all, true liberation comes from inner transformation rather than external actions.

Understanding the Four Noble Truths and the Eightfold Path provides a foundation for how Buddhists approach life's challenges and suffering. These teachings emphasize the importance of cultivating wisdom, compassion, and mindfulness throughout one's life. When it comes to the end of life, these practices become particularly significant. Buddhist teachings not only guide how to live but also how to face death with a transformed perspective. The process of dying is seen as a critical phase where one's accumulated spiritual practices and mental state play a crucial role in determining the nature of the afterlife.

Central to the MAiD debate is an emphasis on the autonomy of the individual and the emphasis on a person's rights. This assertion of the independent self is a post-enlightenment perspective not found in Buddhism, which approaches moral issues from the standpoint of a compassionate, heartfelt wish to support the awakening of everyone rather than defend the autonomy of the individual. Of course you do not want to suffer as you die, do not want to see your family grieve, do not want the pain you presently have or undergo the pain *you imagine* will come. You do not want to move into the end of... you. You do not want to cross the transformative fields of chaos, despair, and sadness. These feel meaningless, yet are highly functional dynamics of change from which we emerge to a completely new state of consciousness.

The Buddhist tradition places significant weight on one's final thoughts and intentions at the time of death. The way one engages with the dying process, influenced by the principles of the Eightfold Path, has profound implications for what follows after physical death. In Buddhism, death is seen as a transition rather than an end, leading to the bardo – a transitional state where one's true nature and accumulated karma come into play. How one faces this transition is critical; engaging with compassion and openness, rather than resistance or fear, aligns with the Buddhist view of navigating this state effectively. Negative or fearful thoughts at the moment of death can result in a turbulent experience in the bardo, potentially leading to rebirth in less favorable conditions. Conversely, maintaining a mindset of compassion and acceptance can help one move through the bardo towards more positive spiritual realms. Thus, Buddhist practices aim to prepare individuals to approach the end of life with a calm, compassionate, and clear state of mind, reflecting the essence of their spiritual training.

HINDUISM

As with the Buddhist tradition, Hinduism teaches that MAiD affects the karma of both the patient and the doctor assisting them. The separation of the soul and body is seen as premature and unnatural, disrupting the natural flow of life and death.[288] This would complicate karma, a Sanskrit word meaning "action," which refers to the law that every action has an equal reaction, either immediately or at some point in the future. This law of karma governs all of life, shaping the ripple effects of virtuous actions on one's life and future incarnations, and the ripple effects of selfish or destructive actions.[289] But how does this impact the person administering MAiD?

Some might argue that MAiD is a virtuous act meant to relieve suffering, a compassionate response to the physical and existential distress a patient may be experiencing. However, Hinduism holds that such an act creates bad karma that will severely compromise the soul of the person assisting in the process on the day they die. It also interferes with the timing of the patient's exit, which is believed to be governed by a cosmic order. According to Hindu tradition, there are specific windows during which it's ideal for a person to leave this world. While it's true that we can never fully know whether a MAiD procedure coincides with such a window, the tradition errs on the side of caution. It trusts that the universe,

---

[288] Harold G. Coward and Julius Lipner, *Hindu Ethics: Purity, Abortion, and Euthanasia* (Albany: State University of New York Press, 1989), 45.

[289] Arvind Sharma, *Hinduism and Human Rights: A Conceptual Approach* (New Delhi: Oxford University Press, 2004), 82.

with its intricate web of cause and effect, is wiser than we are on matters of life and death.

Hinduism is clear in its general disapproval of euthanasia, but the tradition is far from unanimous in its views. This is not a monolithic religion; it encompasses a vast array of traditions, philosophies, and practices. Different schools of thought within Hinduism, such as Advaita Vedanta, Vaishnavism, and Shaivism, might approach the issue of euthanasia differently. While there is a common disapproval of euthanasia across these traditions, the rationale behind this disapproval and the emphasis placed on certain aspects of it might differ. For instance, some schools might focus on non-duality and the illusory nature of suffering, suggesting that engaging in MAiD misunderstands the deeper truth of existence. Others might emphasize devotion to a particular deity, underscoring the importance of submitting to divine will rather than taking matters into one's own hands.

Hinduism teaches that the ideal death is a conscious death, one in which the individual is fully aware and engaged with the process of dying. MAiD circumvents this by preventing the shifts in consciousness and ego-deconstruction. Additionally, the state of mind that leads a person to choose euthanasia could negatively affect the process of reincarnation. One's last thoughts are deeply relevant to the process of rebirth, and choosing euthanasia out of fear or despair might set a troubling course for the soul's next life.

This focus on the state of mind and intention is crucial. As with Buddhism, Hinduism places a strong emphasis on assessing the intention behind an action, often more so than the action itself. The tradition is less interested in abstract ideas of right or wrong as they are understood in Western philosophy. Instead, Hinduism is concerned with the consequences of our actions, particularly how they align with one's *dharma* – one's moral duties and responsibilities. Dharma is always evolving; it is never static. Hinduism, therefore, is a dynamic way of life that adapts to time, place, and circumstances.[290] Even the most important value on which

[290] Shubha Sharma and Rajeev Sharma, "The Ethics of Euthanasia in Hinduism," *International Journal of Hindu Studies* 10, no. 2 (2006): 159.

Hinduism is based, the dharma principle, is applied according to the specific context in which a person finds themselves.

This adaptability is one of Hinduism's strengths, allowing it to accommodate a wide range of beliefs and practices. However, this also means that the views on MAiD can vary. Some contemporary Hindu thinkers might navigate the tensions between traditional teachings and modern ethical considerations differently, particularly those in the Hindu diaspora who may be influenced by the legal and medical frameworks of the West. For instance, the question of whether ending a person's suffering could be considered a virtuous act might be viewed more leniently by those who emphasize compassion as a key aspect of dharma, even if it conflicts with the traditional interpretation of ahimsa.

Nevertheless, the doctrine of karma remains central to how Hindus approach life and death. Because of this, Hindus often try to get their life in order before they die, ensuring that there is no unfinished business and that relationships are restored. This preparation for death is not just a matter of practicalities but is deeply spiritual, aimed at entering the state of a *sannyasin* – one who has renounced everything: all possessions, all relationships, and, most significantly, all self-identity. Herein lies significant tension with MAiD, which stems from the insistence that "it's *my* body, *my* life, *my* choice."

The concept of a conscious death is particularly significant here. For Hindus, the goal is to leave this world in a state of spiritual purity, free from attachments and desires that bind the soul to the cycle of rebirth. But few Westerners receiving MAiD renounce the world and die as religious ascetics. They die as embedded in ego-identity as ever, often seeking to escape dying in any other way. From a Hindu perspective, this is problematic because it suggests that the individual is not only failing to renounce the world but is actively reinforcing their attachment to it. This could lead to accumulating more karmic debts, complicating the soul's journey.

Hinduism also places great importance on the role of the community and rituals, especially during the end of life. The community, along with the family, plays a vital part in supporting a person facing end-of-life decisions. Rituals such as the *Antyeshti*, or last rites, are performed with the belief that they aid the soul's journey after death. These rituals are seen as essential in ensuring that the transition from one life to the next is as smooth as possible. In this context, MAiD might be seen as disrupting these sacred practices, preventing the soul from receiving the full benefits of the rituals that are meant to guide it on its journey.

ISLAM

Just as with Buddhism, many nuances and subtle-yet-significant points are lost in translation when Western Christians explore common ground with their Muslim brethren. While Islam acknowledges suffering, it is often viewed as a test or trial from God, and the response is framed within the concepts of patience (*sabr*) and trust (*tawakkul*). So, before exploring what Islam teaches on MAiD, we first need to appreciate the distinctions that shed new light on Islam's teachings about Allah's love and sovereignty, as well as a person's free will and limits to self-determination.

So many times I've sat with a patient or family member and heard the spiritual cliché, "There must be a purpose in this." Often sighed softly, how it is worded reveals a sense of being lost, of reaching for hope, fumbling for a way forward. Even the more affirming "God has a purpose in this" rings with what the Christian church calls a *theodicy*, the vindication of divine goodness and providence in the face of the existence of evil and suffering. In other words, it's a subconscious defence of God's goodness and providence.

Hear these words from a Muslim patient, and the tone is quite different: an affirmation, even a proclamation of God's will. This is not a defence of God's goodness, nor simple submission to divine whims, but full participation in the will and ways of Allah. There is no searching for the way to go but a commitment to the road ahead. As a result, there is a meaningful engagement with what may be more accurately termed "affliction."

Muslims attribute the moral quality of suffering only to human action.[291] Everything else is under God's absolute sovereignty. The connection between physical agony and inward spiritual pain, which the word "suffering" regularly connotes in the West, is foreign to the Islamic perspective. Therefore the very nature of existential distress is quite different and would not be a significant motivator for something that Islamic culture does not consider: requesting one's life be terminated by a doctor because of distress and the inability to live the remainder of life on one's terms.

Islam's preferred response to such situations is patience and trust. More than that, Muslims should submissively praise God for the experience of affliction.[292] As a result, lament and complaint are far less in the Islamic orientation towards suffering and death.

In light of this, it is no surprise that Islam sees human life as a precious gift from God to be cherished and respected. Suicide, assisted suicide, and euthanasia are forbidden, and that is stated plainly in the Qur'an: "And no person can ever die except by Allah's leave and at an appointed term."[293] The Qur'an and *hadith* (a collection of traditions and sayings of the Prophet Muhammad) are the authoritative sources for the Islamic code of law, which discusses many issues regarding life and death, concluding that a physician carrying out MAiD is guilty of homicide.[294]

If a patient has a terminal illness, withholding or withdrawing futile medical treatment is permissible. The Islamic Code of Medical Ethics states, "it is futile to diligently keep the patient in a vegetative state by heroic means.... It is the process of life that the doctor aims to maintain and not the process of dying." Indeed, this view is agreed upon by most of the world's spiritual traditions.

The adjective most commonly used to describe Allah in the Qur'an is بسم الله الرحيم الرحمن،ال, *the compassionate one, the merciful.* This is what

[291] Griffiths, Paul J. *Problems of Religious Diversity*. John Wiley & Sons, 2015.

[292] Pieper, Christopher. "Why the Hardship? Islam, Christianity, and Instrumental Affliction." *Open Theology* 6.1 (2020): pp. 636–645.

[293] The Holy Qur'an, 3:145 Wordsworth Editions, 2000.

[294] Madadin, Mohammed, et al. "The Islamic perspective on physician-assisted suicide and euthanasia." *Medicine, Science and the Law* 60.4 (2020): pp. 278–286.

the dying bank on as they head to judgment and, hopefully, paradise. Prematurely ending one's life destroys that hope, as it asserts your own will over that of God's in the pivotal moment upon which salvation is imminent. Remaining faithful sanctifies one's inner nature through the storm of illness and into death. Here lies the ultimate moment in which the dying are encouraged to meditate on and repeat the *Shahada*, a profession of faith. "I bear witness that (there is) no god except Allah; One is He, no partner hath He, and I bear witness that Muhammad is His Servant and Messenger." Ideally, these would be the last words upon one's lips before their transformation.

JUDAISM

Respect for life as a gift of God continues to be the core principle by which we engage suffering in our final days. This respect is central to the Jewish faith. Active euthanasia is expressly forbidden, even if the terminally ill patient is suffering. Similarly, suicide is forbidden, although religious martyrdom is permitted in certain situations. Passive euthanasia is more complicated, as expressed in the sixteenth-century Jewish code called the *Shulchan Aruch*: "if there is anything which causes a hindrance to the departure of the soul... it is permissible to remove [it] from there because there is no act involved, only the removal of the impediment." That seems straightforward, but the line blurs as technology advances. Does intravenous hydration prolong death or provide comfort? Well, both, but it depends on the person's metabolism, weight, and disease process. These matters must always be well-measured.

To go deeper, though, let's explore the nature of suffering and how the Jewish faith understands its role in shaping a person's soul, shifting them to share the Ground of Being with their creator. And, I'd like to do this through a person who was not dying, though his brother would soon see to that.

JACOB

He was a despicable, backstabbing selfish fool. He lived for himself, was resentful of his siblings, and was bitter that he always seemed to get the short end of the stick. Jacob decided to take things into his own hands. He betrayed his elder brother by tricking their dying father into giving him the elder's inheritance.

The story is found in Genesis, a book filled with backstabbing and brutal betrayals. (It's not Sunday school material!). Jacob runs from his fate to hide in a distant land, finding employment with his uncle and negotiating a soap opera of relationships. But laying low only works for so long. In a cryptic dream, God tells him that his progeny would be a blessing to the earth. However, to have such a legacy, he would need to reconcile with his past. (The Bible has a pattern of this: God uses the worst in us to bring out the best from us. Which means God is either a fool or very good at the job!) Like anyone negotiating with his enemies, Jacob sends a messenger ahead and prepares elaborate peace offerings, but his brother wants nothing but Jacob's head. And his brother is approaching with an army, the messenger reports. Better run for the hills.

What to do? Destruction is on the way. Jacob has nothing to go on except this abstract promise, a weird vision given in a dream (another preferred method of the Spirit. Nothing is straightforward from their end!) He sends his travelling companions back to safety and turns to face his fate alone. That posse would arrive the next day, so, exhausted, he found a place to sleep by a river. If you're going to lose your life, sleep can be a wonderful escape. And then… you guessed it, another dream. A figure, described as both an angel and a man, wrestles with Jacob through the night. Though the figure is powerful beyond measure, Jacob nonetheless seems to match him move for move until morning, when the opponent wrenches Jacob's hip and stands over him, exhausted. Here's how it reads from Chapter 32:

> 25 When the man saw that he did not prevail against Jacob,
> he struck him on the hip socket; and Jacob's hip was put out
> of joint as he wrestled with him. 26 Then he said, "Let me go,
> for the day is breaking." But Jacob said, "I will not let you
> go, unless you bless me." 27 So he said to him, "What is your

> name?" And he said, "Jacob." [28] Then the man said, "You shall
> no longer be called Jacob, but Israel, for you have striven with
> God and with humans, and have prevailed." [29] Then Jacob
> asked him, "Please tell me your name." But he said, "Why is it
> that you ask my name?" And there he blessed him. [30] So Jacob
> called the place Peniel, saying, "For I have seen God face to
> face, and yet my life is preserved." [31] The sun rose upon him
> as he passed Peniel, limping because of his hip.

Nothing is as it seems when it comes to dreaming or dying. Everything has layers of meaning; everything invites you to dive deeper… especially suffering. Is Jacob wrestling with himself? Is this his shadow, his conscience, or a celestial entity? What it is doesn't matter; it's what it does that matters. Jacob says, only after the wrestling has reached exhaustion, "Enough! Let me go, for the day is breaking." A symbol of emerging from the dark night of the soul? A metaphor of how wrestling with God can only be done alone, without the aid of even seeing your bearings around you? Rabbi Shmuel Klitsner, a lecturer in Biblical Exegesis at Lindenbaum College in Jerusalem, puts it this way: "The things that you're wrestling with are the things you've relegated to darkness… but when the rise of dawn comes, that enlightenment is the most threatening part of this…. Our ways of prevaricating, of lying to ourselves or deceiving others don't withstand the light of day…. This struggle of Jacob's is so intensely human…. He needs his identity to evolve the same way I need my identity to evolve: over time and through struggle."

And what of Jacob's odd request? He asks his nemesis to bless him. Is this, again, his selfish instinct to get anything he can from a situation?

The angel retorts with a question: "What is your name?" Clearly, an angel would know that already. One's name always meant something; it represents your story, the meaning of your life in the world. The Bible is full of this understanding, with the story of Jacob replete with that application. The angel is telling Jacob to examine himself, be authentic in his character, and see the mythologies he has carried about himself for what they are. "Who are you really, Jacob? Do you know yourself?" That question becomes the blessing through the new name God gives him: "Israel," meaning one who has wrestled with God and humans, with life itself, and prevailed.

The heart of the story is this: the only way to get real is to engage with suffering fully. Do not turn away, take a detour, or shrink back. There are no shortcuts. Through struggle, you will be changed… wounded, and the better for it.

Who am I? What is the name I have made for myself, and what is the name I can achieve, especially in my dying? Just asking the question can move us toward a better answer. Just asking the question demonstrates our capacity for growth and introspection. We don't shrink back from the struggle of living or dying. We do not do anything to change the rules, to fix the fight. Instead, we are all called to take God to the mat and will emerge bruised, bloodied, and blessed.

It's the perennial wisdom imparted by countless spiritual traditions: you are not who or what you think you are. What is the name, the essence, the "I" that is asking?

CHRISTIANITY

The majority of christian denominations state that MAiD violates the sanctity of life. The Roman Catholic Church, which comprises over half of Christians worldwide, is clear and firm on this matter: "Whatever its motives and means, direct euthanasia consists in putting an end to the lives of disabled, sick, or dying persons. It is morally unacceptable. Thus an act or omission which, of itself or by intention, causes death in order to eliminate suffering constitutes a murder gravely contrary to the dignity of the human person and to the respect due to the living God, his Creator. The error of judgment into which one can fall in good faith does not change the nature of this murderous act, which must always be forbidden and excluded."[295]

[295] Paul II, Pope John. *Catechism of the Catholic Church*. London: Geoffrey Chapman, 1994. Paragraph 2258

This exhortation stems from the biblical doctrine of *imago Dei*: that we are created in the image of God. It is the basis of the sanctity of life principle in which our dignity and worth are derived from our identity as this sacred image.[296] As much as it may feel like your life is your own, this spiritual position asserts that your consciousness, your life force, arises from another, the Divine Source. You are the steward of this life and this body through this time. And your assignment is to grow into a being that loves, for God is love.

To request euthanasia is to judge that your own life is not worthwhile. Indeed, that's identified in the determination of "unbearable suffering": life is not acceptable on the patient's terms. This placement of the person as the central authority on their own experience seems an obvious truth to most. Still, it runs counter to the sanctity of life principle, which states that your quality of life is utterly irrelevant to the value of your life. That theological assertion will feel like a slap in the face unless backed up by the community's commitment to compassionately walk with and support the dying until their last breath. No wonder Christians were exhorted to "bear one another's burdens" (Gal 6:2a) and to treat "the least of these" (which includes the sick) as if they were Jesus (Matt 25:40). Without such traction, the sanctity of life argument becomes an injury to the dignity of the dying.[297]

Protestant churches tend to agree with the Roman Catholic position, with the more conservative faith groups being most vocal in their opposition to MAiD and the more liberal ones favouring individual choice. Leading the liberal position is the United Church of Canada, stating that

[296] The catechism reads, "Human life is sacred because from its beginning it involves the creative action of God and it remains forever in a special relationship with the Creator, who is its sole end. God alone is the Lord of life from its beginning until its end: no one can under any circumstance claim for himself the right directly to destroy an innocent human being." Ibid, paragraph 2277

[297] The statement from the Atlantic Archdiocese on this matter demonstrates a deeply compassionate response to how the Roman Catholic Church can address MAiD, and minister to those who desire it. Roman Catholic Archdiocese of St. John, Pastoral Letter from Atlantic Episcopal Assembly https://rcsj.org/news/pastoral-letter-from-atlantic-episcopal-assembly. Accessed Feb. 27, 2023.

MAiD "may be chosen as a faithful option in certain circumstances"[298] while emphasizing that

1. the criterion of "foreseeable death" for access to MAiD be maintained
2. ending suffering due to mental illness not be a category for MAiD, and that the church advocates for increased mental health resources
3. advance directives in relation to MAiD not be permitted
4. for mature minors, the capacity to decide for MAiD should be judged on a case-by-case basis by medical professionals in consultation with family and the community[299]

These points were adopted in response to the proposal to allow MAiD for those with mental health and non-lethal conditions. They could see the direction this was taking and implored the government to focus on access to palliative care as the front-line strategy, not medically assisted death.

The Anglican Church, in their 1998 document, *Care in Dying*, concluded that medically assisted death is a failure of the human community and that care cannot include an act whose primary intention is to end a person's life. Euthanasia could not be construed as an act of care. But culture changes. In 2022, Archbishop Linda Nicholls recommended avoiding publicly opposing the expansion of MAiD. This recommendation was based not on shifts in theological insight but on how unpopular it would be. "The mood in Canada" is not "to consider what churches have to say about this," she said, warning against "imposing Christian values." Far better for the church to "focus on providing pastoral care to people

[298] "Medical Assistance in Dying: The United Church opts for a balanced case-by-case approach to medical assistance in dying." The United Church of Canada. May 8, 2017. https://united-church.ca/news/medical-assistance-dying. Accessed April 17, 2022.

[299] "Revised Statement on Medical Assistance in Dying: Guidance for those engaged in discussions around end-of-life decisions." The United Church in Canada. June 1, 2020. https://united-church.ca/news/revised-statement-medical-assistance-dying Accessed April 17, 2022.

who are considering medical assistance in dying."[300] While advocating for greater palliative care the Anglican position concluded that the job of the church is to help the dying "continue to experience meaning, purpose and control over one's life."[301] That's ironic since, for Christians, we are called to live by faith, with an acknowledged dependence upon each other and, above all, on God. Additionally, what death asks of us is the final state of complete surrender to the Enfolding Presence that transforms us. As stated earlier, a bad day for your ego is a great day for your soul.

My own denomination, the Evangelical Lutheran Church in Canada, followed suit, emphasizing pastoral care and accompaniment. In a study guide for its 2019 document, *The Call to Faithfully Journey with Those Who Are Dying: An ELCIC Resolution*, it asks, "If the chief purpose of life is to know God and to enjoy God forever, is it possible to conceive of circumstances where a person might faithfully conclude that this purpose could no longer be furthered by the extension of their life and might choose, not merely to cease to resist the approach of death, but to embrace it actively?"[302] Those circumstances indeed can be conceived, but acceptance at the level of mind and ego is quite unlike the transpersonal state of being that naturally envelops us at the end. Few from the Buddhist and Hindu positions could claim to have achieved a state of enlightenment through which ending life is acceptable. How much more so for the untrained, individualistic Western mind?

Rather than speaking to the moral gravity of euthanasia or the shifts in consciousness through the dying process, the focus is on a "relational theology" that emphasizes self-determination as the ideal at life's end. It's

---

[300] Crosby, Benjamin. "Church Should Not Oppose MAiD Law, Primate Says." *Anglican Journal*, 31 Oct. 2022, anglicanjournal.com/church-should-not-oppose-maid-law-primate-says/.

[301] "In Sure and Certain Hope: Resources to Assist Pastoral and Theological Approaches to Physician Assisted Dying." Anglican Church of Canada. February 2018. https://www.anglican.ca/wp-content/uploads/In-Sure-and-Certain-Hope.pdf. Accessed May 5, 2024

[302] ELCIC Study Guide for Conversations on Medical Assistance in Dying, p. 8. https://eft.elcic.ca/decisions-at-the-end-of-life/documents/MAiDStudyGuide2016_FINAL.pdf Accessed April 17, 2022

disheartening that individual choice would dominate in a tradition that teaches how spiritual growth leads to the disappearance of the self as the revealing of the Christ consciousness. This is at the heart of baptism, one of two central sacraments through which, according to Lutheran theology, we are mystically joined to the death and resurrection of Christ. Living one's baptismal identity is a daily practice of dying to the old self and identifying one's essence as being in Christ.[303] At no point in the human journey is this brought to completion as through physical death and the process of ego deconstruction to which Kathleen Singh refers. Not identifying this is a profound failure in a church that emphasizes the way of the cross, that continually affirms that while God's grace will protect us from nothing, it will sustain us through everything. Not trusting ourselves in complete surrender to that enshrouding grace at the ultimate moment it will manifest is a significant oversight in my church's decision to support MAiD.

Even more, in a surprising interpretation of Martin Luther's teaching on the Fifth Commandment not to kill, my church has concluded that this instruction supports a doctor killing their patient so as not to prolong their suffering. Luther had deepened the meaning of this commandment from a single act of violence to a life-long calling to care for our neighbour: "We are to fear and love God, so that we neither endanger nor harm the lives of our neighbour, but instead help and support them in all of life's needs."[304] In 1529, these words were a call to community, an instruction to rise above avarice towards those who annoy, and to love one's enemy rather than seek revenge. That's a far cry from a 21st-century palliative situation in which the dying are approaching the transcendent states of consciousness just before death but are shut off because of the resistance of the personal self, the ego, what Luther called 'the old Adam.'

We can see a pattern here, just as Richard Rohr stated: all spirituality is about what we do with our pain. Buddhists, Muslims, Jews, Hindus,

---

[303] Matthew 16:24-26, Romans 6:6, 1 Corinthians 15:31, Galatians 2:20, Galatians 5:24

[304] Luther, Martin, and Conrad Dieterich. *The small catechism*. St. Louis, MO: Concordia, 1960.

and Christians... all engage in suffering as inevitable in life and the most potent means of impelling us to become authentic, compassionate, connected to others, and spiritually awake. That's also embedded in the Biblical stories, specifically in how Jesus engaged with these ultimate questions of suffering, meaning and death. I'll be going more in-depth here, as I'm steeped in the Christian tradition and have a greater appreciation of its insights into psycho-spiritual dynamics than those within the other faith traditions. We're going to get Biblical here, so if that doesn't interest you, I encourage you to jump to the next chapter, where we'll explore the mystical aspects of death and its implication for MAiD. But if you'll stay with me, I'd like to begin our exploration of what the Christian scriptures say about suffering and facing death through what many find to be the most entertaining of spiritual dynamics: temptation.

EXERCISE 23: QUESTIONS OF FAITH

FIND A QUIET AND COMFORTABLE SPACE WHERE YOU CAN REFLECT WITHout distractions. Take a moment to centre yourself and prepare for introspection.

1. *Consider the concept of the sanctity of life, which emphasizes the inherent value and sacredness of human life. Reflect on how this concept aligns or conflicts with the practice of Medical Assistance in Dying (MAiD).*
2. *Think about your personal beliefs and values regarding the sanctity of life. Consider how your faith or spiritual perspectives inform your understanding of this concept.*
3. *Write down your thoughts and reflections on the following questions:*
    a. *How do you define the sanctity of life? What does it mean to you personally?*
    b. *How does your faith or spiritual beliefs influence your understanding of the sanctity of life?*
    c. *In the context of MAiD, do you perceive any tensions or conflicts between the sanctity of life and the individual's right to choose the timing and manner of their death? If so, how do you navigate these tensions?*
4. *Take a moment to read through your responses and reflect on the insights you've gained.*
5. *Consider any potential areas of growth or further exploration in your understanding of the sanctity of life and the role of faith in relation to MAiD.*
6. *Close the exercise with a moment of gratitude or prayer, expressing appreciation for the opportunity to explore these complex topics and seeking guidance and wisdom as you continue to navigate these important considerations.*

Remember, this exercise is intended to initiate personal reflection and encourage exploration of the interplay between the sanctity of life, faith, and MAiD. It is valuable to engage in respectful dialogue and seek diverse perspectives to deepen your understanding further.

CHAPTER 24

JESUS IN THERAPY

The opposite of spiritual is not material but egotistical.

– MICHAEL POLLEN

"I'M A DEEP AND COMPLEX PERSON, FULL OF CONTRADICTIONS AND not easy to understand." My wife looked at me straight and said, "No, you're forgetful."

It would be wonderful if life made sense, let alone people, but complexity will always triumph over simplicity, so few matters maintain integrity when they are reduced. Perhaps this is why I'm drawn to Christianity, a faith intentional in embracing contradictions. It espouses a God whose power comes through weakness, whose presence comes through a whisper, who chooses the least among us to be the best example of the sacred within us. Almighty God? More like an all-vulnerable God. The lamb of God, not the lion. This is the way of love, the way of compassion, and the way around our ego's defences to pierce the heart of the matter, now elevated from what we do with our pain to what God does through our pain. This was the tension embedded in the teachings of a desert rabbi from a backwards town in the middle of nowhere we think we are familiar with.

We're going to do some spiritual psychotherapy here on someone we tend to think had it all together: Jesus. We're going to explore the deconstruction of his ego through a situation that threatened his life.

Let's start by identifying three primary instinctive needs at play in ego formation, preservation, and disintegration. These are the need for security (driven by the instinct to survive), the need for power (to have a voice in our community and our world), and the need for esteem (the desire to belong and to be loved).

It's interesting to see how Jesus addressed these subconscious needs through a powerful illustration of engagement with the deepest self: the story of the temptation in the wilderness. It starts in Matthew 3, where Jesus is baptized by his cousin, John. This Jewish ritual of cleansing and dedication is usually a matter of getting dipped and done, but it gets weird as the clouds part and God's voice proclaims, "This is my son, in whom I am well pleased!" Okay, his dad is proud, but this is about more than an overt affirmation and proclamation of God's love for him. (Which is a setup. You know what always happens in the story after a parent says you're the favourite.)

Notice that this occurred at the conscious level (they all heard the voice) through a public ritual (baptism) in the company of his friends and community (the crowd gathered around him). Jesus, at the level of ego-identity, is feeling pretty good. He has security (food, water, shelter), he has esteem (the love and adulation of the people, and even more, of God), and he has power beyond measure, which flows from this astonishing awareness of his connection to that community, to the Creator, and to creation itself.

Now comes the drama. He is *driven* into the wilderness. He doesn't wander off or go for a walk. He is consumed by a compulsion that he must go, with no clue of what will happen when he gets there. Jesus gives himself entirely to the ultimate wilderness survival experience, where these three instinctive needs will be tested. The trip commences by going into solitude – always the place where the emotional scripts and programs of our subconscious run up against the surface level of ego-identification and functioning. He knows God loves him, but that knowledge has to be embedded in the depths of his soul, and the only way to drill that deep is through hardship and challenge. Suffering becomes the crucible of faith. Like Jesus, the wilderness landscapes of our lives (loss and grief, divorce and disaster, suffering and death) challenge the core aspects of our identity. Is my inner security strong enough to sustain me? Do ability and outward circumstances determine my value in this world, or can I source it from within myself? What is my place and my role in this world if I lose my job, my partner, my family, my health, and my body?

Welcome to the wilderness, a place of spiritual revolution, not of personal retreat. It is a place of inner protest, not outward peace. It is a place of deep encounter, not of superficial escape.

We catch up with Jesus late in the ordeal, after he has been fasting in the desert for forty days (a symbolic number reflecting gestation – so deep). He's tired, he's hungry, and he should be desperate. In this vulnerable state, anyone might question how true that proclamation of God's love really is (even when it comes from the clouds above). And there, he faces engagement with his ego through the backdoor of the subconscious self. This is presented in the voice of the tempter, who begins the challenge by first questioning Jesus's sense of security. We find it in Luke 4:3–13:

> 3 The devil said to him, "If you are the Son of God, command
> this stone to become a loaf of bread." 4 Jesus answered him,
> "It is written, 'One does not live by bread alone.' "

Notice this first plays into an instinct we've all fallen for – to manipulate a situation for our benefit. Turning a stone to bread represents a refusal to accept things as they are – we will change them to get what we want, to help ourselves feel better. Here, it applies to the most basic of needs – to eat and stay alive. We can think of MAiD in the same way, but this time it hits the desire to control how we die, to remain comfortable as we go. That's even more basic than bread and water, which makes the need expressed in the request for hastened death entirely understandable and utterly human.

The response of Jesus is cryptic: "One does not live by bread alone." It means many things (these parables always do). He's quoting Deuteronomy 8:3, in which the Israelites were sustained in their wilderness (not for forty days, but forty years!) by mysterious flakes of bread called *manna* that appeared each morning.[305] This renewed their trust that God was with them, despite their hardships, and even through them. By accepting things as they are, Jesus establishes his identity and agency in God, in Source. He doesn't need to change anything external to calibrate his consciousness to comfort.

The second temptation challenges his sense of power:

> 5 Then the devil led him up and showed him in an instant all
> the kingdoms of the world. 6 And the devil said to him, "To
> you I will give their glory and all this authority; for it has been
> given over to me, and I give it to anyone I please. 7 If you, then,
> will worship me, it will all be yours." 8 Jesus answered him, "It
> is written, 'Worship the Lord your God, and serve only him.' "

This one really is ridiculous, marked by grandiosity and a gross distortion. Remember, it's not a literal story but one representing the fundamental dynamics of the ego. Here, forces of darkness promise so much more than they can deliver (always the case). Is Jesus's dignity, role, and identity in the world expressed by power over others or power with others? In other words, is he going to choose power over presence? The people expected the messiah to be a political figure who would drive out the Romans. As such a figure, Jesus must contemplate what kind of leader he would be and how he would use this divine connection. Carl Jung felt this account was Jesus voluntarily engaging with this darkness, not suppressing any aspect of it or being suppressed by it. He consciously let it act on him and assimilated it. He accepted that this was part of his darkness but chose to follow the ways of love. This is the wisest engagement with *the shadow*. Think of the film *The Matrix* in which (*spoiler alert!*) Neo defeats Agent Smith not with power but by allowing Agent Smith to assimilate

---

305 The term can be roughly translated as a question: "What is it?" Interestingly, in Melanesian and Polynesian cultures, mana is the word for the spiritual life force energy or healing power that permeates the universe. Anyone or anything can have mana. It is a cultivation or possession of energy and power, rather than being a source of power.

him, transforming that darkness from within itself. In the final film, we find Neo even allows Agent Smith to develop, grow, and evolve on his own course toward authenticity and self-actualization. The way of love and awareness does not destroy anything, strive for anything, or change anything except by incarnating full presence with all that is… including the aspects of ourselves we deem unacceptable.

This brings us to the final test: esteem. Do you really think God loves you? Why not test it? (Who hasn't done that!) Here it is in verses 9–12:

> 9 Then the devil took him to Jerusalem, and placed him on the
> pinnacle of the temple, saying to him, "If you are the Son of
> God, throw yourself down from here, 10 for it is written, 'He
> will command his angels concerning you, to protect you,' 11
> and 'On their hands, they will bear you up, so that you will
> not dash your foot against a stone.' "
>
> 12 Jesus answered him, "It is said, 'Do not put the Lord your
> God to the test.'" 13 When the devil had finished every test, he
> departed from him until an opportune time.

This last one is so relatable. We've all been there. When life starts unravelling, we may become desperate, using emotional, psychological, or physical manipulation to get our way. We have all, throughout history, doubted that love and compassion could change the world. We've all tested the love of God and others, placing ourselves in dangerous or unwise situations to see if others will rescue us.

Mindfulness is the inner wilderness in which we invite this confrontation, this temptation to occur, so that we may train ourselves in these three core truths:

1. That we are secure, even in the face of death, for we are each localized expressions of the underlying consciousness of the universe.
2. Infinite power and love flow through us, not from us. We do not need to impose it on the world.

3. That we are esteemed. We are infinitely loved, for love is the highest state of consciousness. God is love, and we flow from that.

When applied to MAiD, we find that at the ultimate moment of life, assisted dying is an act that restores our sense of control over the ultimate, our sense of power to act, and our esteem in maintaining dignity on our terms. It makes sense, then, that it brings relief to have MAiD in your back pocket. In this respect, Christianity and Buddhism align nicely, seeing the desire for control at the end of life as an exertion of ego at the moment of one's exit. Spiritual traditions offer another way: to allow these feelings, recognize their role in consciousness, and accept and process them as indicators of something far deeper: that death is a doorway to a distinctly different form of life.

Confession time (always good for the soul): It is difficult to write this as I consider the suffering of my patients. It can seem like a theological thought experiment compared to the brutal reality of dying, especially when pain cannot be well controlled. I witness souls torn between worlds: wanting to leave this one comfortably but refusing palliative sedation because it severs contact with those they love, with life, with the self. The last vestiges of identity are clinging to the thread that ties them to this realm. In that suffering, they share more with the Divine than they realize.

THE CROSS

The message of ego self-preservation is brought to a brutal climax in the story of the Passion of Christ (the word passion comes from the Latin word *passio*, meaning suffering). Here, the deconstruction of Jesus's personal identity, his community of friends, and, finally, his body opens his soul to ultimate surrender. Yes, that word, which is the opposite of control, is essential in the spiritual journey at the end of life. And, if it means anything, the story reveals that Jesus struggled with it as much (I would assert more so) than any of us.

I'm bringing this up aware that many people these days are not familiar with the story, and if they are, they may be too familiar with it, no longer feeling its significance. Yes, I'm going into the heart of the Christian faith, but please stay with me. This is not to persuade you to my religion. There's no need to "get God into you" as you arise from that reality anyway. The story has great value, and its lesson is mirrored in other faith traditions. I'm just drawing on mine as it's the one I'm most familiar with. So, let's have a look.

Jesus has been going about teaching, preaching, healing, and sharing the message that God is Love – a radical notion in such a barbarous age where might was right and mercy was nothing more than a sovereign's whim. The ultimate test of that message occurs in a grove of olive trees in Jerusalem: the garden of Gethsemane. Jesus has gone there to pray for strength, for he knows the Roman soldiers are coming to arrest him. He is in anguish, realizing fully that death is imminent. And it will be excruciating. I'm going to explore that in some detail, as anyone considering MAiD is also imagining the worst ahead: the pain, the helplessness, the anguish, on top of the disintegration of their identity in the world.

Death on a cross was designed to be prolonged torture. Since he had been to Jerusalem, Jesus had seen it just outside the city walls. His body would be nailed to the cross, spikes driven between the forearm bones at the wrist. This would sever the median nerve, which not only caused immense pain but would have paralyzed the victim's hands. (While crucifixes and movie depictions show pierced palms, the body's weight would have ripped the nails through the finger joints.) His arms would then be lashed to the crossbeam, which was raised onto the vertical beam, to which his feet would then be nailed. One dies more from asphyxiation than from blood loss – the weight of the body pulling down allows only shallow breaths to be taken. Prisoners usually passed out from the pain – a small mercy – but the story depicts Jesus remaining conscious to the end. This was an intentionally slow death, so the condemned person experienced maximum agony, and so those who watched learned never to rebel against the state.

This is likely what Jesus envisioned while sitting among the olive trees. The story depicts him alone in contemplation. He turns to pray, plead, implore, and negotiate with God for some other outcome. This was no pious kneeling with hands together, contrary to what is depicted in many paintings. The Greek text says he threw himself to the ground and begged the Almighty, "Let this cup pass from me!" He was writhing in anguish at the thought of it. He was dissolving into fear. We don't usually think of Jesus being overwhelmed, but it's critical to emphasize his humanity, especially if the story is to be relevant for those also facing death. The account from Luke 22:44 helps us do precisely that: "And being in agony, He prayed more earnestly. Then His sweat became like great drops of blood falling down to the ground." A dramatic simile… or perhaps a rare medical condition? Hematidrosis causes one's sweat glands to constrict and then dilate to the point of rupture, resulting in blood pouring into the glands. The cause of hematidrosis? Extreme anguish. The other gospels amplify this, with Jesus moaning, "My soul is overwhelmed with sorrow to the point of death."[306]

It's a powerful and poetic way of expressing the thoughts one might have when facing death from cancer, ALS, or other unbearable diseases. "I don't want to do this!" If you are a Christian in this situation, I invite you to deeply consider how close you may be to this existential nightmare. Perhaps you keep it at bay to protect your family. Perhaps you suppress it to protect yourself. But deep down, as you know how you will die, can you detect a part of you (a large part!) that wants to escape? Can we consider that even the story of Jesus in the Garden of Gethsemane provides insight into the desire for medically assisted death?

This cry reminds me of the story of a monk whose students gathered around him as he approached death. Looking at them, he asked, "Have you come to witness how an enlightened one leaves this world?"

"Yes," they answered.

As the monk kicks and thrashes, he cries aloud, "I don't want to go! I don't want to go!"

At least he had his students by his side. Jesus' disciples, on the other hand, fell asleep. Upon finding them slumbering, his heart sank and he

---

[306] Matthew 26:38; cf. Mark 14:34

didn't hold back. "Couldn't you even stay awake for a short while?" And this occurred not once, but three times! Throughout his ultimate personal struggle, he keeps checking on them only to find that they have drifted off. If compassion and the company of loved ones help us feel safe in the face of death, Jesus didn't even have that support from his friends.

It's comforting to consider, when discussing MAiD, that Jesus also asked if he could skip the torture and proceed directly to the resurrection. "Let this cup pass from me!" How relatable this makes him. How human it is for him to inquire if there's a way to die without the pain, the darkness, and the indignity. I've heard many faithful patients ask the same question and opt for the injection instead, regardless of whether they are Catholic or Protestant. Of course, the Roman Catholics knew it went against the teachings of the church, but that held little sway when faced with what they imagined awaited them. They didn't worry about being judged by God, believing the divine to be more compassionate and understanding than those who established those rules.

So here is Jesus, asking God if there is a path to the glory and vision of Easter Sunday that bypasses the pain and humiliation of Good Friday. It appears that there isn't, but it is impossible to comprehend this before one's own death. It only became clear to him afterwards.

The resurrected Christ is walking along a road and encounters his disciples, who initially do not recognize him. They recount the story of their friend – his teachings, his death, and their grief. And he rhetorically asks them, "Wasn't it necessary for the Christ to suffer in this way?" The road to death necessarily passes through pain and suffering. Kathleen Dowling Singh, among others, proposes this positively: these dark forces are naturally calibrated to move us beyond what is more superficial towards what is more profound. The process of dying is calibrated to open us to deeper dimensions of consciousness.

We know this. If we're honest with ourselves, we must admit that our most significant growth came from what challenged our ego integrity, embarrassed us, terrified us, and stripped us of dignity and control. What we like to talk about generally reinforces or inflates our ego. Dissolving the self is our final spiritual practice, but our ego-identity instinctively sets boundaries to prevent us from going there.

This is typical throughout life and exponentially more intense as we die. That's the modus operandi of suffering: it reverses the entire process that formed our identity to open us up to a reality and consciousness beyond the one we perceive as so convincingly real.

Jesus went through the same thing. As he hung on the cross, despair engulfed him, ultimately tearing at his being in connection with the Ground of Being with which he was so intimately connected throughout his life. The anguish poured from his lips, "My God, my God, why have you forsaken me?" (Luke 23:46) He was quoting from Psalm 22, a plea for deliverance from suffering and persecution. This poem pulls the tension tight between utter abandonment and the affirmation of God's providence without diminishing either. It is a profound example of how one can hold hope and hopelessness simultaneously in the heart. The authenticity of that irreconcilable wrestling leads to resignation, a complete surrendering of self. This goes far beyond accepting that one is dying. That intellectual and heartfelt recognition can bring peace, but it does not bring ecstasy. This resignation is seen in Jesus crying out, "Father, into your hands I commend my spirit." It was not a faint whisper on a dying man's last breath. The Greek word used is "megalē," meaning tremendous or fierce. It was a bellow from the depths of despair, the final release of self before resignation. He breathed his last, and the ecstasy was given. We know nothing about the inner dimensions of his being at that moment of transition. The soul's journey from here to there seems forever shrouded in mystery if it were not for a fascinating phenomenon reported by millions dying under far less violent circumstances.

EXERCISE 24: SECURITY, SELF-DETERMINATION AND DIGNITY

Find a calm and quiet space where you can reflect without interruptions. Take a few moments to settle into a comfortable position and focus on your breath.

1. *Begin by contemplating the concepts of security, self-determination, and dignity in the context of the end of life. Reflect on your own understanding and beliefs about these aspects.*
2. *Write down your thoughts and reflections on the following questions:*
   a. *Security:*
      - *What does security mean to you? How do you define it?*
      - *How has your ego-identity served you throughout your life?*
      - *Are there any fears or concerns you have about letting go of your ego, or personal identity, as you approach the end of life?*

   b. *Self-Determination:*
      - *How do you understand self-determination? What does it mean to you in the context of the end of life?*
      - *What are your desires or preferences regarding decision-making and autonomy during this phase of life?*
      - *Are there any conflicts or tensions between maintaining self-determination and embracing the natural process of transformation?*

   c. *Dignity:*
      - *How do you define dignity? What does it mean to you personally?*
      - *What factors contribute to a sense of dignity in your life?*
      - *How might the deconstruction of ego-identity impact your perception of dignity, and how can you cultivate a sense of dignity during this transition?*

3. *Take a few moments to read through your reflections and contemplate the insights you've gained.*
4. *Consider any emotions or concerns that arise as you explore these topics. Allow yourself to sit with these feelings and offer yourself compassion and understanding.*
5. *Reflect on ways to release your personal identity as a process of giving yourself to something greater, to the mystery at the end of life. Consider any shifts in perspective or adjustments that may support a sense of inner peace and acceptance.*
6. *Close the exercise with a moment of gratitude for the opportunity to reflect and explore these significant aspects of your end-of-life experience.*

Remember, this exercise is intended to support personal reflection and self-exploration. It can be helpful to share your insights and reflections with a trusted loved one, spiritual guide, or healthcare provider who can provide support and guidance. Additionally, consider seeking additional resources or professional assistance to further explore and navigate the complexities of ego-identity, self-determination, and dignity during the end-of-life journey.

Chapter 25

NEARING-DEATH AWARENESS

I regard consciousness as fundamental.
I regard matter as a derivative of consciousness.
– Max Planck

Anne was dead when I entered the room. The air was infused with a density that slowed time. I sensed the stillness of her body right away, as if some primal instinct, accustomed to the breath of another, was immediately alerted by its absence. A soft and gentle smile was upon her lips, and she looked radiantly beautiful.

Harry sat at her side, holding her hand. He looked up, nodded, and quietly motioned for me to enter. Then I noticed Tina, Anne's nurse, sitting on the other side of the bed. She was holding Anne's other hand, who had clearly left this world in the presence of deep love and good care. I took my place behind Harry, by the open window. A few minutes passed before he spoke, and what he said was astonishing. "I never expected at this moment to feel so overwhelmed with such love and gratitude." His tears softly flowed down his face. "If there is such a thing as a good death, then this is it!"

She had passed not five minutes ago, and the story Harry shared lives on in me as an example of how astonishing and sacred death can be when managed well. It began, as most love stories do, with how they met, how they loved, and how they lost.

This was an exceptional couple. Together for 33 years, they had travelled the world and raised a son. Lyell was an old soul, for, at the age of 20, after completing two years studying art, he wanted to expand his horizons and ventured to exotic lands, ending in an Indian ashram to study meditation. Then tragedy struck – one day, he came home from the ashram, washed a shirt, and flung it over the balcony to dry. It blew up against a high-tension wire, and he was electrocuted.

Devastated, Harry and Anne rushed to the end of the world to sit with their son on the edge of life. There he lay for two weeks in the ICU, suspended over the abyss. It felt like forever until the doctors shared the words parents long for in these situations: vitals were improving. Lyell seemed to be recovering.

How fragile hope feels when so much rests on such few words. It's as if one's entire world could disintegrate like a dream, which is what came to Harry in the dark hours before the final dawn. It was a vivid apparition – Lyell in his hospital bed, propped up by pillows, facing his father. Lyell didn't say anything, but a man's voice resonated within Harry's being: "He wants to give you his life." Immediately, electricity shot out of Lyell's shoulders into Harry's feet. It felt like a wonderful, gentle, warm energy bubbling up his legs, through his body, all the way to the top of his head. How strange. Then morning came, and the doctors summoned Anne and Harry to share that Lyell had passed sometime during the night.

Grief is strange. It undulates through the currents of life, sometimes swamping you in great waves, other times carrying you gently to your tomorrows. Harry confided that it often felt like Lyell helped them with this, sometimes in the most amusing ways. For example, six months after he passed, a lone duck landed in their backyard. It felt strange; they had never had ducks on their property before. It would waddle up the driveway and stand at the bottom of their steps as if waiting for food to be offered from this puzzled couple. It would fly away for the summer and autumn, only to return every day from November to May, for years on end. The coincidence was that Anne's term of endearment for Lyell was "Little Duck"!

In the last days, Anne descended to the unconscious depths, where the water is still and dense and dark. But Harry was confident she felt no fear, for they were familiar with this stillness, having practiced meditation together since Lyell's death. This continued as she died, with each morning marked by contemplative practice. And on this, the last day, while Harry was holding Anne's hand in meditation, she suddenly squeezed his, and her lips moved with the word "goodbye." Then she smiled and stopped breathing. He was confident that what she saw was Lyell. And he knew that, as much as her body suffered, as much as their hearts broke at the idea of her death, as much as they shared a long and loving relationship, he somehow knew that all was well. That she was well. That she was transformed and no longer inhabited that lovely shell lying there before us.

For philosophical materialism, this simply should not be. The prevailing model of reality in the Western world, materialism is a perspective summed up in the phrase, "what you see is what you get." It asserts that the mind arises from the brain's activity – consciousness is a side-effect, an illusion, an epiphenomenon of the neural activity from the three pounds of fat between your ears. The mind, in this model, does not continue to exist after the brain shuts off. We come to the final breath of life and call it a dead end, yet what we see in "real" life is utterly different – an awakening to wonder. And it begins weeks before you go.

Dr. Christopher Kerr, a palliative physician at Hospice & Palliative Care Buffalo in New York, found that over 80 percent of his dying patients experienced end-of-life dreams and visions in which they perceived their welcoming party, shifted to transpersonal states of consciousness, were apprehended by a mystical wonder and love that felt utterly safe. These are described as more real than any experience they had had in life.[307]

Dr. Kerr is cautious not to imply any paranormal framework of spiritual meaning to these phenomena, but, instead, presents them without

[307] Nosek, Cheryl L., et al. "End-of-life dreams and visions: a qualitative perspective from hospice patients." *American Journal of Hospice and Palliative Medicine* 32.3 (2015): 269–274.

interpretation. His main concern, and indeed the primary concern of the patient and family, is in their lived effect here and now as the person dies. That effect is an unexpected grace, elimination of death anxiety, greater sense of gratitude and purpose, reconciliation and forgiveness, and great expectation of whatever awaits after the last breath.

Other researchers are more adventurous in their speculations. Dr. Kenneth Ring, researcher and world expert on near-death experiences, confirms this is very common. He shares the story of Susan, a forty-four-year-old woman who died of breast cancer. Being a worrier made her treatment an even rockier road, so when cancer worsened, she sank into depression, hanging on to her family, crying and sobbing, "I don't want to die." Her existential suffering surpassed even her physical pain until the remarkable happened. She said she had seen and talked with her uncle, who was dead, and also a friend who had died of breast cancer. She told her family that her deceased uncle and friend were "waiting for her" and that she was ready to die. Her entire persona changed as if a huge weight had been removed. Suddenly, impossibly, she was not afraid. Sharing this with others helped them not be scared and opened up healing conversations that were so needed in her family. She died healed in the deepest dimensions of her being, confident that she was part of a greater mystery.[308]

It seems fantastic. Something out of a movie, the stuff of fantasy or foolishness. Surely not compatible with the rational mind. How can so many around us glimpse the other side but don't talk about it? How can nearing-death awareness be reported by most people who are conscious as they die, yet we hear nothing of this from nurses and doctors?[309] If this is going on, what does it say of the mystical and, frankly, "out there" stuff like psychic phenomena, mediumship, and after-death communication? Are these universal? Well, a study by the Institute of Noetic Sciences

---

[308] Horacek, Bruce J. "Amazing grace: The healing effects of near-death experiences on those dying and grieving." *Journal of Near-Death Studies* 16.2 (1997): 149–161.

[309] Mazzarino-Willett, A. "Deathbed Phenomena: Its role in peaceful death and terminal restlessness." *American Journal of Hospice and Palliative Medicine*, 27(2) (2010): 127–133.

indicates they are. It found that over 90 percent of people, including scientists and engineers, reported exceptional experiences that transcend the everyday boundaries of space and time, such as perceiving someone's thoughts from a distance.[310] If we do, indeed, arise from the spiritual realm, then it makes sense that everyone, at some point, would experience something that defies the physical laws that govern this material plane; that spiritual phenomena would be universal. So why don't we talk about it? You know why. People will think you're weird, unprofessional, or worse. This is the stuff your eccentric aunt talks about, the stuff of psychics and mediums and charlatans. For many medical professionals and scientists, seriously proposing consciousness continues after death risks undermining their credibility.

In addition, the phenomenon is often so fleeting that it leaves one wondering, "did that really happen?" This defies rational explanation; it shatters the boundaries of everyday life. It creates not only cognitive but existential dissonance. We try to make sense of it, but it is beyond the ego's capabilities to integrate. However, it is not beyond the heart's wisdom or the soul's longing to gasp as one is grasped by that realm. This is captured well in the words of one of the greatest scientists, Erwin Schrödinger:

> It is relatively easy to sweep away the whole of metaphysics, as Kant did. The slightest puff in its direction blows it away, and what was needed was not so much a powerful pair of lungs to provide the blast as a powerful dose of courage to turn it against so timelessly venerable a house of cards. But you must not think that what has then been achieved is the actual elimination of metaphysics from the empirical content of human knowledge. In fact, if we cut out all metaphysics it will be found to be vastly more difficult, indeed probably quite impossible, to give any intelligible account of even the most circumscribed area of specialization within

[310] Wahbeh, H., et al. (2018). "Exceptional experiences reported by scientists and engineers." *Explore,* 14(5) (2018): 329–341.

> any specialized science you please. Metaphysics includes, amongst other things… the unquestioning acceptance of a more-than-physical – that is, transcendental – significance in a large number of thin sheets of wood-pulp covered with black marks such as are now before you… A real elimination of metaphysics means taking the soul out of both art and science, turning them into skeletons incapable of any further development.[311]

Schrödinger is saying that the sublime spiritual reality underlying ours is beyond rational understanding yet is fundamental to our existence and the experience of anything genuinely significant. I appreciate this may be upsetting or offensive to those who hold fast to a material framework of reality or reject any notions of spirituality. As we explore this, I want you to consider the real question: not "Is there a God?" but "What is consciousness?"

Exploring this is critical when considering the spiritual dimensions of medically assisted death. I am not asserting in any way that euthanasia compromises one's state of being in the afterlife, even though several religious traditions warn against it, both for the one leaving and for the one who assists death. I do assert, though, that MAiD prevents loved ones and caregivers from witnessing that final transcendent state. Even more significantly, MAiD prevents patients from experiencing it while still with those they love. As that state of being eliminates the fear of death and dying by dissolving ego-identity, it integrates all aspects of the unconscious self. It heals the existential distress driving the request for MAiD. It places one in a state of pure openness to the true nature of reality. Most of all, it calibrates one to Spirit, to the highest form of consciousness. It tunes one to love.

All the world's spiritual traditions point to this: that dying is the process by which we experience natural liberation from the state of separation that is so convincing to our world. We move from a dualistic state,

---

[311] Schrödinger, Erwin. Translated From the German by Cecily Hastings *My View of the World*. Cambridge at the University Press, 1963.

in which "I" am separate from "you" and everything around us, to non-dual awareness, in which there is only consciousness. All wisdom traditions state that the purpose of physical life is to awaken to one's essential nature, an expression of this mysterious Oneness. Plutarch, the Greek philosopher who was a priest at the Temple of Apollo in Delphi, put it this way: "At the moment of death, the soul experiences the same impressions and passes through the same processes as are experienced by those who are initiated into the Great Mysteries."[312]

What of the person who dies by MAiD? I can only trust and hope that the grace of the Ground of Being is more than enough to receive the dying patient and the one who causes death with utmost compassion and understanding when their day comes. I also feel that what happens to a person after death is beyond my scope of practice. Yes, I'm clergy, a chaplain, and a near-death experiencer, but all that does is help me acknowledge when to hand off those ultimate affairs to the team on the other side. It does not give me the authority to judge what happens when anyone gets there. And I'm confident those celestial entities are very good at what they do! I do feel, though, that a moral weight is left on us who remain to transform our understanding of death, to heal our fear of mortality, and to coordinate our compassion in the health care system. After all, that's why I wrote this book.

Nearing-death awareness is an enigmatic yet extraordinary phenomenon in which a person seems to drift from this reality to another and back with relative ease. Their attempts to share the wonders of these experiences are often obstructed by our lack of understanding of their symbolic language. For example, speaking of having to get a suitcase, catch a train, and have a sense of urgency about it. Often they are surprised and filled with joy to perceive the spirit of a loved one who died or even a gathering of several souls, human and angelic alike. They may reach out, or up, to unseen forms. Their expression during this is astonishing, with eyes wide, even

[312] These were the Eleusinian Mysteries, secrets enacted through ritual traditions for over 1,000 years. These insights on the fundamental nature of the human soul, indeed of reality itself, are what you and I are let in on through the dying process. Singh, Kirpal. *Mystery of Death*. Ruhani Satsang, 1975.

with strength returning to limbs long left flaccid and drained by disease. Unlike hallucinations, however, the patient can comprehend our reality concurrently with the other. They are not confused. They are not distressed. They are at peace, cryptically coherent, even rapturous with wonder. I've seen this myself, with the patient looking at me, looking to the unseen presence, pleasantly perplexed as to why I could not perceive them. Also, unlike hallucinations, these experiences do not fade. They remain vivid, a living memory that dispels the fear of death, replacing it with anticipation and confidence. And no wonder, as the dying describe heavenly realms, and often know the day or hour they will die. Such was the case with my father, who even called his landlord to say he would not renew his lease, as he would be dead the following week! This can be upsetting or confusing for family, then, as it occurs, it is astonishing and, in hindsight, comforting. Their grief flows far smoother in the process.

The dying person often exercises a strange power and clings to life, even when their body is frail, waiting for a particular person to arrive or leave. What a surprise it is to realize that death may be more within our control than we ever imagined, without the need to exit before the body naturally shuts off. This wisdom cannot be accessed directly. It cannot be planned, but is instead intuitively activated with sublime timing. Maggie Callanan, author of *Final Gifts: Understanding the Special Awareness, Needs, and Communication of the Dying,* states she was shocked to discover that dying is in our control more than we could ever expect it to be. "When I started at hospice, because I came from critical care where we were in charge of everything, suddenly, patients are behaving in a way that said, 'I'm doing this my way.' And as long as we keep them physically comfortable, which hospice and palliative care do better than anybody else in the world, as long as we keep them comfortable and peaceful, they can show us their strength and choose the moment. It's pretty powerful!"[313]

[313] "Final Gifts | On Call with the Prairie Doc." YouTube video. Uploaded August 30, 2018 by the Prairie Doc. https://www.youtube.com/watch?v=4b-YAGZICFQ. Accessed January 17, 2022.

In *Final Gifts*, she relates the story of Jose. "He was a forty-five-year-old man dying of kidney failure, a complication of unmanaged diabetes. When I visited Jose to admit him to palliative care, he asked me if I could find his tuxedo and get him dressed. His family told me, 'Don't worry about that. He's been asking us to do that all day. He's just confused.'

"I asked Jose what he needed his tuxedo for. 'Are you planning to go somewhere special, Jose?'

"Jose replied, 'Yes, I need my tuxedo on. It's time to go and I want to look my best. My bags are packed, and I just need my tuxedo.' "

Several hours later, Jose died. He was preparing for his "journey" toward death and wanted to look his best. What his family thought was confusion turned out to be something much more special.

For many years, there have even been reports of patients with severe end-stage dementia experiencing an unexpected return of mental clarity for a short period, especially near the end of life. People who have been unable to recognize loved ones or recall memories from their past for many months or years may suddenly and unexpectedly regain mental clarity. This includes speaking complete sentences, appropriately responding to questions, recovering physical movement, recognizing family members, and even describing seeing deceased loved ones. Your welcoming party awaits.

TRANSCENDENCE

ANNE, WHO SAW HER DECEASED SON AT THE FOOT OF HER BED THE NIGHT before she died, had achieved a state of consciousness often referred to as transcendence, rising above self and connecting to a greater reality. It's critical to note that she didn't achieve this state herself, but rather it came upon her or emerged from her when her construct of self and attachments to this world were sufficiently dismantled by suffering. Not only was she filled with peace, but she also had foreknowledge of her impending death and a state of expanded consciousness through which she could perceive the spirit of her deceased son. Transcendence is not something we achieve through our own efforts, but rather a state of being that naturally resides at our core, but one that is often covered by the layers of ego construction that begin at birth, as explored in Chapter 5.

This natural and final state of consciousness represents a developmental stage marked by a deep sense of purpose, vulnerability, well-being, and an acceptance of the reality of what is. It correlates with movement into the causal state of awakening in integral theory. Here, we are able to engage with and consolidate the deepest dimensions of the self, which encompass our fears and our shadow.

If you are considering MAiD, ask yourself what lies beneath the statements about dignity or the "right to die without suffering." What scares you most about dying? What do you imagine it will be like to lie there, unable to speak, unable to move… descending while your family sits at your side, descending while you are alone in the room, vitality and volition evaporating with the days of waiting for it to happen. One must take serious time to explore this. We do it best through contemplation, opening to the darkness of our imagination, staying with our need for control and avoidance of suffering, and then going beneath it through stillness, waiting, not-knowing, and ambiguity… by becoming lost to ourselves so that we may be found. Transcendence requires that we get out of our own way.

Such is the insight of several thought leaders in nursing, psychology, and palliative care. Among them are Dr. Martha Rogers, whose theory is known as the Science of Unitary Human Beings, and Dr. Pamela Reed, whose theory is of self-transcendence. Reed described transcendence well, as an "expansion of self-conceptual boundaries multidimensionally: inwardly (e.g., through introspective experiences), outwardly (e.g., by reaching out to others), and temporally (whereby past and future are integrated into the present)." She later added another type: transpersonal expansion, in which the individual connects "with dimensions beyond the typically discernible world."[314] She even asserted that this state is a developmental imperative; it is the completion of the human experience, the ultimate fulfilment and final realization of who we are in the world and

[314] Reed, Pamela G., and Nelma B. Crawford Shearer. *Nursing Knowledge and Theory Innovation: Advancing the Science of Practice*. Springer Publishing Company, 2017.

what we are in reality itself. This is not possible with MAiD. Yes, the person may feel at peace, may feel grateful, may feel love and that they are loved. They certainly feel relief. But this is from the all-too-human aspects of our need to feel safe, out of danger. It is still embedded in the ego. That may be enough for many, but compared to ultimate fulfillment, "enough" falls far short of what we would experience through natural death just before leaving this realm.

There is nothing, of course, to prevent us from thinking that the transcendent state waits for everyone, no matter how we die. We are, after all, talking about the ultimate mystery: the nature of consciousness. I would assert that it is precisely because it is the final mystery that we do our best to trust its natural process, and I'm emphasizing again that the moral weight of MAiD remains here with us on this side of the grass. We have created a situation that, for an increasing number, is too attractive for the ego. When it comes to our final transformation, MAiD is the epitome of our culture's spiritual poverty.

Transcendent experiences have been referred to as peak experiences, clear light, objective consciousness, and many other names. Religious traditions equate them with an infilling or being apprehended by God's spirit, while non-religious people tend to feel it as unity with the world around them. Transcendence is also accessed through various forms of meditation and, of course, psychedelics.

Dr. Paul Wong, a clinical psychologist who has written extensively on death acceptance, emphasizes that this existential orientation animates compassion, moral excellence, resilience, and eudaemonic happiness (that is, well-being as a process of realizing one's true nature). This is a radical shift from self-focus to meaning-focus as the most promising way to lift individuals from the dark pit of despair to a higher ground of flourishing.[315]

This has great significance when exploring the existential distress driving most MAiD requests. If only it could come upon us earlier in the

---

[315] Wong, Paul TP. "Viktor Frankl's Meaning-Seeking Model and Positive Psychology." In A. Batthyany & P. Russo-Netzer (Eds.), *Meaning in Positive and Existential Psychology*. Springer, New York, NY, 2014, pp. 149–184.

dying process! If only it could come upon us at all throughout life. But the sad reality is that this is a state the vast majority of modern people never reach in their ordinary days. Their level of self-awareness remains very low. People, for the most part, are driven by their thoughts and feelings, convinced by their attachments and perceptions, confusing them with objective reality. As a result, terminal illness tends to make us regress psychologically and emotionally; the need for survival, safety, belonging, and esteem becomes paramount. That's exactly the formula fed by the rhetoric of dignity, autonomy, and self-determination over the dying process. We are back at the temptation of Christ, an archetype for the pivotal point at which we must decide to bow to the ego's demands for self-preservation or rise to a new level of our humanity: transcendence. Fortunately, amazingly, this is the one stage that, if we hang on through the wilderness, comes upon us as part of the natural process of dying, and is marked by an ease and opening to all that is best summed up in the word "grace."

A remarkable quality in this state is the absence of any concern for the future, including concern for how death will feel when it comes. There is no fear, no anxiety, only this moment, this connection, this awareness. There is also an understanding that goes beyond traditional forms of knowledge. It can only be imparted through the language of music and mystics, poets and seers. This certainly reaches fulfillment in nearing-death awareness, wherein the final expansion of consciousness before death is into something wholly other, something fundamental to reality itself. I know from speaking with hundreds who've had a near-death experience and say it is the most meaningful experience of their lives. What a contrast to those who request MAiD.

It's such a paradox. How could this flourishing of consciousness even be possible when you're withering away? How could it be possible that the state we most desire at the end of life – to feel safe, to feel loved, not to be afraid, to not add to our suffering through our anticipation of it, to have more than comfort, but dignity – how could it be possible that all this is already within us? Well, we are human creatures, afraid and unfamiliar with dying. We want to feel safe, especially as we leave. And I appreciate that so many receiving MAiD are deeply loving and deeply loved, but what we are exploring is not a human level of love. It is transcendent. In the Christian tradition, it's called *agape*, one of four types of love. The others are *philia*, or friendship; *eros*, sensual or romantic love; and *storge*, or familial love. Agape is an unconditional love that transforms the very nature of your being. It is divine love. These nuances are even more diverse in the Sanskrit language, which has ninety-six words for love. Persian has eighty. English, only one. Odd, considering it is the most powerful and significant emotion and state of being we are capable of.

Here is hope. We all have the wisdom and ability to experience this state of being. It requires acceptance of what is, of not knowing how death will feel, of opening and giving oneself fully to its wisdom within us, not to our control over it. This vulnerability is marked by astonishing stability as if we have been apprehended by grace. Indeed, that's precisely what happens. I want to assure you that a gentle wonder guides our days, a delightful deep in which we are held by love, from which we emanate in joy – the wisdom beneath dances with astonishing dexterity. There is something approaching that sustains us, that gives us breath even as ours fades from this world. Our surrender to it yields nothing less than awakening. The ride is wild and perfectly safe.

EXERCISE 25: EXPLORING THE MYSTERY

FIND A QUIET AND COMFORTABLE SPACE WHERE YOU CAN REFLECT WITHout interruptions. Take a few moments to centre yourself and create a calm atmosphere.

1. *Take a few deep breaths to relax your body and bring your focus to the present moment.*
2. *Reflect on the concept of nearing-death awareness, which refers to the potential for heightened awareness and extraordinary experiences as one approaches the end of life. Consider that these experiences may include visions, encounters, spiritual insights, or a sense of peace and acceptance.*
3. *Write down your thoughts and reflections on the following questions:*
    a. *Have you had any personal experiences or observations related to nearing-death awareness? If so, describe them briefly. If not, what are your thoughts or beliefs about this phenomenon?*
    b. *How do you feel about the possibility of experiencing or encountering something extraordinary as you approach the end of your life? Are there any hopes, fears, or uncertainties that arise for you?*
    c. *Reflecting on your spiritual or existential beliefs, how might nearing-death awareness align with or challenge your current understanding of life, death, and the nature of consciousness?*
    d. *If you were to encounter or experience nearing-death awareness, what impact do you think it might have on your sense of meaning, purpose, or preparation for the end of life?*
4. *Take a few moments to read through your reflections and contemplate the insights and emotions that arise.*
5. *Consider sharing your thoughts and reflections with a trusted loved one, spiritual guide, or healthcare provider who can provide support*

and guidance. Engaging in open and respectful conversations can deepen your exploration of this phenomenon.

6. *Close the exercise with a moment of gratitude for the opportunity to reflect and explore the potential for extraordinary experiences as you approach the end of life. Embrace a sense of openness and curiosity about the mysteries that may unfold.*

Remember, this exercise is intended to support personal reflection and exploration of the concept of nearing-death awareness. It is important to approach this topic with an open mind, allowing space for personal beliefs and experiences to shape your understanding. Seek support from others who can provide guidance and a safe space for discussing these profound aspects of the end-of-life journey.

CHAPTER 26

NEAR-DEATH EXPERIENCES

Consciousness cannot be accounted for in physical terms,
for consciousness is absolutely fundamental.
It cannot be accounted for in terms of anything else.
– ERWIN SCHRÖDINGER

HE SPOKE WITH MEASURED WORDS, AS IF INCREMENTALLY ASSESSING my acceptance of his story. He described himself as an agnostic, a businessman, a pragmatic person with no comfort for the private matters of people's hearts. He was to be discharged the next day, yet for some reason requested a chaplain to drop by. The nurse stated he was healthy and that his operation went well. His account, though, indicated otherwise. Something significant had happened.

He lay in bed with his wife at his side. She was holding his hand, with that expression that tells you she's pouring in her love, that she's so grateful to have him awake and well. The formalities of introductions and arranging space for the chaplain to sit felt like too much fussing, but that's part of the encounter. I was glad they couldn't offer me a cup of tea.

"I want to talk about something personal," he said. Clearly, this would be unfamiliar territory for him. I wondered if his wife had suggested he speak with me. She was leaning forward slightly, stroking his hand in encouragement. I remained quiet to allow him space to find his words. "I had the strangest experience, or dream, or something. But it felt so real, so calm… I don't know what to make of it. I came in because of a bowel obstruction… needed a section cut out. Cancer. I'm glad they could do something about it, and that I don't have a bag stuck in my side. So, I recall being put to sleep, and then, at some point, I was above my body. I could see my body, and the operating room and, the surgeon, the nurses. I know that was me on the table, but didn't really care. I felt so calm."

I nodded, said, "Yes." My expression and body language demonstrated safety and acceptance while my heart and mind leapt in anticipation of what would come next. I'm privileged to hear of these accounts frequently, each time a glimpse into the ultimate mystery.

"I wasn't afraid. I wasn't excited. I was just… calm. And happy. Really happy! It felt perfectly natural. And then there was this light, this place… beautiful. I was in the presence of this love. Not like I can describe, but this love, this place was so natural, like a mountain meadow, like I was in nature and it was full of life, but I was the only one there, in this Presence. I think it was God. But it didn't feel religious, it didn't feel anything but perfectly natural. I was so calm and happy."

I nodded my head. "Sounds like you had a near-death experience. A mystical shift in consciousness. Sounds wonderful!"

"Yes, I've heard of those! That's it! But I thought it would feel extraordinary. Mine felt ordinary… I mean, like it's the most natural thing in the world. I don't know how long I was there. It's not like it felt like a long time. There was no time. There was just this… being there. And the voice, the message… not like we're talking now, but a knowing. It was so clear. Absolute love. I understood. Everything. It all made sense. And then I was told I had to come back. Now, none of this makes sense." He looked at his wife, lowered his voice as his eyes got teary. "Is it wrong for me not to want to be here? I love you, I love you, Mary, I'm not saying I don't want to be with you. But this all feels… so much less…" His words were whispered. I could almost feel the sharp lump in his throat. "Was it real?"

I nodded, sat forward, and shared what always seems astonishing to people when they don't work in the trenches of mortality – that these are common. One in ten who have a brush with death, and one in five who have a cardiac episode, report these mystical shifts in consciousness.[316, 317] Perhaps the only thing more amazing than that they occur is that they occur with such frequency!

Zach Bush, an intensive-care unit and emergency room doctor, reports that one night, he and his team brought back three people from death. All reported near-death experiences, all resented being pulled back, for all stated they had never felt so loved and accepted as when they died. They let go of the ideas of who they thought they were and awakened to what they were. Waking back in this world left them angry, but oddly enlightened. His insight into this experience is profound. "They all said they felt completely accepted for the first time in their life. So, I think we're all walking around lonely as hell. This is our opportunity to rebirth, because death is not an endpoint; it's a transformation moment. It's an expansion beyond the limits of this frail, biological shell that we carry around. And the instant we step out of that, we find out the universe embraces us in every single second of our existence… We are enough, in and of our own identity of 'I am' at every second of every point of our existence."[318] Here is that intrinsic dignity we all crave, we all have, and that we all will awaken to. Unfortunately, it often takes death to make that happen.

Normalizing this ultimate event is the best first move in supporting its integration. Otherwise, one is left in an existential dissonance that never fades. The incongruity of living in the mess of this world compared to the complete awakening in the "other" can result in higher addiction, depression, and a restless search for completion. The orphaned heart is looking for its home.

---

[316] Tucker, Reed. "5% have had a near-death experience – and they say it made life worth living." *New York Post* (Feb. 20, 2021). https://nypost.com/article/five-percent-have-had-near-death-experiences-research/. Accessed Nov. 13, 2022.

[317] Henderson, Jennifer. "One in Five May Recall Near-Death Experience After CPR." *MedPage Today* (Nov. 11, 2022). Accessed Nov. 13, 2022.

[318] "Best Monologue EVER: Zach Bush, MD | Rich Roll Podcast." YouTube video. Uploaded by Rich Roll Jan. 9, 2019. www.youtube.com/watch?v=aLaVutWXju0. Accessed Dec. 21, 2022.

So, what's a near-death experience like? Most commonly, there is an initial out-of-body experience in which the person perceives themselves floating above their body. Some go through the now cliché dark tunnel and encounter a divine light or celestial beings. As with nearing-death awareness, often there is a reunion with loved ones who have died. Sometimes, information about one's life is imparted, then they return to the body.

The event is so profound that it often alters the experiencer's life, transforming priorities and values, eliminating the fear of death, and strengthening belief in the afterlife.[319] These have been reported throughout history in all cultures and demographics. They are independent of faith, universal in their manifestation but particular in their details; everyone moves to the expanded state of consciousness in a reality more real than this material plane, but how this manifests will be specific to the individual's culture, language, and life story.[320] All is contextualized according to one's cognitive and existential framework. Hence, as you drill down to specific cases, the details become more diverse, from species to culture to family and, finally, one's individual story. There is great hope here, as near-death experiences help us consider that the experience of death is far different from the appearance of death.

My own near-death experience was the result of my second tumour. I was conducting a Sunday service in a hospital chapel when it kicked in – public speaking is an anxiety-provoking experience, and this is no less true for clergy. I was a student at the time, still finding my legs. Well, they gave out immediately when the paraganglioma released hundreds of times the usual dose of powerful hormones (catecholamines, including norepinephrine) directly into my femoral artery. I passed out before my head hit the floor.

---

[319] "Near-Death Experiences (NDEs)." University of Virginia Division of Perceptual Studies (Feb. 24, 2023). med.virginia.edu/perceptual-studies/our-research/near-death-experiences-ndes. Accessed Apr. 1, 2023.

[320] "Near-Death Experience and the Origins of Afterlife Beliefs" with Gregory Shushan. YouTube video. Uploaded by the IanRamseyCentre. Nov. 19, 2012. www.youtube.com/watch?v=QVeoV14J2dY. Accessed Apr. 1, 2023.

Suddenly, effortlessly, I was in another realm that sounds so simple when I describe it, yet was utterly extraordinary: a grassy hill, a tree at the top, an expanse of sky. The light was not shining upon everything; it was streaming from within everything. And I was one with that light infused with love itself. Everything about me was recognizable: the grass, the clouds, my body. And yet it was so much more real than anything I've experienced here. Most significant for me was my state of being, my consciousness. There was no aspect of myself that was suppressed or that I was blind to – no ego, no persona or subconscious, no shadow, no critical or scattered thoughts. I was congruent, integrated, completely authentic, and completely present. No past, no future, only the Now. It was a realm saturated with the sacred and grounded in joy, as was the entity that greeted me.

"It's good to see you, David. Welcome!" He seemed to be someone who had known me all my life and who I had always known. His character was the embodiment of peace and love, compassion and power, wisdom and clarity. Despite his remarkable character, I remember him being so casual and relaxed, just like a best friend. Our conversation was straightforward and reassuring. He told me that my life was going well, but there was still much work for me to do. How did I react to this? I simply shrugged it off and challenged him to run with me to the tree. Every part of me longed to reach the top of that hill and see what was on the other side. I was fully aware that once I did, there would be no returning to this place. However, my legs refused to comply with my desire. Something about his presence held me captive. There was an undeniable authority and power that I couldn't ignore or treat casually. I had to listen and let his words sink in: I could not stay. Naturally, I protested. Why would I leave this joy? Why would I go back to the physical world, which felt like a mere shadow compared to where I currently resided? But there was no room for debate. He placed his hand on my shoulder, filled me with peace, and said, "We'll be with you. See you later."

To describe this is to reduce the experience drastically. Words are simply inadequate, even woefully insufficient, in capturing the essence of it all. All I can say is that the memory still lives within me to this day and leaves me secretly homesick for what I saw. It has forever transformed my understanding of God, faith, heaven, and reality itself. I can't help but wonder what the experience is like for those who choose MAiD. Unfortunately, the only comparison we have are the experiences of those who take their own lives in a very different manner.

SUICIDE

My experience was undeniably positive and uplifting. You might assume that those who have a near-death experience as a result of a suicide attempt would have a contrasting experience – one marked by torment, darkness... or worse. However, the data may surprise you. (I want to make it clear that I recognize people who attempt suicide are not in the same existential state as those who choose MAiD. The only similarity is the desire to escape – one to escape an unbearable life and the other to escape an unbearable death.)

Dr. Bruce Greyson, professor emeritus of psychiatry and neurobehavioral sciences at the University of Virginia, is one of the world's leading researchers on near-death experiences. In his analysis of the phenomena among those who attempted suicide, he found no correlation between the incidence or type of near-death experience and those who had a near-death experience from other causes of death.[321] Nancy Evans Bush, perhaps the leading authority on distressing near-death experiences, also reminds us that no evidence shows a correlation between a person's character or means of dying and the nature of their near-death experience.[322]

This echoes the work of Drs. Kenneth Ring and Stephen Franklin, who found that among thirty cases of attempted suicide, the incidence

---

[321] Greyson, Bruce. "Near-death experiences and attempted suicide." *Suicide and Life-Threatening Behavior* 11.1 (1981): pp. 10–16.

[322] Bush, Nancy Evans, and Bruce Greyson. "Distressing Near-Death Experiences: The Basics." *Missouri Medicine* 111.6 (2014): p. 486. https://med.virginia.edu/perceptual-studies/wp-content/uploads/sites/360/2017/01/NDE-78-Distressing-NDEs-the-basics-2014.NDE-MoMed.pdf. Accessed April 3, 2022.

and type of near-death experience recall were not significantly different from that among victims of illness or accidents. However, their experiences tended to be of shorter duration and did not include a reunion with deceased loved ones or realms of incredible beauty.[323]

Though the research on this is still minimal, generally, the desire for suicide disappeared as a result of their near-death experience. Not only was there no more fear of death, but there was also no more fear of living. Many returned feeling that if they had a pulse, they had a purpose.[324] That's significant, but even more so was the deep sense that all moments have perfect timing – a profoundly difficult concept for us to grasp when we see the world's suffering.

Suicide accounts are, of course, even more emotionally laden than "standard" near-death experience stories, and this is where we can observe one difference. Researchers found that the existential states that drove people to attempt to take their life often became the homework they were confronted with on the other side. They were told they could not die in that way, as it was not their time. This is not a reprimand, but the message is delivered with both immense compassion and authority. Based on the limited research available, we cannot draw any further correlation between the type of near-death experience and the means of death. However, all researchers did find that, whether a near-death experience was incredibly positive or distressing, there was a strongly anti-suicide orientation among those reporting them.[325]

Most individuals receiving MAiD are not as distressed or clinically depressed as with suicide cases. Distress certainly drives them to request MAiD, but, once approved, they are far *less* distressed, thanks to knowing how they will die and that it will be handled by a professional. This may correlate with the calm sometimes experienced by people as they

---

[323] Ring, Kenneth, and Stephen Franklin. "Do suicide survivors report near-death experiences?" *OMEGA-Journal of Death and Dying* 12.3 (1982): pp. 191–208.

[324] Taylor, Steve. "The confrontation with death and the renewal of life." *Suicide and Life-Threatening Behavior* 8.2 (1978): pp. 89–98.

[325] Greyson, Bruce. "Near-death experiences and attempted suicide." Suicide and Life-Threatening Behavior 11, no. 1 (1981): 10-16.

consider suicide,[326] especially as MAiD is institutionally condoned by the government, the health care system, and the public, to an extent greater than suicide. The frame of mind of those dying by MAiD appears to be no worse, and often better, than those who die naturally under good nursing care, with the exception of two significant factors that remain unexplored by MAiD assessors, the doctors performing the procedure, the families, and the patients.

First is a state called cognitive constriction. This is an inability to engage in "meaningful thought." Cognitive constriction is characterized by black-and-white thinking – seeing things as all or nothing, good or bad, one way or the other. In other words, it's like tunnel vision. According to Dr. Christine Moutier of the American Foundation for Suicide Prevention, certain areas of the brain's functioning change when a person is seriously considering suicide. Their ability to imagine or consider multiple solutions to solving the problem of their despair is drastically diminished, resulting in a limited range of coping options.[327] We all know that it's difficult enough to think clearly when one is stressed. That becomes exponentially more challenging as cognitive constriction takes hold.[328] Alternate ways of thinking can become inaccessible as the person can only perceive their current circumstances and feel that their pain will never dissipate. So, stresses we normally would bend to, we break to.

It begins with ruminative thinking, builds through brooding, and results in hopelessness to fix or escape the situation – which is not death in this case, but the experience of dying. That's a significant distinction, and one remedied by the process of surrender explored earlier. However, I propose that the person choosing MAiD can no longer consider that because society has failed in its responsibility to cultivate spiritual intelligence

---

[326] Crane, Catherine, et al. "Comfort from suicidal cognition in recurrently depressed patients." *Journal of Affective Disorders* 155 (2014): pp. 241–246.

[327] Murray, R. "What Is It Like to Survive a Suicide Attempt?" Today. Aug. 31,2013. www.today.com/specials/suicide-attempt-survivors. Accessed Apr. 14, 2023.

[328] Miranda, Regina, et al. "Cognitive inflexibility and suicidal ideation: Mediating role of brooding and hopelessness." Psychiatry research 210, no. 1 (2013): 174-181.

around death and dying. Even more, our culture has rendered that far more difficult by placing a functional option before the dying that:

a. distorts the issue from a mystery to engage with to a problem to be solved,

b. is aligned with the function of the ego's instinct for self-preservation and, therefore, is too tempting for many experiencing greater death anxiety.

Cognitive constriction is why suicide-attempt survivors often express that they felt it was their only way out. It debunks the myth that those who die by suicide are selfish or weak, as these traits become irrelevant during a state of cognitive constriction. For the one attempting suicide, this temporary distortion results in a permanent action to escape life circumstances.

Here is where we have overlap. The same can be said of those desiring MAiD. They can imagine no acceptable option to the suffering they imagine lies ahead – becoming weak and frail, breathing in a bed and little more until there is nothing more. Cognitive constriction is so intense at death that it is unlikely to be alleviated without a trained therapist, a wise and compassionate guide familiar with the valley of the shadow of death. No one should judge a person choosing MAiD as weak, wrong or selfish. They are doing the best they can with what they've got. But what they've got has been given to them by experts who should know better and a culture that could know better. This book is an investment in that knowledge; a single deposit in a vast bank that may not recognize the currency I deal in. After all, we are talking about an entire population cultured to cling to concepts like autonomy, empowerment, and avoidance of struggle. That makes the alternative to MAiD a tough sell.

The second factor unexplored in deliberations about MAiD is that the final stage in human development – transcendence – is not experienced by the one dying by injection. At least, not on this side of the grass. Instead, the ego's primacy in the MAiD process is enshrined as the last word at the final moment. Here, Kathleen Dowling Singh's insight that suffering into death deconstructs ego-identity as a functional process that calibrates us for transformation has significant weight. The final attunement takes place in the wilderness of waiting, of stillness, of not knowing. This is the opening to the deepest realms of the Ground of Being. It cannot be reached without first traversing the transformative fields of chaos, but, when reached, it is a sublime, radiant state of quiet wonder and even joy. I recall one man who, from the depths of intermittent comatose states near the end of his life, kept surfacing back to awareness, telling his family and any lucky nurse who happened to be at his side, "I cannot describe the beauty and peace of this."

The transcendence that follows is beyond anything the ego could attain, beyond any description or frame of reference to this world. This astoundingly graceful transition dissolves the person you used to be as a process of awakening to the Ground of Being that has always been. It is well described in the classic guides the *Ars moriendi,* the *Tibetan Book of the Dead,* and thousands of other texts and traditions. However, it remains unfamiliar to the medical world as these mystical stages are inaccessible to empirical understanding. They are characterized by expansion, luminosity, and disconnection from physical form. Mind, identity, fear, anxieties, concerns, and attachments are all unravelled. Surrendering to this process in the earlier stages of dying positions us for the infilling of grace. Resistance, on the other hand, reinforces our struggle against the inevitable. So, from a spiritual perspective, it implies that MAiD patients are leaving this world while still tied to the baggage we are never meant to take with us: the ego. Is that true even when one's heart is filled with gratitude and release? I don't know. Perhaps it will be as simple on the other side as a baggage check at the airport – items not permitted will be confiscated. Will that result in significant delays? A missed flight? Would it be better to travel light?

I am still carrying too much baggage. Awakening from my near-death experience did not leave me instantly evolved. It left me longing for what I had become. It left me in a mess, feeling even more like a stranger in this world. It took me years to integrate the event and decades to grow from its effects. But I'm still ridiculously human. My ego is as evident as ever. And yet I know that when the bell tolls and I'm taking off, grace will jettison what is not of love, what is not of my true nature. Every patient I have had the privilege of escorting to the gate has reminded me of the same. And as they fly, I quietly send a final thought: "Say hi from me. See you on the other side."

EXERCISE 26: CONSIDERING TRANSFORMATION

Find a quiet and comfortable space where you can reflect without interruptions. Take a few moments to relax your body and clear your mind.

1. *Take a few deep breaths to centre yourself and bring your focus to the present moment.*
2. *Reflect on your own knowledge, beliefs, and experiences related to NDEs. If you have never personally experienced an NDE, consider your thoughts and perspectives on this topic.*
3. *Write down your thoughts and reflections on the following questions:*
    a. *Have you heard or read about specific NDE accounts that have intrigued or resonated with you?*
    b. *If you were to have an NDE, how do you imagine it might impact your perspective on life, death, and the nature of consciousness? Are there any specific elements or themes that you hope to encounter or explore?*
    c. *Reflecting on your own spiritual or existential beliefs, how might NDEs align with or challenge your current understanding of the nature of existence and the possibility of an afterlife?*
    d. *Consider how awareness of NDEs may influence your thoughts or attitudes towards death and dying. Do you find comfort, inspiration, or curiosity in the accounts of those who have had NDEs?*
4. *Take a few moments to read through your reflections and allow yourself to absorb the insights and emotions that arise.*
5. *If you feel comfortable, you may choose to share your thoughts and reflections with a trusted loved one, spiritual guide, or healthcare provider. Engaging in open and respectful conversations can deepen your exploration of NDEs and provide an opportunity for further growth and understanding.*

6. *Close the exercise with a moment of gratitude for the opportunity to reflect and explore the profound phenomenon of near-death experiences. Embrace a sense of openness and curiosity about the mysteries and transformative potential of these experiences.*

Remember, this exercise is intended to support personal reflection and exploration of near-death experiences. It is important to approach this topic with an open mind, allowing space for personal beliefs and experiences to shape your understanding. Seek support and guidance from others who can provide a safe and nurturing environment for discussing these profound aspects of the human experience. You can explore more at the International Association for Near-Death Studies, iands.org and the Near-Death Experience Research Foundation, nderf.org

Chapter 27

REALITY CHECK

Science advances one funeral at a time.

– Max Planck

DOWN THE RABBIT HOLE

In the dim light of his dusty library, the esteemed psychologist and philosopher William James reclined on a worn leather couch. Sunlight filtering through the tall curtains illuminated specks in the air, which floated like plankton in ocean depths... not so unlike the realm his consciousness had traversed to, a dimension as alien as any abyssal world. It was 1900, the dawn of a new century, and his explorations of the mystic realms reserved for shamans and seers of old would result in a pivotal publication, *The Varieties of Religious Experience*. As a key figure in Western psychology, he was trying to present essential insights that modern medicine has, nonetheless, largely ignored. In doing so, it severed itself from the spiritual foundations of what it is to be human, a particular expression of the underlying unity of life.

James emphasized that as fantastic as mystical states are, they are available to everyone. These experiences are staggering in their scale, disruptive in their power, and utterly transformative in their ability to deconstruct, then reconstruct identity. As esoteric as that sounds, James emphasized that mystical states are valid experiences to study, even though they are subjective and immune to observation. This experience, James wrote, is marked by four qualities. First, it is *noetic* – relating solely to the mind and how it places structure and meaning upon perceived reality. As much as physical sensations and forms can mark the experience, these are all in the mind; there is no "external" world to interact with. One can hear Dumbledore's admonishment to Harry Potter's questioning mind: "Of course, it is happening inside your head, Harry, but why on earth should that mean that it is not real?"[329]

Second, it is *ineffable*, or beyond description, which makes it challenging to study. The description is not the experience itself but an inadequate representation. The poverty of words cannot convey the profundity of the event. Everything related is symbolic, imparted through one's linguistic and cultural framework of self and reality.

Third, it is *transient*. Due in part to the inability to place the experience within a coherent cognitive understanding, it descends to the core of one's being. There it lives nonetheless, with the same transformative power and significance for years to come, sometimes permanently. This is not the transience of a dream but of an encounter, a love, an ascension to another reality for which the tools of this one are grossly inadequate to convey. So, while specific details fade, enough remains to permanently change the foundations of identity for the person: no longer separate from others, no longer apart from the universe – one with all. Adjectives employed often include amazement, awe, joy, timelessness, ecstasy, ineffability, ultimate reality, and freedom from the limitations of the personal self. This is a direct experience with something sacred, alive, holy, and all-encompassing. No wonder many have said it was the most significant experience they have ever had. No wonder patients report that their psychedelic sessions were invaluable experiential training for dying.

This is similar to the effects of nearing-death awareness and near-death experiences. With nearing-death awareness, all anxiety around death evaporates, and is replaced with expectant anticipation. With a near-death experience, one is reoriented to the continuing journey here on earth. This is often accompanied by permanent physiological changes, such as increased sensitivity to medications and synesthesia, and psychological

---

[329] The reference is Rowling, J.K. *Harry Potter and the Deathly Hallows.* New York: Arthur A. Levine Books, 2007, 723.

shifts, such as sensitivity to violence, increased compassion, and an elusive yet inescapable sense of purpose in life. So, nearing-death awareness prepares us for death, and near-death experiences teach us how to live.

Finally, mystical experiences are those in which you are *passive*. You are the object, not the subject in the experience. As you give yourself to it, it flows and you are opened to new dimensions of being. As you resist, torment and even terror can ensue, for the journey entails the disintegration of the perceived self, the ego. The ego's defence mechanism to automatically protect the perceived self is resistance to this more profound process that calibrates you to a deeper identity. All that was compressed in the subconscious is opened for integration. That requires the "you" you think you are to cease to exist. You have no choice in this, no willpower or agency, no say in the matter at all. Sounds a lot like dying.

William James goes on to suggest that these experiences expand our "field of consciousness." Boundaries of the self dissolve and remain permeable thereafter. This applies to what resides within as well as to the external world.

That sounds great, except when you do not have a strong sense of self, when you have baggage you beat yourself up over, and when you cannot forgive the mess you made in the wake of your journey. Holding to those personal mythologies (a term that describes meaning-making) can enrich or compromise the health of your ego, your perceived identity. A healthy ego functions much like a chalice. It is meant to be a structure of self that contains spirit (or unity, source, love, etc.). But inevitably that sacred stuff gets mixed with the mess: pain, separation, injury, how we have not been well loved, how we have not loved well. So, the ego erects structures of self-defence, sometimes functional, often dysfunctional. The chalice is no longer healthy and filled with *the everything*. It fills itself with itself. It becomes a solid container, sealed off by fear from that which is meant to overflow it with wonder. That's going to cause existential pain, for truth is self-eviscerating. Diving into the fundamental state of self demands raw authenticity, for it will expose what lies in the shadow, all that fights to remain hidden.

Distressing aspects of the mystical experience, as explored through a questionnaire developed at Johns Hopkins University, can include anxiety, despair, isolation, loneliness, panic, and a real sense that you are dying. There can be intense emotional and physical suffering. Even worse is the fear that these sensations will last forever.

William James found that mystical experiences, for the unhealthy ego, are distressing not because they unearth what is suppressed (they do that for everyone) but because the ego resists its deconstruction, resists surrender to that which is greater and not only unknown but unknowable. (Let's remember that you are the object, not the subject, here. You are the one known in this experience, not the one who seeks to know. It is not, ironically, about you, for there is no "you," not in any way you imagined.) One wonders if, in its defence, the ego cannot bear to see anything other than itself, so the reality we experience is one projected. We see the world as we are, not as the world is.

James called these experiences *diabolical*, not because they are evil but because they are frightening and confusing. He is careful not to place any judgment upon the experience, good or bad. Those value labels compromise our ability to see all mystical experiences as helpful, for they all reveal information about the self. They all invite awareness and can facilitate existential integration.

We've heard all this before, of course. As much as mystical experiences point away from the self, they are the claim to fame for seers and sages over thousands of years. Let's touch upon their insights to enrich our hope and address our hesitancy about what we will become.

Lutheran theologian Rudolf Otto wrote on this in his idea of the holy, something he called the *numinous*. This is marked by an intoxicating quality that devours you, a terrifying obliteration that you strangely long for, a shattering silence, a deep beyond description. This, for Otto, was an apt description of what it's like to feel the Divine, of grazing the edge of the Infinite, to which we exclaim both "Yikes!" and "Yes!"

MEDICAL RESISTANCE

Bring such esoteric topics as transpersonal states of consciousness or mystical experiences up with most doctors, and you'll get a guarded response. Why the resistance? Even more, why, if most people at the end of life have mystical awareness, is it not part of our medical model of care or the conversations around MAiD? Is it really that common?

Well, a research paper from the Institute of Noetic Sciences indicates that unusual paranormal phenomena are surprisingly common and staggeringly so. The study entitled "Exceptional experiences reported by scientists and engineers" sought to evaluate the prevalence of extraordinary human experiences (EHEs) that transcend everyday boundaries of space and time, ranging from from intuition and dream insights to perceiving someone's thoughts from a distance, near-death experiences, and extrasensory perception. Because these phenomena are associated with suspicion, as they violate material conventions of reality, the researchers thought the most critical thinkers among us, scientists and engineers, would be far less likely to have or report such events. Volunteers were divided into three groups: the scientists and engineers, the enthusiasts, and people from the general public. The results surprised everyone.

Among the 175 scientists and engineers surveyed, 93.2 percent reported having at least one experience, a level comparable to the 94.0 percent reported by the 283 participants from the general population. In comparison, 99.3 percent of the 441 enthusiasts reported at least one instance of an extraordinary experience.[330] While the majority of these experiences were subtle, such as feeling another person's emotions or knowing something you would otherwise have no ability to perceive, the researchers note that "these numbers stayed above 80 percent when items that could potentially be construed as normally perceived with the traditional five senses were removed."[331]

If this is so common, why is it discussed in hushed tones among friends, and dismissed by the institutions that could explore it further? The fact that EHEs are not considered empirically attested to the satisfaction of the majority of the scientific establishment, plus long-standing academic taboos that restrict open discussion about these experiences and lack of research funding, likely conspire to discourage scientists and engineers from publicly

[330] Wahbeh, H., et al. "Exceptional experiences reported by scientists and engineers." *Explore* 14 (5) (2018): pp. 329–341.

[331] Ibid

expressing their beliefs about or describing personal EHEs. Opinions in the scientific community about EHEs are usually skeptical, often passionately so.

While there are many factors that hinder acceptance of these strange phenomena, let's examine the four main reasons for this resistance, specifically regarding nearing-death awareness.

First, for most deaths, let's acknowledge that while family members are often present, and hospice or palliative care nurses are sometimes present, most medical professionals rarely have the opportunity to witness death and certainly do not have the consistency of presence to witness nearing-death awareness. The stories of these amazing moments then tend to remain stories – anecdotal information beyond verification by the scientific method.

Second, these intensely personal moments are held close to the chest for fear of ridicule, reduction, and rejection. These are sacred moments of wonder, astonishing epiphanies that have the power to radically alter one's very view of reality itself. To share it with someone who has never experienced such things is to invite them to the shore of an entirely new dimension of being while you are still trying to integrate the implications. And yet, I am continually surprised at how frequent the experience is. Even in our culture, where most people have not witnessed death, many still quietly confess the sacred secret of strange synchronicity around a loved one's passing or subliminal signs of after-death communication. That may be because of where I work, of what I do. But I cannot help but wonder if you, the reader, have not experienced the same.

Third, we are uncomfortable discussing death. It is often viewed as depressing and difficult, as it forces us to confront the pain and suffering that comes along with the final stages of life. It is not a casual topic for dinner conversation! We struggle to express our sympathies and are unfamiliar with the raw emotions that come with death until we are faced with the loss of a loved one or our own declining health. Nowadays, most people pass away in hospitals or nursing homes, so death is no longer a part of everyday life. Children are shielded from its harsh reality, and adults are primarily exposed to it through entertainment such as movies, music, and fictional stories.

Fourth, the medical model screens students for their scientific mindset and deductive reasoning skill. Medicine is detective work: deciphering clues, recognizing patterns, finding solutions. And it is based on material evidence, not metaphysical speculation. Students are also groomed to be biological engineers: understanding how the body's systems work and specializing in specific aspects due to their complexity. And death, in this model, is the enemy. It's what we're fighting against and is the ultimate failure in a practice focused on sustaining life. This is why it's important to discuss goals of care when facing advanced disease – optimal health of the whole person as they move toward death, not optimistic dreams of restoring life as it was before the illness.

This medical model, unfortunately, assumes nearing-death awareness is a hallucination or due to hypoxia (oxygen starvation to the brain), or metabolic and chemical aberrations affecting perception, effects of pain medication, or psychological instability. The same biological explanations are used for near-death experiences, in which a person is temporarily transformed into an expanded state of being and glimpses the afterlife. However, as with nearing-death awareness, the result is not confused hallucination or disturbing apparitions but heightened peace, paranormal perception, and, most significantly, the elimination of the fear of death.

Even though most patients engage serious illness as a spiritual experience,[332] most physicians see themselves primarily as scientists and secondarily as health managers rather than primarily as healers attentive to the whole person.[333] So, while patients want to discuss the spiritual dimensions of their illness with their doctor, that rarely happens or has any depth when it does, even though the majority of doctors also, of course, have spiritual beliefs and religious practice.[334]

---

[332] Koenig, Harold G., David B. Larson, and Susan S. Larson. "Religion and coping with serious medical illness." *Annals of Pharmacotherapy* 35.3 (2001): pp. 352–359.

[333] Shanafelt, Tait D., et al. "The Impact of Organizational Leadership on Physician Burnout and Satisfaction." Mayo Clinic Proceedings 89, no. 3 (2014): 396–406. https://doi.org/10.1016/j.mayocp.2013.11.016. Accessed Feb. 19, 2022

[334] Robinson, Kristin A., et al. "Religious and spiritual beliefs of physicians." *Journal of Religion and Health* 56.1 (2017): pp. 205–225.

Given how common nearing-death awareness is and that one in ten people who've had a brush with death has a near-death experience (one in five who've had a cardiac episode![335]), it's likely that many doctors have had, or know of, a case. To share it may risk professional integrity. The medical model, their entire education, and the culture in which they practise may not allow it.

Peter Fenwick gets that. He's a neuropsychiatrist and neurophysiologist known for his studies of epilepsy and end-of-life phenomena. He used to see mystical accounts as rubbish until they turned up in his consulting room. A patient had an arrest while getting a cardiac catheter. He left his body, watched the resuscitation, experienced that classic tunnel, the divine light, and felt that connection to a wider consciousness beyond description. This led Fenwick to seriously study the phenomena, specifically the mental states of the dying in the weeks and days before death. It was a five-year retrospective and one-year active examination with a palliative care team, thirty-eight nurses, doctors and end-of-life carers from two hospices and a nursing home. Interviewees' reports (first-hand and second-hand accounts from relatives, patients, and residents) found the phenomena were quite common. Nearing-death awareness included visions, coincidences, and, most significantly for the living, resulting in the desire to reconcile with estranged family members. The report goes on to say, "these experiences seemed to comfort both the dying and the bereaved. Interviewees described other phenomena such as clocks stopping synchronistically at the time of death, shapes leaving the body, light surrounding the body, and strange animal behaviour."[336,337]

---

[335] Van Lommel, Pim, et al. "Near-death experience in survivors of cardiac arrest: a prospective study in the Netherlands." In *Parapsychology*. Routledge. 2017. pp. 91–97.

[336] Fenwick, Peter, Hilary Lovelace, and Sue Brayne. "Comfort for the dying: five year retrospective and one year prospective studies of end of life experiences." *Archives of Gerontology and Geriatrics* 51.2 (2010): pp. 173–179.

[337] Brayne, Sue, and Peter Fenwick. "End-of-Life Experiences: A Guide for Carers of the Dying" McGill. https://www.mcgill.ca/council-on-palliative-care/files/council-onpalliative- care/nearing_end_of_life.pdf. Accessed Feb. 19, 2022

What an impoverishment when care providers misinterpret these sacred moments. Family, friends, nurses, and doctors may respond with annoyance, treat the patient condescendingly, discounting the experience or, worse, medicating them to prevent further "delirium." But once caregivers are equipped with the knowledge to recognize this type of communication, they benefit from participating in this transformative process. It is the ultimate experience at the end of life, one that medically assisted death prevents from occurring just as it is about to manifest. MAiD curtails the cumulation of what it is to be human, the fulfillment of the long years of struggle and joy, of hardship and triumph, by sabotaging our experience of the transcendent. Can there be any loss more significant than that?

When it comes to MAiD, this is even more significant for the patient. Nearing-death awareness can bring profound assurance that something of great significance is waiting on the other side of the wilderness before them. The rough ground between here and what they imagined to be the end blooms unexpectedly with the hope that their death is actually the beginning of a great adventure. How, then, will they prepare for the trip? How can they return their borrowed stardust to the universe with gratitude and trust that the universe knows how to receive it in its time? One might think the best way would be to talk to a chaplain, a priest, or another religious leader. Surprisingly, that may not be such a good idea.

RELIGIOUS RESISTANCE

There's an odd tension at play with religious leaders on this matter. While I've found most are open to nearing-death awareness, few clerics are open to near-death experiences. That's ironic, especially in the Christian church, since it could be said this is the bread and butter of Sunday proclamations. The miracles of Jesus, the resurrection at Easter, the assurance of God's love – these all seem to be acceptable ancient events, but to think an average person in the pew could glimpse heaven and directly talk with God in a near-death experience or be taken up into the initial stages of a loved one's death can make even the clergy question the veracity of the event. This is even more so with after-death communication and other paranormal phenomena. There are three main reasons for this resistance.

First, of course, is how this has become part of pop culture. Television shows, psychic fairs, and spiritual entrepreneurs have all undermined the credibility of the exceptional. They have taken what used to be reserved for the saints and seers of old and divorced it from the church's structure and discipline, doctrine, scripture, and the centrality of Jesus Christ in the salvation story. As such, it is viewed as a corrupt spirituality, or worse, a demonic deception meant to lead one away from God's grace.

Second, clergy are all too aware of how the ego will hijack any spiritual endeavour for its gain. That's the nature of the beast, one religious leaders too often succumb to – the more spiritual you are, the greater the temptation to enjoy the respect and admiration of others. You begin to believe you are unique, different, and blessed with a higher purpose. Which, as clergy, you are… but no more than anyone else.

Finally, and most significantly, when considering the future of religion, mystical experiences threaten the established order. In the beginning, this was to ensure everyone's egos did not hijack the whole enterprise of awakening (as it is prone to do). Yet as the authority of the church grew, it, too, was taken over by power. Policies and creeds ensured access to the almighty was mitigated through the priests and procedures laid out only by the faith. Church was empire, and citizens must behave. So, the church moved away from direct mystical awareness and toward narrative doctrinal order; a direct connection to unconditional love is not good for politics. In the cause of empire, no one could come to God except through Mother Church. Fortunately, despite the church's best efforts, these connections continue, for no one has a copyright on love.

Research on exceptional human experiences bears this to be true; mystical states at the end of life are universal. For thousands of years, across all cultures, people have had visions of their welcoming party, a sense that the spiritual realm lies immanently underneath this one, and that what we do here, how we love here, and how we leave here has great significance.

When it comes to near-death experiences, there is no correlation between belief, behaviour, age, gender, sexual orientation, economic status, how the individual came close to death, or religious practice and the chance of having a peek at the other side.[338] It's universal. That can threaten doctrine and belief systems which claim an exclusive truth about God and salvation, even more so when Christian denominations refer to Jesus saying in John 14:6, "I am the way and the truth and the life. No one comes to the Father except through me."

(Theological detour: I invite you to consider that 1 John 4:8 states, "Anyone who does not love does not know God, for God is love." Then, in verse 16, "We know how much God loves us, and we have put our trust in his love. God is love, and all who live in love live in God, and God lives in them." Since the creeds of the church state that God and Jesus and the Spirit are one Being (the Trinity), then one can accurately state John 14:6 as "Love is the way, the truth and the light. No one comes to God except through love." With this, the denominational and doctrinal doors are blown wide open.)

The universality of these experiences also challenges specific beliefs, such as on baptism, which some denominations hold as essential for salvation. I recall in my parish ministry how many wanted their kid "dipped" because that's just what you did – you had your child baptized to ensure they were good to go in the right direction should any tragedy befall them. For so many, clergy were there for the three essential rites of passage: baptism, marriage, and funerals – hatch, match, and dispatch.

(Another theological detour: This stems from the centuries past when child mortality was so high. The doctrine that baptism ensured their soul would go to heaven was a gross misunderstanding of what baptism is about. It's not a warranty or stamp of approval but an affirmation of a relationship. Baptism is a community ritual, not a private ceremony, that affirms one's identity as a child of God, an identity the community promises to cultivate as that child grows. It becomes an affirmation throughout life that you are loved and restored by the divine consciousness from which you

[338] Greyson, Bruce. "Getting Comfortable With Near-Death Experiences: An Overview of Near-Death Experiences." *Missouri Medicine* 110.6 (2013): p. 475.

emanate and by which you are sustained, even when you don't love yourself. It's not required for life after death; it's a ritual manifestation of one's mystical connection, grounding your identity in God as you live this life.)

Nearing-death awareness and near-death experiences have also not been part of theological education or pastoral care training. Clergy are simply unfamiliar with the phenomena. We are trained in church history, parish administration, systematic theology, biblical interpretation, presiding at worship, and some counselling. Prayer was something we did "by the book." The nature of our direct connection to the divine was assumed, but not formally explored, even more so for meditation and models of consciousness.

I recall one patient sharing her pastor's response when she told him of her near-death experience. "That's of the devil," he said. "You must be careful to discern the spirits and not be fooled by dark forces masquerading as beings of light." She was struck by how, as incredible as near-death experiences sound, what he was espousing sounded like primitive superstition compared to the loved and expanded consciousness she briefly touched upon. These events are life-changing, especially in terms of a person's faith. However, when church leaders fail to affirm and process the experience, people simply leave. She never went back to church again.

It's such a loss, especially as these phenomena speak to the meaning of life, the mystery of our purpose, and so radically change the trajectory of grief. It's not that sadness is supplanted with joy but that grief and gratitude are discovered to be companions in the heart. Wonder washes away despair, and the world is once again enchanted by hope. How ironic that people gather for worship to experience the divine, but when that manifests so directly, it's often dismissed by the faith community. If religious leaders don't take the lead in raising awareness of this, as one imagines they should, then who will?

A NOTE OF CAUTION

Caution must be exercised when considering mystical experiences not to assume that they are extraordinary: in nature, yes, but not in frequency. If we believe in them at all, we tend to feel it is only the exceptional among us, the mystics and saints, or at least anyone other than ourselves, who will experience them. But the evidence from palliative and hospice nursing, the research from Dr. Christopher Kerr, the Institute of Noetic Sciences and many others indicate these are universal as we die. Everyone will have a transcendent experience at some point, especially their endpoint. We who sit on the safe side of the bed will be fortunate to witness some, but most will be shrouded from observation and analysis. Don't dismiss them, thinking they won't happen to you. They will happen to everyone.

A second caution speaks to the modern medical mindset to dismiss such things as delusions, or worse. It's understandable that mystics would be viewed with suspicion of having psychosis. However, the inflated egoism of the manic-depressive or psychotic is always conspicuous, whether in the elated phase, wherein they think they are God, or in the depressed phase, in which they think they are irredeemable. The genuine mystic, however, interprets their experience as an unexpected gift, a grace that comes upon them and in which they have no ego or sense of self, let alone the significance of self. There is genuine humility, beauty, and wonder.

The final and most vital caution speaks to our ego's tendency to hijack any spiritual experience: having a mystical experience does not make you special, for "special" is the ego's affirmation of being chosen, of being different. And it does not make you a mystic. You wouldn't want that anyway; mystics tend to be challenged by some form of lifelong affliction that, while it may consistently rub the ego raw enough for the spiritual dimensions of being to filter through, results in more struggle than most of us would ever want to manage (and I say this clearly from my ego's enjoyment of relative comfort and stability!).

EXERCISE 27: INTO THE MYSTIC

Find a quiet and comfortable space where you can reflect without interruptions. Take a few moments to centre yourself and bring your focus to the present moment.

1. *Begin by considering the range of mystical experiences, from the mild and common to the more dramatic. Reflect on experiences such as synchronicities, meaningful coincidences, intuitive insights, moments of awe, and extraordinary states of consciousness like nearing-death awareness or near-death experiences. Acknowledge that these experiences can challenge or support religious beliefs or beliefs about reality.*
2. *Write down your thoughts and reflections on the following questions:*
    a. *Reflect on any personal experiences you've had that fall within the spectrum of mystical experiences. Consider experiences that challenged or supported your existing religious beliefs or beliefs about reality. Describe these experiences and their impact on your worldview.*
    b. *Explore how these experiences have influenced your understanding of the nature of reality, spirituality, or the divine. Have they challenged or expanded your beliefs? How do they relate to your religious or spiritual framework, if applicable?*
    c. *Contemplate the potential conflicts or tensions that arise when mystical experiences challenge established religious beliefs or conventional notions of reality. How have you navigated or resolved these conflicts? Have these experiences led to a reevaluation or refinement of your beliefs?*

   d. *Consider the broader implications of mystical experiences on religious and spiritual traditions. How do they shape or challenge traditional doctrines, practices, or interpretations? Reflect on how mystical experiences can contribute to a more nuanced and inclusive understanding of spirituality and the nature of existence.*

3. *Take a few moments to read through your reflections and contemplate the insights and emotions that arise.*

4. *If you feel comfortable, share your thoughts and reflections with others who may have had similar experiences or who are open to discussing mystical experiences and their impact on beliefs. Engaging in respectful conversations can provide new perspectives and deepen your exploration.*

5. *Close the exercise with a moment of gratitude for the opportunity to reflect and explore the profound aspects of mystical experiences and their connection to beliefs about reality and spirituality.*

Remember, this exercise is intended to support personal reflection and exploration of mystical experiences and their relationship to religious beliefs and beliefs about reality. Each individual's experiences and beliefs are unique, so embrace your own perspective and allow for open-mindedness as you engage with this exercise. Seek support, guidance, and further exploration from trusted individuals or communities if you desire a deeper understanding of these experiences and their implications.

Chapter 28

A New Model

And as imagination bodies forth
The forms of things unknown, the poet's pen
Turns them to shapes and gives to airy nothing
A local habitation and a name.

– William Shakespeare

Does it seem unreal? Do my concerns and ideas about the afterlife sound fanciful, misguided, or an irrational delusion? Perhaps you are a medical professional trained to be skeptical of all this, a critical thinker suspicious of anything spiritual, or someone who has faith but feels that these mystical phenomena ended with the saints of old. In that case, I will first make an effort to animate your imagination through the creative process, then touch your heart with insights on love, and finally integrate it for your mind with a simple scientific model of reality to consider.

Every act of creation is first an act of destruction. It's a brutal truth from which the raw materials of thought, form, and being are brought together again and again in new ways, rendering the ever-ongoing expressions of coherent energy, of life itself. This is what creation does – it creates. Stars are born and burn to create ever-heavier metals which descend to their core and, after eons, release those concoctions into the universe with a supernova explosion. For millions of years, they travel the expanse of space to somehow coalesce and eventually appear… as us. All the matter within our bodies is derived from such cataclysms. We are the universe, staring back upon itself, now conscious, now self-aware.

Plants transform this same starlight into energy-rich organic compounds, which serve as fuel for growth and food for animals. Eventually, these animals die and return their nutrients to the earth through decay and the astonishing activity of fungi… some of which you can ingest to experience your unity with the stars once again.

This is creation at play, not as a sentient form but as a coherent process of creation, destruction, and metamorphosis. Creation practices all this through evolution; the processes that produce life are as numerous as the trillions of combinations offered by protein folding and genetic mutation. But only the viable will survive; only the most masterful will endure.

We participate in this magic. A musician, after decades of practice and discipline, knowing her instrument so instinctively, need not think about finger placement or breath. She can intuitively be one with the music, one with the moment. When you're in that zone, there is a sense that something wants to be created through you. It appears as a thought, an image, a longing from within. From this, the artist begins to plan, but this is so much deeper than anything the ego could orchestrate. This is a dance between intuition and awareness, between sense and skill. And, fundamentally, this is a spiritual process.

Inspiration, the artist's fuel, comes from the root words "spirit-breathed." The ancient Israelites emphasized this connection by using the term Yahweh as God's name. Yet that name was considered so sacred that it should not be spoken. This would bring one too close to the Divine; you risk obliteration in that presence! (Think of the film *Raiders of the Lost Ark.*) To prevent this, they removed the vowels from all sacred texts. The name is expressed in four letters: ,הוה. When spoken, they're pronounced Yod, Hey, Vah, Hey. But these are actually vowel sounds… breathing sounds. Prolonged inhalation and exhalation…Yawh… Heah… Ahhhh… Heah. Our very breath is the name of God, the first utterance of new life, the last word on one's lips as they leave. Do we die because we can no longer breathe or because we can no longer say the name of God?[339]

[339] Bell, Rob. *Nooma Breath 014.* DailyMotion. www.dailymotion.com/video/x3d5q6_nooma-breathe-014_creation. Accessed March 1, 2023

This gives us insight into whether ending a life is the wisest way to go, for creativity calls on us to put ego aside and be part of this cosmic flow. Death, after all, is not the end but an ultimate and essential moment in reality's ongoing, transformational nature. By contrast, the ego only wants to create that which serves itself. Its plans are limited by its need to enhance itself, and they are deeply flawed, especially in the ultimate matters over which it has no insight. It could not be involved in entering this world, for your birth was the universe, even life expressing itself into being through you. How much more so at death. Can you step aside at this critical event and let the universe take control? After all, it does so through all the billions of life forms on this planet. We are the only kind that tries to grab the wheel in this process. Ironic since at no point in life can we participate so fully as channels of universal energy as at our death. At no point save birth is something so fundamentally greater than ourselves expressed through us to open us to the field of consciousness that is behind what many think is life's end.

In this, death is much like love – not something you understand, but a force that apprehends you. Not anything you can rationally explain, but certainly an aspect of your humanity you can refine and become familiar with. With death, the rehearsal comes through compassion and meditation, gentle manoeuvres of grace that help you dissolve in order to connect and awaken. With love, it comes through self-understanding, for all the times love seemed to fail, it also provided us with the greatest lessons in growth. All the love we've ever known prepares us for the love to come.

Social psychologist, psychoanalyst, and philosopher Erich Fromm wrote in his classic *The Art of Loving* that love is not a sentiment anyone can easily indulge in, regardless of maturity or experience. Fromm asserts that love is a skill, a way of being that shifts one's relationship with life itself. Such a fundamental orientation to expansion and connection requires decades of practice, just as artists hone their skill in portraying their inner reality. Yes, some are innately gifted, but most of us stumble along, sabotaging and sacrificing our growth in love in various ways. We treat it as something that comes upon us. We fall into love, are smitten by it, look for it, and desire to be the object of it. "All these attempts for love are bound to fail," he asserts, "unless a person tries most actively to develop their total personality with humility, courage, faith and discipline."[340] No wonder the great Zen teacher Thich Nhat Hanh admonished that to love without knowing how to love wounds the person we love. To truly love, the effort must be focused on becoming love itself. This echoes my assertion that if God is love, then love is not merely an emotion, but rather the highest state of consciousness.

Who among us could ever claim to have achieved such a state? Perhaps only the dying, in their final hours or moments. They become this; they realize this because they have been worn raw enough to cease resisting it as their true nature. They are apprehended by the Ground of Being. They are transformed into wonder. With this in mind, can we consider that the loss of dignity feared by those who desire assisted death is a loss of connection to love itself, not the human kind of love, not only the role in family or community, but a detachment from the foundational reality of who and what the person is?

Fromm continues, "If two people who have been strangers, as all of us are, suddenly let the wall between them break down, and feel close, feel one, this moment of oneness is one of the most exhilarating, most exciting experiences in life. It is all the more wonderful and miraculous for persons who have been shut off, isolated, and without love. This miracle of sudden intimacy is often facilitated if it is combined with, or initiated by, sexual attraction and consummation."[341]

How much more united are we with the essence of existence, with that from which we originate? Once again, we can hear the ecstatic bliss of the mystics as they surrender to the transcendence and penetration of rapture. However, this is not only a union with the Divine but also a reunion with oneself. Richard Wagamese, the remarkable Ojibwe poet and journalist, expressed it this way: "There are times in your life you are flung into the undiscovered country of being, a place beyond time and tide and detail,

---

[340] Fromm, Eric. *The Art of Loving*. HarperCollins.1956 (Reprint. 2006).

[341] Ibid

the full magical breath of you heaving with the indescribable joy of being, and you realize then that parts of you exist in exile, and completeness is journeying to bring them home."[342]

Can you do this? Can you do this as you die? The only way to navigate this well is by being enfolded in the support of community, of family, and of the wise application of medical care. Through sharing our story; through saying the four most important phrases of thank you, I love you, forgive me, and goodbye; through developing the skill to sit with discomfort and not knowing; or giving oneself to the ambiguity of everything, and letting go of control; to let it go into the wisdom of nature's way... this is the ideal, eloquently described by theologian and mystic Teilhard de Chardin:

> To become unified and concentrated upon itself, the being must break many sensible attachments. To make itself one with others and give itself to them, it must encroach upon those intimate personal intellectual and emotional reserves that it most jealously guards. To enter into a higher life, by centering itself upon another self, it must destroy its own preliminary unity. This can mean only one thing: at all levels of the formation of being, creative synthesis involves detachments – every aggregation being accompanied by segregation. The moral effect is necessarily accompanied by suffering and sacrifice. That is why, in every moral condition, perfection is inseparable from suffering, and the highest life is attained through a dying. Death (which means disintegration) accompanies every change for better or worse. However, while in the case of some (which it leaves permanently disintegrated and diminished), the death is *ad mortem*, in the case of others (those it reintegrates as it disintegrates them), it is a transition... that leads to a new life.[343]

---

[342] Wagamese, Richard. *Embers: One Ojibway's Meditations*. D & M Publishers, 2016.

[343] De Lubac, Cardinal Henri. *The Religion of Teilhard de Chardin* (quoting L'union créatrice). Image Books. December 1917, p. 53.

MAiD is a denial of this experience because of an endemic cultural ignorance of it. For the individual, it is demonstrated in the inability to imagine or trust the wisdom of death, which is the wisdom of creation itself, for death is the most pivotal moment of existence that sits with birth as the bookends to our life story. If only we had learned to read it better, for the final chapter has a great surprise, which is based on an astonishing truth: we are incapable of perceiving reality as it is.

Our biological sensory organs are designed to perceive only a sliver of the electromagnetic spectrum – that of visible light – and our brains are designed only to process that information in such a way as to facilitate our biological survival. That's the limit of what evolution produces on this material plane. Every species has likewise developed perceptual and processing wetware (as opposed to biological hardware) over millions of years to facilitate its unique survival parameters. Insects perceive ultraviolet through hundreds or thousands of individual lenses that detect the sun's position through the polarization of that light. Whales communicate over thousands of miles through ultra-low frequencies. We are limited to what we perceive, and what we perceive is so convincing as to be all there is. And yet science tells us that beneath perception are the subatomic and quantum realities in which matter ceases to exist. This is an esoteric realm of potential energies and gravitic waves. Even more, cosmology now understands that what we perceive as real – material form – makes up only 0.004 percent of the universe. That's the visible spectrum of light. All the matter in the universe, all the atoms we cannot see, make up 4 percent of the cosmos. The rest is roughly divided into two esoteric categories: dark matter (27 percent) and dark energy (68 percent).[344] What you see is not what you get.

Additionally, the greatest mystery to science is not the nature of the universe but the nature of ourselves: What is consciousness? Either it is an epiphenomenon arising from the brain's electrical and chemical neural substrate or an underlying principle of reality mediated through the

[344] "Dark Energy & Dark Matter." NASA Science. https://science.nasa.gov/astrophysics/focus-areas/what-is-dark-energy/. Accessed Feb. 19, 2022.

brain. The former is the dominant view of medicine, but the latter is actually a serious contender in science. It's called simulation theory, which proposes that we live in a projection from a higher dimensional reality. This perspective arises from the only model that reconciles Newtonian physics with quantum physics. "It's not considered some wild speculation among most theoretical physicists," says Leonard Susskind, the Stanford physicist who first formally defined the idea decades ago. "It's become a working, everyday tool to solve problems in physics."

Simulation theory provides us with a contemporary model of ancient spiritual truths found in the world's wisdom traditions: that there is another realm, one of pure consciousness, from which this reality emanates and by which it is sustained.[345] When applied to Kathleen Dowling Sing's insights on ego formation through differentiation, contraction, and attachment, we gain a shocking insight: we are grieving and gripped by anxiety at the idea of leaving an illusion. Everything we have thought of as real… is not. The "real" world, that which we can touch, see, and sense in every way (including the reality of our body), is a representation. True reality, the electromagnetic field and the quantum level from which that arises, is presented to us through our biological senses, which are designed to drastically filter the information, to reduce, distort, and compress it in such a way as to ensure only our physical survival. That may also be the design of the brain – a reducing valve, a reality sieve that strains the field of consciousness to a trickle sufficient for physical functioning and survival. At the end of life, however, we need no such apparatus. At the end, we drop the instrument through which the song of life has played or perhaps step up an octave beyond which our physical form could produce. Could we ever not be part of the music?

Sounds idealistic? It is, as that is the name of the philosophical theory which claims that the universe arises from consciousness. Now the scientific instruments of our modern era finally support the assertions of sages throughout time. It is the second spiritual reformation so desperately

[345] Bagchi, Arjun, et al. "Entanglement entropy in Galilean conformal field theories and flat holography." *Physical Review Letters* 114, 111602 (2015).

needed, and to which British scientist James Jeans referred when he said, "I incline to the idealistic theory that consciousness is fundamental and that the material universe is derivative from consciousness, not consciousness from the material universe… In general, the universe seems to me to be nearer to a great thought than a great machine. It may well be… that each individual consciousness ought to be compared to a brain cell in a universe mind."[346]

Here is the Ground of Being, once again. And here, as abstract and philosophical as it may sound, as arbitrary to your daily life as it may seem, here is the mystery and absolute nature of reality you are headed to. You are not an object made of matter but an activity of mind. That mind, that underlying consciousness from which we and all reality emanate and by which it is sustained, has been called by many names: Allah, God, Brahma, Aum, Shekinah, Ik Onkar, Source, Manitou, Aengus, Tao, Tianzhu. Whichever one you choose, or none at all, the fact remains that you will die, which means all illusions of what is real and what you are will fall away. It is unfortunate, to say the least, that death is required for that transformation into a reality that remains abstract until it moves from head to heart. Then it hits home. And yet, even the trust that we all will awaken to a realm of wonder will not stop the tears.

[346] Jeans, James. The Mysterious Universe (Cambridge University Press, 1930), 136.

EXERCISE 28: YOU ARE THE WONDER

As you read this sentence, notice the voice in your head speaking the text, reading the sentence. Continue to listen to that voice which is understanding and interpreting the black marks on the page or screen. That voice you hear is your mind. It is designed to receive information through your senses and either send impulses to your body to respond to this information or store it for later use. But who is the one listening to these words right now? Step back once again and observe your own thinking. Who or what is that which is observing? It is consciousness. Consciousness is that which is aware of existence; it is that by which you can observe the mind, or ego-state of identification and experience. Consciousness, the mind, and the body are separate entities. The mind and body are limited by the confines of their physical nature, while consciousness is all-pervading. This simple meditation will assist in opening you to a state of awareness and the wonder of what is universally available to you in every moment.

1. *Find a quiet and comfortable space where you can sit undisturbed. Close your eyes and take a few deep breaths to relax your body and mind.*

2. *Bring your attention to the present moment, allowing any thoughts or distractions to gently fade into the background. Shift your focus inward, directing your awareness to the depths of your being.*

3. *Begin by contemplating the mystery and wonder of your existence as an individual expression of consciousness. Reflect on the notion that you are a unique manifestation of the underlying consciousness or the Ground of Being from which reality arises.*

4. *Visualize yourself as a distinct, luminous presence within a vast and boundless field of consciousness. Allow this image to fill your mind with a sense of awe and reverence for the mystery of your existence.*

5. *Shift your attention to your breath. With each inhale, imagine that you are drawing in the essence of the underlying consciousness, filling your entire being with its infinite potential and wisdom. With*

each exhale, release any tension, resistance, or limiting beliefs that hinder your connection to this deeper truth.

6. *As you continue to breathe, bring your awareness to different aspects of your being. Reflect on your body, mind, emotions, and the subtle energy that animates your existence. Observe them as temporary and ever-changing phenomena arising within the vastness of consciousness.*

7. *Gradually let go of any identification with thoughts, emotions, or external labels that define your sense of self. Instead, embrace the spaciousness of awareness itself, recognizing it as the essence of who you truly are.*

8. *Rest in this state of pure awareness, allowing any insights, intuitions, or sensations to naturally arise. Be open to the profound interconnectedness of all things and the unity underlying apparent diversity.*

9. *With a sense of gratitude and wonder, affirm your connection to the underlying consciousness or the Ground of Being. Silently repeat a simple mantra or affirmation, such as "I am one with the infinite mystery of existence" or "I embrace the boundless nature of my true self."*

10. *Take a few moments to simply be, allowing yourself to bask in the expansive, peaceful, and awe-inspiring nature of your being. When you're ready, gently bring your awareness back to your surroundings and slowly open your eyes.*

Remember, this meditation is designed to help you contemplate the mystery and wonder of your individual expression of consciousness. Embrace the sense of awe and reverence that arises as you delve into the depths of your being. Each experience during this meditation is unique and personal, so allow yourself to fully immerse in the exploration of your true nature as an expression of the underlying consciousness. For a longer guided experience of this exercise, go to https://soundcloud.com/david-maginley/exercise28

Chapter 29

GOODBYE

I am not afraid to die; I am only afraid
of saying goodbye to you forever.

– Shannon Alder

Finally… my mother is dying. It's been four years of this disease imprisoning her in a cell of flesh and bone. Even with excellent, compassionate care, even with lovely elderly nuns (some also swimming in the abyss of Alzheimer's or dementia), even with family visiting daily and luxury accommodations, the palace is still a prison. Yet never did she complain. Never did she project her frustration or anger. And now, she couldn't if she tried. The seizures had increased in frequency. She descended deeper into the abyss, occasionally roused as the nurses turned her, as she heard the voices of her children and grandchildren gathered around. These moments were like breaks in the clouds. Her eyes would open, if only slightly, and someone would instinctively rise to gaze into them directly to assure her we were there. Our anxiety and sorrow were thinly veiled as much as we tried to offer comfort. Our faces were the manuscript of grief. It was written upon our movements, our voices, our restless sleep through the night, listening for that last breath.

There are eight of us, so to prevent crowding and fatigue, we agreed we would take shifts of two hours each. We had learned from our father's passing a year earlier not to insist on camping out permanently at the bedside but to coordinate moments of respite. That turned out to be wise, for, as is often the case, Mom's final journey took far longer than we anticipated

– weeks, not days. I recall that while sitting in pairs allowed us to play cards and reflect, it was the moments of solitude with Mom I cherished most, especially as it allowed me to be straight-up with her.

"You know, Mom," I said to her sleeping form one evening, "as much as we hesitate to say the words in your presence, you are, in fact, dying. It is happening, and we are right here at your side. You are comfortable, you are loved, and you have excellent care. And you know how to do this. It's written in your soul as was the ability to be born. You knew how to come into this world, and you know how to leave it. The love of God will take you home to the music, to the ones waiting. Your welcoming party will be huge; your parents, your brothers, everyone who's passed on. And Dad will be there too. Open arms, everyone. They will embrace you and kiss you… it will be wonderful."

I gave this assurance as it is so commonly reported by the dying. Recall the study mentioned earlier by Dr. Christopher Kerr. Over 80 percent of his dying patients perceived their welcoming party, which eliminated the fear of death. This nearing-death awareness is what my father experienced. Oh, how I longed for my mother to have it as well.

Interestingly, just as I said they would kiss her, she turned her head and puckered her lips, kissing unseen forms in the air. It was… adorable. It was so sweet. Was it a mystical moment? Frankly, I believe it was simply that she heard me. It was her humour, that mischievous wit. How beautiful that she would expend such precious strength to blow a kiss. Well, since I had her attention…

"Mom, there's also a few ground rules I want to cover with you." An odd foray in the conversation, yes, but our mother always joked about the psychic world, calling herself "witchipoo" with a wink and a smile whenever she "manifested" a phone call from someone at just the right time or banked on her intuition in navigating life, instead of logic or common sense (which often worked out beautifully). I continued with a warm but firm tone. "No haunting. No orbs, no flashing lights, no moving objects. No freaking us out. You are to behave yourself over there, follow the rules, and stay out of trouble. There's no need to mess around. Now, if you can guide your daughters and grandchildren, that would be fine. But don't worry about us boys. We'll be fine. I'm sure you'll have plenty of connections and be given grand projects to play with, so just have a good time. Bask in God's love, explore the light, and say 'hi' to Dad from us when you get there."

She did not stir during the lecture. Good. I had more to say.

"Finally, and I mean this: no reincarnation. If that's a thing, then just don't get in line. This place is going to get even crazier, from the looks of things, and you don't need to come back for more struggle. You're done. You're just fine. You've loved beautifully, amazingly, in fact. No more lessons here for you. Go off; it's a great big universe. I'm sure there's plenty to do. And know we love you."

Right. With that off my chest, I sat back, gazed at her, and sat in gratitude until my sister arrived for the night shift.

"You'd think I would be good at this stuff." That was my thought the next day as I found myself in a particularly foul mood. The longer Mom was still and seemingly stable, the more restless I became. I've seen this in other families with countless patients. The edge in the voice, the short replies to other family members. The pacing. The desire for a doctor to give a precise prophesy of when the end will come... at least to the day, if not the hour. She was dying, wasn't she? Shouldn't this be a steady progression to the end? What if she remained held in this suspension for weeks, after all the years of waiting for the worst to come? I found my own impatience surprising and shameful. This was my mother, and I was the chaplain who had sat with hundreds as they were dying. I have seen it stretch on far longer than the family thought it would. I have seen loving company agitated and aggravated by... dare I say it... the delay.

There we were, classic figures in the tragicomedy Waiting for Godot, awaiting the ironically compassionate Grim Reaper who, like in the play, never arrives. The result was a sense of futility and existential absurdity. And here I was, twisting in the torment of God's silence, when what I wanted was God's action. Set my mother free, dammit! She's been trapped in this too long.

Stuck in frustration, I decided to go to the beach with my son and older sister. She had told me of a beautiful stretch strewn with multicoloured stones not far from the nursing home. It was popular for its orange, crystal-like rocks and a vast sandy seabed. The three of us walked silently, feeling the wind and watching the clouds. It was just what Mom would want, one of her favourite family pastimes when we were small. Melancholy washed over me as sandpipers chirped near the rippling waves. The walk helped a bit, but we became anxious that Mom might die while we were away.

My younger sister, who had taken the morning shift, was amused when I returned and shared the instructions on the afterlife I had given Mom the previous night. And then she made a wonderful but impossible request. "Dave, why don't you do some Therapeutic Touch® on her? I was speaking with a friend who does massage, and she asked if anyone had grounded Mom."

Therapeutic Touch is an energy treatment in which the practitioner passes their hands over, but does not touch, the recipient. It's been shown to interface the two bioenergetic fields and facilitate the biological and non-physical aspects of the ill patient.[347] At the end of life, grounding facilitates the dying to release their connection to this earthly plane. "I'll spend some time rubbing her feet," my sister encouraged, "but if you gave her a treatment, maybe that would help."

"I'm in no shape to do energy work," I confessed. "I'm a wreck, all twisted up inside. Didn't sleep well, and I feel… impatient. Me! I'm impatient with Mom's death!"

"Yeah, I get that. We all are," came her reply. "We're all messed up."

That was so good to hear. In my heart, I had to admit that I rarely allowed myself to be upset or be anything other than calm. Which means I am a mess far more often than I realize! But, like everyone, I am unable to see myself accurately from within my own experience. So, I need others

---

[347] Giasson, Marie and Louise Bouchard. "Effect of Therapeutic Touch on the Well-Being of Persons with Terminal Cancer," *Journal of Holistic Nursing* 16, no. 3 (September 1998): pp. 383–398. See also Joines, William T., et al, "Electromagnetic Emission from Humans During Focused Intent," *The Journal of Parapsychology* 76, no. 2 (2012): p. 275.

to let me know. That's what family is for – to see through your facade. So annoying!

I went for another walk. When in doubt, use the body; move. That gave me space to wrestle with something that had sat with me since Mom was first admitted to the hospital – her request for MAiD. Had I known these long years of dementia lay ahead, would I have dissuaded her? Would it have been more kind to surround her with love and prevent the suffering by stopping her heart with a simple injection? Then she could have said the important words. Then she could have felt our support. Then we could have protected her from this wilderness. She could have avoided all this! It would have been... easier. So much easier.

I had to think this through. Was she not surrounded by love? Yes, every day. Nurses and nuns, family and friends poured in heartfelt compassion and care... until the pandemic. That shut us out, with only one, sometimes two, able to visit. And only from a distance of six feet! We could not enter the building, only talk with her... to her... in a porch area: no touching, no hugging, no way to hold and comfort. The pandemic amplified the whole matter of her suffering, for she had become a ghost in the shell, unable to speak or move, a frozen witness in a flowing world.

I could feel my heart beating as I considered this. The pulse in my neck was met by a sharp lump in my throat, and I began to weep. I let the tears flow, knowing they were temporary, knowing grief was just as important as understanding. More so, in fact. I paused, took a deep breath, and thought it through. OK, was she bearing up through the suffering? Was she able to cope? It seemed so from her brief interactions, but imagining her inner world only made me appreciate the desire to avoid such a life through MAiD. I had no clear answers, only love for my mother as we sat with her suffering.

My explorations of the grounds led to a fortunate discovery. The nursing home was built where Bethany Motherhouse used to be. As part of the development, a beautiful garden was made for the Marian Community, with a pond, a fountain, trails through the woods and a *via dolorosa* – the stations of the cross. One walks this path mindfully, contemplating the suffering and crucifixion of Jesus. The name means "the way of grief." Perfect.

I plodded the steps and dragged my cross along – an emotional bag filled with irritability, frustration, agitation, sadness… and regret. Staring at the images along the way was sobering. Jesus stumbling, receiving assistance from others, being beaten, stripped, hung…. It didn't minimize my sorrow but opened me more fully to that of my mother's, to that of my siblings, even to the suffering of the world. In that solidarity, I was not alone. In that solidarity, compassion was energized, and I could have my pain instead of it having me. Finally, I got out of my own way. This was about her, and my role, as her son and as a chaplain, was to walk with her every moment I could and incarnate the love from which everything flows. Ultimately, fundamentally, this is what is meant by the way of the cross, the passion of Jesus: to enter into the inevitable suffering of life without resistance or resentment for how it both deconstructs our ego as individuals and reconstructs our purpose as community. It awakens the transformative power of compassion, calling us to be those warriors mentioned in the Buddhist tradition – bodhisattvas. This is not a passive, empathizing witness but a heroic dive into darkness without hesitation to transform suffering from within. It is the most powerful state of consciousness possible. This is what love does: heals what can be healed and abides with what cannot. Through that vulnerability, in that connection, we are held and not alone. And in that connection, I knew my mother would be transformed.

So, what of her question about MAiD? The procedure certainly would have fixed her suffering, an empathetic and utilitarian answer to her question, "What's the point?" Yet, as explored earlier, it was a medical solution to a spiritual issue – existential, not physical pain. This is why, as I stared up into the face of the crucified Christ, it was not the words of Jesus that came to mind but the writings of Albert Camus, once again. Nothing has meaning on its own. Meaning is made; it is forged in the fire of experience. The hotter the flame, the deeper the meaning. So, my question became, what has suffering made of her and of us? What did we do with it?

Well, from what I could see, our mother met the suffering she dreaded with humour, kindness, even wit. I have no way of knowing her inner world, but I sense she adapted to it, to discover she did not transform into the violent monster her mother became, nor did she completely disappear into a murky realm. Yet, I could not imagine it. How do you adapt to this experience? How, when it stretches on into years? I suppose the same could be asked of any trial in life: poverty, abuse, imprisonment, war, illness… death. The only thing one wants to do is escape the imagined suffering ahead. Yet, most discover they endure. Perhaps this is the living example of Victor Frankl's thesis "a person who has a 'why' to live can endure any 'how.' "[348]

What was Mom's "why"? I searched for it, but she had descended too far to articulate such a complex notion. (I would say most of us have enough difficulty with that when we're well!) All I could do was ask, at every visit, if she felt lonely, if she was suffering. Her responses were minimal. Most of the time, an affirmation: "I'm good." Sometimes, a confession: "I'm ready." The rest, silence.

All I could know was that my heart was breaking every time. I felt sad and powerless. I grieved as the disease took a bit more of her away every month. But instead of snuffing it out, we used this suffering as fuel to deepen our humanity, demonstrate our steadfast love, delve into the ambiguity and eternal waiting, to sit and shine at her side. In that effort, we (imperfectly!) became Christ in disguise. Along with the nurses and nuns, we were the manifestation of the mercy of God. Bodhisattvas. As I made my way back to the room, head clear and heart open, I felt ready to do what had been requested.

It was interesting to give a treatment with family present. My sisters had never seen me do Therapeutic Touch and seemed slightly restless. Often those in the room benefit from the session, feeling the relaxation response along with the patient. The energy fields in the local environment are affected, and I've even had nurses and family members almost fall asleep! It certainly would be interesting if they did too.

---

[348] Frankl, Viktor E. *Man's Search For Meaning*. Simon & Schuster, 1985. This quote was originally spoken by Nietzsche.

The treatment was simple, as it should be. A few breaths to clarify my awareness and relaxed perception to settle into what is within and around me. Feel the space just beyond the fingertips... I placed my hands lightly upon her feet to initiate, then moved to the head with gentle, sweeping gestures to assess her field. Brushing the air, it looks like smoothing energetic ripples as I move down her body. This initial assessment is a quick pass through her biofield in which I sense energy active at the head, suppressed and weak through the body, a slight peak at the base chakra near the tailbone, and then heaviness and density at the feet. Yes, this makes sense. Congestion. It needs a bit of help to flow into the ground, into the earth, and in the flow, there is release. It's as if the energy at the head, the crown chakra, is preparing to flow out, to leave, but the roots are still tied to the earth. This energetic attachment can parallel our attachment to this world, to our relationships. "Time to let go," I thought.

A few more passes through her biofield with flowing light brought me to her feet again. I sat on the cot and held them, closing my eyes and breathing into the earth. I don't know how long I was there, but when I looked up, my sister was smiling.

"I spent time massaging Mom's feet while you were out. Nice to see we're on the same wavelength! Did you feel anything?"

"Oh, yes. I feel great! So relaxed."

"Not you!"

"I know, I know. Energy at the head, flowing out, but soft. Along the body, it's weak, suppressed, but there's a lot of congestion at the feet. It feels clear now. I think we grounded her. Certainly grounded me!"

They seemed more settled, too. We decided my older sister and I would run my son back to the house, grab a coffee, and return for the 4 p.m. shift so our younger sister could go home to prepare a large family meal. This, also, would have pleased our mother. Nothing made her happier than a good feed with everyone around the table. It was a Sunday tradition – roast beef with Yorkshire pudding, or ham and scalloped potatoes, always with at least three vegetables. This would be the first time since we arrived for the vigil that we would have a feast together. So immersed in the pattern of presence now established, we didn't clue into this subtle sign of its ending.

Tables turned. Now, instead of me being restless, my older sister found herself twisting with tears, intensely agitated that Mom would die. It did feel closer – her breath was yet again softer, and there had been no movement since she blew a kiss. My sister wept. I held her as the grief flowed, as her love poured out along with the fear of the void soon to come. Mom had been the central figure in her life, that special kind of mother-daughter relationship marked by both friction and affection. We spoke of navigating grief, of allowing it, accepting the void ahead, for in there would grow gratitude for ordinary things and awareness of the gift of life, even as sadness would become a familiar companion.

"But how?" She cried, holding herself while leaning into me.

"Well, by ironically allowing all of it. Your body will hold it, so listen to the physical sensation of sorrow with acceptance, with kindness. You have these feelings; they don't have you… well, not all the time. Why don't you go down to the pond, to the fountain? Breathe in the beauty, connect through your body to Mom, and find your calm spot so you can be deeply present when she goes."

My sister sighed. "OK, that sounds good. I can do that. That sounds good. Just a short time."

"Right. You can get a coffee from the kitchen when you're back, and I'll be right here."

I lay on the cot after she left, breathed deeply, and tried to practise the advice I had just given. The room felt different with me as the solitary witness once again.

Grief has such energy, such power. It can lay mute beneath the thin crust of the composed self, pulsing and throbbing occasionally when an incident or sympathetic word penetrates us. Our eyes register the wave like a seismograph, dilating, then darting away. It can also be an explosion, in which the raw and fundamental aspects of our identity are hurled into the world, fragments of our story raining down upon the landscape of life.

Closing my eyes, I descended into my grief, more familiar now with its pressure. Listening for my mother's breath, hearing only my own. I checked; her chest was rising and falling almost imperceptibly, a subtle wave on a deep ocean. Life lay there, far beneath the surface, somewhere in the dark, in a form now unfamiliar to us. Images flickered through my mind, memories of her laughter, her nurturing, her terrible cooking, her wonderful love, and her astonishingly resilient spirit. Our mother had faced significant challenges, bouncing back, ever buoyant, from each of them. As turbulent as some years were, she rose, again and again, on the one raft she knew how to construct: community. Mom was a leader in the performing arts – a piano teacher, an opera and theatre producer, an adjudicator, a cultural festival organizer… there seemed to be no end. She established a school, advocated for government funding, and nurtured talent wherever she saw it. In universities and small communities, at local, provincial, and national levels, Mom brought her passion to bear to lift others up, having great fun along the way. It made me wonder what creative endeavours lay ahead when the curtain closed on this stage and opened on another.

A change: something like sea foam was on her cheek as if blown out from her nose. Strange, her breath was hardly strong enough to do this. I wiped it away, then paused, realizing this was it. The calls were calmly made to my family making supper, to my sister by the pond. "She's going now. It's very gentle, but you should come." Their distress felt like a gale-force wind high above these deep waters, where there was no sound, no death rattle, only the soft signs of one evaporating from this world. Skin became pale; breath simply ceased, wisps of life fading like the edge of a wave, hissing softly on the golden sand.

"Thank you, Mom. Thank you for everything. You are free. You are free from all this: no more body, no more limits. Go be with Dad. Be with God. We love you. We love you." My voice was so quiet. I did not want to disturb her flight. I simply sat, one with the air about me.

Siblings arrived with lightning speed. My older sister, of course, was the first. "I was just coming up to the building; I was so close. So close!" She burst into tears, not torrential, but the deep sobbing that catches you like a gust of wind. She heaved and gasped as she brushed Mom's hair back from her forehead. "She's gone! She's really gone." When one hangs on the edge of a precipice this long, you would think the fall would be accepted, but we have committed ourselves to the grasp. It is all we know for days, for weeks on end. When the loved one dies, it is not that we have let go, but that they have taken wing.

The rest arrived, a storm of pent-up sadness let loose into the room. Again, the words echoed, "She's gone, she's gone!" Brothers sat quietly, grandkids embraced their parents, and the sky, so long greyed with clouds, seemed to suddenly break with unfamiliar light. My younger sister gazed deeply at Mom's still form. Her tears streamed like gentle rain upon the body, and she said something wonderful.

"I'm so relieved. So sad but so relieved for her. It's been so long. So incredibly long, Mom. You never complained. You endured this awful disease with such grace."

I moved to let her sit close, to step back so others could touch her cheek, kiss her lightly, and begin the final contact with her frail form. "We shouldn't have left… but I'm glad you were with her," she said, looking at me.

"I know; I was just on my way back from the pond," said my other sister, still weeping. "I shouldn't have gone, but when I was there, I did what you said, David. I listened to my body. I breathed. I felt calmer, and then I talked to Mom. I told her it was OK to go."

"I bet she heard you," I said, smiling. "I bet that enabled you to connect in a way you couldn't do here. Perhaps that helped."

"I think your Therapeutic Touch helped, too," my younger sister commented. "You did that at four. After you left, the nurses came and turned her. They said her body was always tense, kind of stiff whenever they moved her, but this time she was much more relaxed. Her limbs could be placed easily; her head turned on the pillow without resistance."

"Really!" I exclaimed. "Hmm. Well, if it helped, I'm grateful. With your massage and the connection at the pond… that would be wonderful." I sat back, marvelling.

"We loved Nana well," said my niece. This perfect pronouncement was medicine for our souls and helped our grief merge with gratitude for the long, difficult years that lay behind us. What our mother could not imagine enduring had transpired. She faced the wilderness, often lost for hours, for days, until the familiar voice of compassion reached out through a nurse, a nun, a grandchild, a son, or daughter, a hand of love to grasp with no rescue other than the voice that says "I am here with you." This is the incarnation, the manifestation of the Christ, a word which means the consciousness through which we live and move and have our being, from which all emanates, to which our mother had returned. How oblivious we are to this mystery. Caught up in the drama of our days, the costume of identity is worn for a few decades, only to fade and wear out; so convincing, so fragile, a shell in the end. Yet, it is no less sacred than the soul that continues, for all of it flows from God in the end.

The conversation that flowed through us, though, took a cheeky turn that felt anything but sacred. It centred on sibling competition that had developed over the years between my older brother and sister: who was the favourite? A claim would be made whenever they'd share a story of time with a parent. My brother had taken a kindhearted jab earlier in the week, stating he was Mom's favourite because she responded so well to his voice, while our older sister was simply… persistent. Burn. And who was I? Well, I was always the quiet one, the one who survived cancer, the one who got ordained. I was the angelic one… until now.

Gazing at my grieving family, I shared how peacefully Mom died. "There was no apnea, no struggle. I just noticed this foam from her nose, wiped it away, and then her breath faded, her skin changed. I told her we loved her, and to go to her welcoming party, to Dad, to God. It was so gentle, so graceful. I guess this means, since she had me at the end… that I'm her favourite."

"Piss off!" exclaimed my sister, incredulous but impressed by my wit all the same. The others roared with unexpected laughter, releasing their grief and tension in the best possible way.

"Too soon?" I asked, looking over at my brother. He was grinning ear to ear.

"Perfect," came his response. "Perfect."

As with our father, our two sisters washed Mom's body, selected the clothes, brushed her hair. We thanked the nurses and the Sisters of St. Martha, we gathered for the family meal our mother would so love us to share. And we felt the strange space ahead of us, no longer having a generation to buffer us from our own mortality. Is this the completion of becoming an adult – when your parents die? It certainly drew us together with a more profound appreciation for each other. And we all agreed with my niece's assessment: we had loved her well.

What a mixture of emotions churned within us: relief and freedom for her, emptiness and grief for us, gratitude and growth for the love. All this amidst a world that did not stop. The sun set, the sun rose, the day lay ahead as ever before. How strange. We embraced after breakfast, packed our cars, and set out for home. My younger sister, for whom the sorrow seemed especially heavy, decided not to hang around the house they shared. A quick camping trip seemed in order (just the thing our mother would have done!). Tents and kayaks, coolers and kids all piled in the car to set off for the highlands. But her tears were not fooled by the change in scenery. Their wet trail marked the distance gained beneath humming tires. And then... the phone rang, the caller's name briefly flashing on the car's screen... Mom's name. Impossible. It went silent as soon as her finger touched the screen. There was no record of it in the list of missed calls, and her name was not among the contacts in the phone's directory. Time seemed to slow, tears paused in wonder, as love whispered, "Eh, none of that! Pull up, my girl." I'm sure she smiled.

Epilogue

SUDDEN SATORI

For now we see only a reflection, as in a mirror,
but then we will see face to face. Now I know
only in part; then I will know fully,
even as I have been fully known.

– 1 Corinthians 13:12

Dying will be the hardest experience of your life, especially if you see it coming. I pray that I have honored that fact in these pages and honored your profound struggle as you face the end of your days. If I have also helped prepare you for the journey home, then I can rest knowing that these words were written not only for my healing, but for yours.

To die wise is not common. It requires discernment to balance length of life with quality of life. It requires a complete reorientation to the story we tell ourselves about ourselves. And it requires our willingness to be both broken by grief and opened by it to a state the mind is incapable of comprehending but which the body and soul instinctively know.

In the Zen tradition, it is called *Satori*, or sudden awakening. In the Christian tradition, it is to take on the mind of Christ. In secular terms, it is direct awareness. All of them mean to know yourself as you truly are. It is a transformation of consciousness in which you are so clearly aware of the nature of self, and therefore the nature of reality, that you are no longer defined by the world of ideas and words and concepts and inherited social notions like individuality, dignity, agency, and identity. Those concepts reveal how we are utterly convinced that we are a separate self, an ego, and that our body and life are owned by us. MAiD arises from marinating in such notions, all amidst a consumer mindset of anxiety and utility. Yet, when we step out of the world of conventional ideas into the clear daylight of reality, and with open eyes look for ourselves, what do we find? Something so vast and yet so simple: unclouded awareness. This is the reality behind a term few dare to claim yet is our baseline: enlightenment.

When a person is in an extreme situation and accepts it, there is a possibility of a natural satori. This leads to peace. It is the acceptance that there is nothing you can do, which allows detachment from outcomes and identities to dissolve. Suddenly, everything becomes clear. This is always the opportunity presented by death – to surrender before passing, to give oneself over to the process. It is an act that the ego cannot comprehend.

To the degree that you are flowing with a stream, you are still. And to the degree you resist the stream, the current becomes whitewater. When you act as a rock, not a leaf, the water always wins. Can you float with the current, even when the stream will sweep you away? You can only die well when you understand that your disappearance as this form is simply part of the flow. You can't hang on to yourself. It cannot be done. And in that paradox lies your freedom. Attachment to all, including the self, dissolves as you realize that all will pass. It sounds so gloomy because we have designed a culture that resists death. Yet death is natural, the most natural thing in the world. It's leaving that is brutal until blessed with gratitude and well-said goodbyes. You have this opportunity to let go of everything, and most central to this is letting go of you. MAiD is movement in the opposite direction of this final assignment of life – it is the preservation of the self due to the mind's anxiety of losing itself, a self which was, ironically, all imagined in the first place. And that deception has been central to the process of creation itself. Here's why:

The world can only be known in duality, in the relationships formed by there being a subject and an object, a self and anything other. The

Ground of Being, God, Consciousness, Source… whatever you call it, had to sacrifice the unity of its own infinitude, had to sever its indivisible being to manifest a form of self far denser. It becomes a separate self in a world, a universe, that seems to acquire its own independent existence. At least, that's how it appears from the finite mind. From the perspective of the infinite, there never was a division. All is manifest *within* that which we call God, through which we live and move and have our being, seemingly separate selves, particular manifestations of this underlying consciousness. We, and the universe, are that through which God has experience. So, what is invisible is made visible. And that creative process is shared by us, for we participate in it every day, little creative forms of life swimming in the sea of consciousness but masked by amnesia.

Think of life as a movie playing on a screen. The screen is our awareness. It is unaffected by the light that flickers on its surface for a brief two hours. Indeed, this is what the screen is designed for – that the movie may be played. And who wants to watch a movie without getting caught up in it? Such is our dilemma – we identify with the drama and sound of the film, with the characters, the triumphs, and the tragedies. Then, when the end of the movie nears and the story is about to reach its resolution, when the character that is us is about to be awakened by a process called grace… we shut off the projector. The story has become too terrifying, too heartbreaking. In our anxiety, we forget our lines which, ironically, would liberate us from suffering and help us remember that we are not just the actor in the story, we are the screen upon which it is played. MAiD becomes an act that further solidifies, in the final moment, the apparently separate self. Just as we are about to wake up, we cling to the dream.

It is no one's fault. There is no fault, only a mistake. But it is a huge mistake, the consequences of which will only be realized over time. Therefore, I pray that MAiD will play some part in increasing our spiritual intelligence and that we will learn from it how to deal with our pain. Until then, I leave you with some difficult questions, and I do so with the hope that you have good medication, good nursing, and good love.

Can you, when you are facing a life-threatening disease, ask how best to balance length of life with quality of life? Can you share your grief and be compassionate with your sorrow? Can you allow your children and loved ones to be embedded at your side while you descend to realms of silence we are incapable of comprehending? Can you imagine that in your dying, you will be completing your final responsibility as a parent, partner, or simply one person among eight billion? Yes, responsibility. As much as you imagine you are protecting your family from suffering and avoiding the suffering ahead, as much as you want to leave on your terms, or at least in a way that seems much smoother and safer, this is not about what you imagine, or your dignity, or your safety. This is about owning your humanity and giving yourself to a process as natural as birth. You will be teaching the living how to live, how to be aware of the gift of ordinary days, how not to reject suffering or any moment of this ultimate event but to navigate it without knowing, controlling, or resisting, only allowing this moment, this truth. You will be teaching them about their mortality. You will be preparing them for their own transformation. They will become both broken and beautiful through the fullness of their humanity.

Can you step back and observe your thoughts and feelings, observe your imagination, however painful it may be, and relate kindly to that frightened part of you? Can you give yourself to this wisdom wired into you at birth, that your body knows how to die? Can you consider that surrendering your control, your identity, and your story is not giving up, but giving yourself to the universal story. Yes, you are one small speck of life, insignificant in the eons, yet infinitely significant as a manifestation of that which you will awaken to through your dying. Can you accept medication to stay ahead of the pain, even if that means losing consciousness and communication? Can you say, in simple ways, thank you, I love you, forgive me, and goodbye? Can you negotiate with mortality and be surrounded by some form of community sufficient to carry you to the end? Can you imagine that your purpose now is greater than it has ever been through life: to increase the social capital of our culture and raise the spiritual intelligence of our species by dying wise?

Can I do this? I don't know. Yet, from what I have learned from the thousands I've cared for as they die, I trust I can. I hope I will. And I'll find out when it happens, for MAiD will be an option for me then as much as it is now for you. It's not going away. Our sense of individual autonomy and dignity is too saturated with death anxiety for that to change. Until that day, I leave you with a promise of hope (certainly a good thing in a book like this!). What waits to be discovered through the final surrender is within you already. It is your fundamental nature: Satori. Grace. Peace. This is why, at the end of every church service and every life, I say the ancient words that have been exchanged for thousands of years as both a greeting and a farewell. I say them to you now with deep gratitude that you have stayed with me through this difficult conversation:

Peace be with you.

HOW WE SQUANDER OUR HOURS OF PAIN

by Rainer Maria Rilke

Duino Elegies and The Sonnets to Orpheus

Someday, emerging at last from the violent insight,
let me sing out jubilation and praise to assenting angels.
Let not even one of the clearly-struck hammers of my heart
fail to sound because of a slack, a doubtful,
or a broken string. Let my joyfully streaming face
make me more radiant; let my hidden weeping arise
and blossom. How dear you will be to me then, you nights
of anguish. Why didn't I kneel more deeply to accept you,
inconsolable sisters, and surrendering, lose myself
in your loosened hair. How we squander our hours of pain.
How we gaze beyond them into the bitter duration
to see if they have an end. Though they are really
our winter-enduring foliage, our dark evergreen,
one season in our inner year –, not only a season
in time –, but are place and settlement, foundation and soil and home.

SUMMARY

If you are the one suffering, dying, bedridden, and bereft of strength, this summary is for you. You may have little energy to read and comprehend, so I'm glad you jumped to the end. Perhaps you picked up this book because you are considering or have decided to end your life through MAiD. Know that there is no personal judgment in these pages regarding that decision. I appreciate that you may be experiencing profound suffering that can result in days of utter misery. I extend to you my heartfelt compassion and hope you have love at your side and peace in your heart. While I encourage you to accept medical care that can alleviate your suffering, even if it prevents you from communicating with those you love due to sedation, ultimately, MAiD is your choice. May your life and its end be part of the mosaic of experiences that help humanity awaken and mature in its spiritual development.

If you are a healthcare professional providing MAiD or considering how you might support it, I am grateful that you are willing to engage with this material and discern the deeper dimensions at play. I also extend to you my heartfelt compassion and honour your desire to alleviate suffering, which comes from your good heart. May these pages help you consider how to engage wisely with the most challenging experience of life.

Here are my thoughts, summarized in four points:

1. Research shows that existential distress, not physical suffering, drives most MAiD requests. People are scared of the dying process, cannot identify meaning in suffering, and want to maintain

control.[349] At the end of life, existential distress is synonymous with spiritual distress - the inability to find sources of meaning, purpose, hope, agency, comfort, strength, and connection. It is our reaction to the threat death poses to the integrity of our identity.[350]

2. As explored in several psycho-spiritual paradigms, dying deconstructs ego-identity (the story we tell ourselves about ourselves) in the reverse order it formed.[351] This calibrates us to the final stage of the human experience: transcendence.[352] It is observed frequently in hospice and palliative care,[353] where research shows that over 80% of those dying exhibit this state.[354] Significantly, it manifests through expansive states of consciousness, lucid dreaming, and nearing-death awareness. In this, one perceives the spiritual realm and the comforting spirits of loved-ones or celestial entities coming to welcome them. This manifests days, hours or moments before death. It is independent of culture or belief.[355]

3. As we open to the dying process, our distress becomes functional, releasing ego-identity and the story of our life and opening to transcendence as the final stage of human development. As we resist

---

[349] Fourth Annual Report on Medical Assistance in Dying in Canada 2022 - Canada.ca. https://www.canada.ca/en/health-canada/services/publications/health-system-services/annual-report-medical-assistance-dying-2022.html

[350] https://bmcnurs.biomedcentral.com/articles/10.1186/1472-6955-10-2

[351] Singh, Kathleen Dowling. The grace in dying: How we are transformed spiritually as we die. New York: HarperSanFrancisco, 1998.

[352] Brayne, Sue, and Peter Fenwick. "End-of-Life Experiences: A Guide for Carers of the Dying" 2008 https://www.mcgill.ca/council-on-palliative-care/files/council-on-palliative-care/nearing_end_of_life.pdf Accessed Feb. 19, 2022

[353] Family Caregiver Perspectives on End-of-Life Dreams and Visions during Bereavement: A Mixed Methods Approach at https://www.liebertpub.com/doi/full/10.1089/jpm.2019.0093.

[354] Nosek, Cheryl L., et al. "End-of-life dreams and visions: a qualitative perspective from hospice patients." *American Journal of Hospice and Palliative Medicine* 32.3 (2015): 269-274.

[355] Shushan, Gregory. Conceptions of the afterlife in early civilizations: Universalism, constructivism, and near-death experience. Continuum, 2009.

this process, our suffering becomes destabilizing and can result in the request for MAiD.[356]

4. MAiD becomes the ultimate act of ego-preservation in the face of the process that deconstructs it for our transformation. Therefore, we are using a medical procedure to treat a spiritual condition.

[356] Singh, Kathleen Dowling. The grace in dying: How we are transformed spiritually as we die. New York: HarperSanFrancisco, 1998. p. 114

ACKNOWLEDGEMENTS

THIS WAS A DIFFICULT BOOK TO WRITE, DUE AS MUCH TO THE emotional cholesterol that accumulates when you swim in suffering as to the gravity of the topic. Yet the discipline of discerning and distilling one's vocabulary to render insights as accurately as possible has left me grateful and satisfied with what you now hold. It would not have been possible without the support and critical eye of people I deeply respect.

To ensure the integrity of my perspective, I've consulted with leading experts in bioethics, philosophy, theology, law and medicine, MAiD practitioners and advocates both for and against, even with those facing the end of life. These assessors counselled and challenged me, illuminating bias and blessings along the way.

To Prof. Megan Best, Prof. Margaret Somerville, Prof. Deanna Hutchings, Dr. Ann Marie Krueger-Naug, Dr. Cynthia Wimberly and Braydon Mills, thank you for your honesty and insights. You took considerable time to dissect this work, and your meticulous critique has been invaluable.

To Martin Rutte, Sue Douglas, Margery Nea, Connie Evans, Freeman Patterson, David Puxley, John Hayward, Barbara Morningstar, and Rev. Kimber McNabb, your support and encouragement gave me fuel to wrestle with this material and faith to trust it was worth the struggle.

To my reviewers, Dr. David Pfrimmer, Dr. Kristine Lund, Dr. Bruce Greyson, Dr. Drew Bethune, Dr. Theo Boer, Dr. Janeta Tansey, Dr. Arne Schelling, and Rebecca Austill-Clausen, thank you not only for your endorsements but for your leadership in speaking to critical issues of our time, issues of meaning and hope, of faith and resilience.

I am profoundly honoured that Dr. Robert Twycross, a hero in the field of palliative care, confirmed the quality of this work and wrote the foreword. Dr. Twycross's collaborations with Dame Cicely Saunders, the Oxford Medical School, and the World Health Organization led to significant advances in palliative care. Sadly, his passing a few weeks before publication meant he could not hold in his hands what you now have in yours. None of the words I have written here seem adequate to express my appreciation for his contribution. That he considered my book an essential addition to this challenging discussion is humbling. A simple 'thank you' hardly seems enough.

To the medical staff in the cancer, palliative and intensive care units of the QEII Health Sciences Centre, it was an honour to work with you. You taught me more than you will ever know. I reflect on my career among your teams and count myself a lucky man. Your expertise was matched only by your compassion and gracious hearts. Your dedication to supporting those who suffer and die was, and continues to be, an inspiration to me. Even more, thank you for incorporating spiritual care as a fundamental aspect of whole-person care. You really understand what we do!

Thank you to my wife, Erika, for all your support for this book and for being the buoyancy I needed when flooded with suffering. I would have drowned were it not for you.

Finally, to those who have died by MAiD while under my care. Your spirits live on in my heart and mind. Given the inadequacy of our culture to prepare you for your final days, I witnessed you face them in the only way you could. You have deepened my humanity, you have demonstrated love and forgiveness, and your choice has clarified my resolve to engage MAiD insightfully, respectfully and honestly. It was an honour to support you.

ABOUT THE AUTHOR

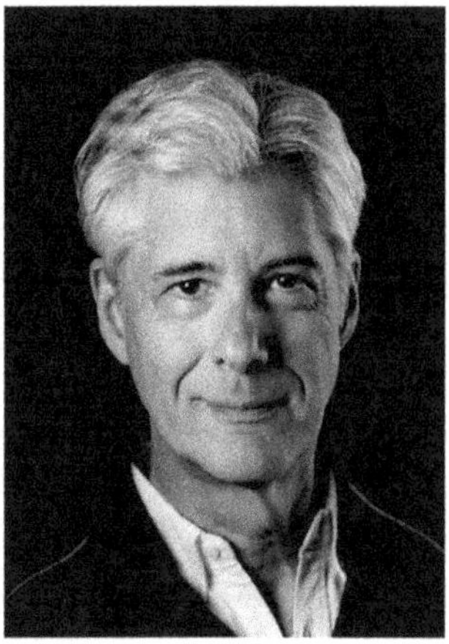

For over 25 years, Rev. David Maginley, MDiv, CSCP, provided psychospiritual care in the cancer, palliative and intensive care units of the QEII Health Sciences Centre in Halifax, Nova Scotia. He has a private practice as a psychospiritual specialist with the Canadian Association for Spiritual Care. His first book, *Beyond Surviving: Cancer and Your Spiritual Journey,* won the 2017 Silver Nautilus Book Award. David also survived cancer four times, which led to a profound near-death experience and explorations in the nature of consciousness.

In addition to being an author, David is an avid photographer. His writing and images explore mortality, compassion, resilience, and hope.

www.ingramcontent.com/pod-product-compliance
Lightning Source LLC
LaVergne TN
LVHW052016200926
848481LV00005B/1504